Pearls and Pitfalls in Head and Neck Surgery

Pearls and Pitfalls in Head and Neck Surgery

Practical Tips to Minimize Complications

Editor

Claudio R. Cernea, São Paulo

Associate Editors

Fernando L. Dias, Rio de Janeiro
Dan Fliss, Tel Aviv
Roberto A. Lima, Rio de Janeiro
Eugene N. Myers, Pittsburgh, Pa.
William I. Wei, Hong Kong

3 tables, 2008

KARGER

Basel · Freiburg · Paris · London · New York ·
Bangalore · Bangkok · Shanghai · Singapore · Tokyo · Sydney

Claudio R. Cernea
Department of Head and Neck Surgery,
University of São Paulo Medical School,
São Paulo, Brazil

Library of Congress Cataloging-in-Publication Data

Pearls and pitfalls in head and neck surgery : practical tips to minimize complications / editor, Claudio R. Cernea ; associate editors, Fernando L. Dias ... [et al.].
p. ; cm.
Includes bibliographical references and index.
ISBN 978-3-8055-8425-8 (hard cover : alk. paper)
1. Head--Surgery. 2. Neck--Surgery. I. Cernea, Claudio R. II. Dias, Fernando L.
[DNLM: 1. Head--surgery. 2. Head and Neck Neoplasms--surgery. 3. Neck--surgery. WE 705 P359 2008]
RD521.P38 2008
617.5'1--dc22

2008015976

Bibliographic Indices. This publication is listed in bibliographic services, including Current Contents® and Index Medicus.

Disclaimer. The statements, options and data contained in this publication are solely those of the individual authors and contributors and not of the publisher and the editor(s). The appearance of advertisements in the book is not a warranty, endorsement, or approval of the products or services advertised or of their effectiveness, quality or safety. The publisher and the editor(s) disclaim responsibility for any injury to persons or property resulting from any ideas, methods, instructions or products referred to in the content or advertisements.

Drug Dosage. The authors and the publisher have exerted every effort to ensure that drug selection and dosage set forth in this text are in accord with current recommendations and practice at the time of publication. However, in view of ongoing research, changes in government regulations, and the constant flow of information relating to drug therapy and drug reactions, the reader is urged to check the package insert for each drug for any change in indications and dosage and for added warnings and precautions. This is particularly important when the recommended agent is a new and/or infrequently employed drug.

www.karger.com
Printed in Switzerland on acid-free paper by Reinhardt Druck, Basel
ISBN 978–3–8055–8425–8

Contents

1 **Preface**

Thyroid and Parathyroid Glands

2 **1.1 How to Avoid Injury of Inferior Laryngeal Nerve**
Jacob Moalem, Orlo H. Clark (San Francisco, Calif.)

4 **1.2 How to Avoid Injury of the External Branch of Superior Laryngeal Nerve**
Claudio R. Cernea, Alberto R. Ferraz (São Paulo)

6 **1.3 Recurrent Laryngeal Nerve Monitoring in Thyroid and Parathyroid Surgery: Technique for the NIM 2 System**
David J. Lesnik (Boston, Mass.), Lenine Garcia Brandao (São Paulo), Gregory W. Randolph (Boston, Mass.)

8 **1.4 How to Preserve the Parathyroid Glands during Thyroid Surgery**
Ashok R. Shaha, Vergilius José F. de Araújo Filho (New York, N.Y.)

10 **1.5 Completion Thyroidectomy**
Eveline Slotema, Jean-François Henry (Marseille)

12 **1.6 Surgery for Intrathoracic Goiters**
Ashok R. Shaha (New York, N.Y.), James L. Netterville, Nadir Ahmad (Nashville, Tenn.)

14 **1.7 How to Decide the Extent of Thyroidectomy for Benign Diseases**
Jeremy L. Freeman (Toronto, Ont.)

16 **1.8 Minimally Invasive Video-Assisted Thyroidectomy**
Erivelto M. Volpi, Gabrielle Matterazzi, Fernando L. Dias, Paolo Miccoli (São Paulo)

18 **1.9 Video-Assisted Parathyroidectomy**
William B. Inabnet (New York, N.Y.)

20 **1.10 Limited Parathyroidectomy**
Keith S. Heller (New York, N.Y.)

22 **1.11 Practical Tips for the Surgical Management of Secondary Hyperparathyroidism**
Fábio Luiz de Menezes Montenegro, Rodrigo Oliveira Santos, Anói Castro Cordeiro (São Paulo)

24 **1.12 Reoperative Parathyroidectomy**
Alfred Simental (Loma Linda, Calif.)

26 **1.13 Paratracheal Neck Dissection: Surgical Tips**
A. Khafif (Tel Aviv), L.P. Kowalski (São Paulo), Dan M. Fliss (Tel Aviv)

28 **1.14 Management of Lymph Nodes in Medullary Thyroid Cancer**
Marcos R. Tavares (São Paulo)

30 **1.15 How to Manage a Well-Differentiated Carcinoma with Recurrent Nerve Invasion**
Patrick Sheahan, Jatin P. Shah (New York, N.Y.)

32 **1.16 Management of Invasive Thyroid Cancer**
Thomas V. McCaffrey (Tampa, Fla.)

Neck Metastases

34 **2.1 Preoperative Workup of the Neck in Head and Neck Squamous Cell Carcinoma**
Michiel van den Brekel, Frans J.M. Hilgers (Amsterdam)

36 **2.2 N0 Neck in Oral Cancer: Wait and Watch**
Yoav P. Talmi (Tel Aviv)

38 **2.3 N0 Neck in Oral Cancer: Elective Neck Dissection**
Fernando L. Dias, Roberto A. Lima (Rio de Janeiro)

40 **2.4 Sentinel Node Biopsy in the Management of the N0 Oral Cancer**
Francisco Civantos (Miami, Fla.)

42 **2.5 Selective Neck Dissection in the Treatment of the N+ Neck in Cancers of the Oral Cavity**
Jesus E. Medina, Greg Krempl (Oklahoma City, Okla.)

44 **2.6 How to Manage the XI Nerve in Neck Dissections**
Lance E. Oxford, John C. O'Brien, Jr. (Dallas, Tex.)

46 **2.7 Preservation of the Marginal Mandibular Nerve in Neck Surgery**
K. Thomas Robbins (Springfield, Ill.)

48 **2.8 Bilateral Neck Dissections: Practical Tips**
Jonas T. Johnson (Pittsburgh, Pa.)

50 **2.9a How to Manage Retropharyngeal Lymph Nodes** 1. Transoral Approach
James Cohen (Portland, Oreg.), Randal S. Weber (Houston, Tex.)

52 **2.9b How to Manage Retropharyngeal Lymph Nodes** 2. Transcervical Approach
Randal S. Weber (Houston, Tex.)

54 **2.10 Management of the Node-Positive Neck in Patients Undergoing Chemoradiotherapy**
Rod P. Rezaee, Pierre Lavertu (Cleveland, Ohio)

56 **2.11 How to Avoid Injury to Thoracic Duct during Surgical Resection of Left Level IV Lymph Nodes**
Gary L. Clayman (Houston, Tex.)

58 **2.12 What Are the New Concepts in Functional Modified Neck Dissection?**
Bhuvanesh Singh (New York, N.Y.)

Oral/Oropharyngeal Tumors

60 **3.1 How to Reconstruct Small Tongue and Floor of Mouth Defects**
Remco de Bree, C. René Leemans (Amsterdam)

62 **3.2 Reconstruction of Large Tongue and Floor of Mouth Defects**
Neal D. Futran (Seattle, Wash.)

64 **3.3 How to Evaluate Surgical Margins in Mandibular Resections**
Richard J. Wong (New York, N.Y.)

66 **3.4 How to Reconstruct Anterior Mandibular Defects in Patients with Vascular Diseases**
Matthew M. Hanasono (Houston, Tex.)

68 **3.5 Adequate Surgical Margins in Resections of Carcinomas of the Tongue**
Jacob Kligerman (Rio de Janeiro)

70 **3.6 Practical Tips to Manage Mandibular Osteoradionecrosis**
Sheng-Po Hao (Taoyuan, Taiwan)

Laryngeal Tumors

72 **4.1 Practical Tips for Laser Resection of Laryngeal Cancer**
F. Christopher Holsinger, N. Scott Howard (Houston, Tex.), Andrew McWhorter (Baton Rouge, La.)

74 **4.2 Practical Suggestions for Phonomicrosurgical Treatment of Benign Vocal Fold Lesions**
Steven M. Zeitels, Gerardo Lopez Guerra (Boston, Mass.)

76 **4.3 Glottic Reconstruction after Partial Vertical Laryngectomy**
Onivaldo Cervantes, Márcio Abrahão (São Paulo)

78 **4.4 Suprahyoid Pharyngotomy**
Eugene N. Myers, Robert L. Ferris (Pittsburgh, Pa.)

80 **4.5 Intraoperative Maneuvers to Improve Functional Result after Supraglottic Laryngectomy**
Roberto A. Lima, Fernando L. Dias (Rio de Janeiro)

82 **4.6 Practical Tips for Performing Supracricoid Partial Laryngectomy**
Gregory S. Weinstein, F. Christopher Holsinger, Ollivier Laccourreye (Philadelphia, Pa.)

84 **4.7 Intraoperative Maneuvers to Improve Functional Results after Total Laryngectomy**
Javier Gavilán (Madrid), Jesús Herranz (La Coruña)

86 **4.8 How to Manage Tracheostomal Recurrence**
Dennis H. Kraus (New York, N.Y.)

88 **4.9 Stenosis of the Tracheostoma following Total Laryngectomy**
Eugene N. Myers (Pittsburgh, Pa.)

90 **4.10 How to Prevent and Treat Pharyngocutaneous Fistulas after Laryngectomy**
Bhuvanesh Singh (New York, N.Y.)

Hypopharyngeal Cancer

92 **5.1 How to Treat Small Hypopharyngeal Primary Tumors with N3 Neck**
Abrão Rapoport, Marcos Brasilino de Carvalho (São Paulo)

94 **5.2 Practical Tips to Reconstruct a Total Laryngectomy/Partial Pharyngectomy Defect**
Dennis H. Kraus (New York, N.Y.)

96 **5.3 Practical Tips for Voice Rehabilitation after Pharyngolaryngectomy**
Frans J.M. Hilgers, Michiel van den Brekela (Amsterdam)

98 **5.4 How to Choose the Reconstructive Method after Total Pharyngolaryngectomy**
William I. Wei, Jimmy Y.W. Chan (Hong Kong)

Nasopharyngeal Cancer

100 **6.1 Indications for Surgical Treatment of Nasopharyngeal Cancer**
William I. Wei, Rockson Wei (Hong Kong)

102 **6.2 Practical Tips to Perform a Maxillary Swing Approach**
William I. Wei, Raymond W.M. Ng (Hong Kong)

104 **6.3 Management of Neck Metastases of Nasopharyngeal Carcinoma**
William I. Wei, W.K. Ho (Hong Kong)

Salivary Gland Tumors

106 **7.1 Practical Tips to Identify the Main Trunk of the Facial Nerve**
Fernando L. Dias, Roberto A. Lima (Rio de Janeiro), Jorge Pinho (Recife)

108 **7.2 Retrograde Approach to Facial Nerve: Indications and Technique**
Flavio C. Hojaij, Caio Plopper, Claudio R. Cernea (São Paulo)

110 **7.3 Intraoperative Decisions for Sacrificing the Facial Nerve in Parotid Surgery**
Randal S. Weber, F. Christopher Holsinger (Houston, Tex.)

112 **7.4 When and How to Reconstruct the Resected Facial Nerve in Parotid Surgery**
Peter C. Neligan (Seattle, Wash.)

114 **7.5 Approaches to Deep Lobe Parotid Tumors**
Richard V. Smith (Bronx, N.Y.)

116 **7.6 Recurrent Parotid Pleomorphic Adenoma**
Bruce J. Davidson (Washingston, D.C.)

118 **7.7 How to Overcome Limitations of Fine Needle Aspiration and Frozen Section Biopsy during Operations for Salivary Gland Tumors**
Alfio José Tincani, Sanford Dubner (Campinas)

120 **7.8 Practical Tips to Spare the Great Auricular Nerve in Parotidectomy**
Randall P. Morton (Auckland)

122 **7.9 Indications for Elective Neck Dissection in Parotid Cancers**
Roberto A. Lima, Fernando L. Dias (Rio de Janeiro)

124 **7.10 Indications for 'Tactical' Parotidectomy in Nonsalivary Lesions**
Caio Plopper, Claudio R. Cernea (São Paulo)

126 **7.11 When Not to Operate on a Parotid Tumor**
Jeffrey D. Spiro (Farmington, Conn.), Ronald H. Spiro (New York, N.Y.)

128 **7.12 Practical Tips on Excision of the Submandibular Gland**
Kwang Hyun Kim (Seoul)

Skull Base Tumors

130 **8.1 Practical Tips to Perform the Subcranial Approach**
Ziv Gil, Dan M. Fliss (Tel Aviv)

132 **8.2 Facial Translocation Approach**
Fernando Walder (São Paulo)

134 **8.3 How to Manage Large Dural Defects in Skull Base Surgery**
Eduardo Vellutini, Marcos Q.T. Gomes (São Paulo)

136 **8.4 Which Is the Best Choice to Seal the Craniofacial Diaphragm?**
Ziv Gil, Dan M. Fliss (Tel Aviv)

138 **8.5 Contraindications for Resection of Skull Base Tumors**
Fernando L. Dias, Roberto A. Lima (Rio de Janeiro)

140 **8.6 Practical Tips about Orbital Preservation and Exenteration**
Ehab Hanna (Houston, Tex.)

142 **8.7 Practical Tips to Approach the Cavernous Sinus**
Marcos Q.T. Gomes, Eduardo Vellutini (São Paulo)

144 **8.8 How to Reconstruct Large Cranial Base Defects**
Patrick J. Gullane, Christine B. Novak, Kristen J. Otto (Toronto),
Peter C. Neligan (Seattle, Wash.)

146 **8.9 Surgical Management of Recurrent Skull Base Tumors**
Claudio R. Cernea (São Paulo), Ehab Hanna (Houston, Tex.)

148 **8.10 Management of Extensive Fibro-Osseous Lesions of the Skull Base**
Claudio R. Cernea (São Paulo), Bert W. O'Malley, Jr. (Philadelphia, Pa.)

Vascular Tumors

150 **9.1 Practical Tips to Manage Extensive Arteriovenous Malformations**
Gresham T. Richter, James Y. Suen (Little Rock, Ark.)

152 **9.2 How to Manage Extensive Lymphatic Malformations**
James Y. Suen, Gresham T. Richter (Little Rock, Ark.)

154 **9.3 How to Deal with Emergency Bleeding Episodes in Arteriovenous Malformations**
Eduardo Noda Kihara, Mario Sergio Duarte Andrioli, Eduardo Noda Kihara Filho (São Paulo)

Congenital Tumors

156 **10.1 Practical Tips to Manage Branchial Cleft Cysts and Fistulas**
Marcelo D. Durazzo, Gilberto de Britto e Silva Filho (São Paulo)

158 **10.2 How to Avoid Surprises in the Management of the Thyroglossal Duct Cyst**
Nilton T. Herter (Porto Alegre)

Parapharyngeal Space Tumors

160 **11.1 How to Manage Extensive Carotid Body Tumors**
Nadir Ahmad, James L. Netterville (Nashville, Tenn.)

162 **11.2 How to Manage Extensive Neurogenic Tumors**
Ziv Gil, Dan M. Fliss (Tel Aviv)

164 **11.3 How to Choose a Surgical Approach to a Parapharyngeal Space Mass**
Kerry D. Olsen (Rochester, Minn.)

Infections of Head and Neck

166 **12.1 Practical Tips to Approach a Deep Neck Abscess**
Flávio C. Hojaij, Caio Plopper (São Paulo)

168 **12.2 Management of Necrotizing Fasciitis**
Dorival De Carlucci Jr. (São Paulo)

Tracheotomy

170 **13.1 Minimizing Complications in Tracheotomy**
Eugene N. Myers (Pittsburgh, Pa.)

172 **13.2 Emergency Upper Airway Obstruction: Cricothyroidotomy or Tracheotomy?**
Carlos N. Lehn (São Paulo)

174 **13.3 Avoidance of Complications in Conventional Tracheotomy and Percutaneous Dilatational Tracheotomy**
David W. Eisele (San Francisco, Calif.)

Reconstruction

176 **14.1 Practical Tips to Perform a Microvascular Anterolateral Thigh Flap**
Luiz Carlos Ishida, Luis Henrique Ishida (São Paulo)

178 **14.2 Practical Tips to Perform a Deltopectoral Flap**
Roberto A. Lima, Fernando L. Dias (Rio de Janeiro), Jorge Pinho Filho (Recife)

180 **14.3 Practical Tips for Performing a Pectoralis Major Flap**
José Magrim, João Gonçalves Filho (São Paulo)

182 **14.4 Practical Tips to Perform a Trapezius Flap**
Richard E. Hayden (Scottsdale, Ariz.)

184 **14.5 Latissimus Dorsi Myocutaneous Flap for Head and Neck Reconstruction**
Gady Har-El (New York, N.Y.; Brooklyn, N.Y.), Michael Singer (Brooklyn, N.Y.)

186 **14.6 Transverse Rectus Abdominis Flap**
Julio Morais Besteiro (São Paulo)

188 **14.7 Practical Tips to Perform a Microvascular Forearm Flap**
Adam S. Jacobson, Mark L. Urken (New York, N.Y.)

190 **14.8 Mandible Reconstruction with Fibula Microvascular Transfer**
Julio Morais Besteiro (São Paulo)

192 **14.9 Practical Tips to Perform a Microvascular Iliac Crest Flap**
Mario S.L. Galvao (Rio de Janeiro)

194 **14.10 The Scapular Flap**
Julio Morais Besteiro (São Paulo)

196 **14.11 Reconstruction of Pharyngoesophageal Defects with the Jejunal Free Autograft**
John J. Coleman 3rd (Indianapolis, Ind.)

198 **14.12 Practical Tips to Perform a Gastric Pull-Up**
William I. Wei, Vivian Mok (Hong Kong)

Miscellaneous

200 **15.1 Indications and Limitations of Fine Needle Aspiration Biopsy of Lateral Cervical Masses**
Paulo Campos Carneiro, Luiz Fernando Ferraz da Silva (São Paulo)

202 **15.2 When and How to Perform an Open Neck Biopsy of a Lateral Cervical Mass**
Pedro Michaluart Jr, Sérgio Samir Arap (São Paulo)

204 **15.3 Practical Tips in Managing Radiation-Associated Sarcoma of the Head and Neck**
Thomas D. Shellenberger (Orlando, Fla.; Houston, Tex.), Erich M. Sturgis (Houston, Tex.)

206 **15.4 Practical Tips for Performing Transoral Robotic Surgery**
Gregory S. Weinstein, Bert W. O'Malley, Jr. (Philadelphia, Pa.)

209 **Corresponding Authors**

213 **Subject Index**

Preface

The main objective of this book is to give the reader very concise and useful information on what should and should not be done when dealing with specific diagnostic and therapeutic situations in head and neck surgery. This is not a conventional textbook, containing a comprehensive collection of all material available, nor is it an atlas of anatomy or surgical techniques. Instead, a highly selected group of top world experts was invited to share their personal experiences about key subjects in the different areas of our specialty. All agreed to discuss, in a very succinct chapter, their view, emphasizing useful tips and particularly warning against potentially hazardous pitfalls that could affect the diagnosis and treatment of our patients. Moreover, all contributors were asked to recommend practical guidelines to help all of us in our everyday practice.

The different sections of this book include the vast majority of the diseases encountered by the head and neck surgeon in his or her everyday practice: (1) thyroid and parathyroid glands; (2) neck metastases; (3) oral and oropharyngeal tumors; (4) laryngeal tumors; (5) hypopharyngeal cancer; (6) nasopharyngeal cancer; (7) salivary gland tumors; (8) skull base tumors; (9) vascular tumors; (10) congenital tumors; (11) parapharyngeal space tumors; (12) infections of the head and neck; (13) tracheotomy; (14) reconstruction, and (15) miscellaneous.

I would like to thank all authors for their efforts to efficiently address their respective subjects in the limited space available. I believe that they have done a terrific job.

I would like to extend my deep gratitude to the co-editors Dan Fliss, MD, Eugene N. Myers, MD, Fernando L. Dias, MD, Roberto A. Lima, MD and William I. Wei, MD, whose participation was vital for this book, not only because of the number and quality of their contribution but also because of their invaluable suggestions concerning revisions, topics and authors.

Also, I would like to thank the publishers Steven Karger (in memoriam) and Thomas Karger, who believed in this project and have made it reality. My special recognition goes to Mrs. Elisabeth Anyawike, the extremely efficient Production Editor who assisted me in dealing with all the difficulties during the editing process.

Finally, my eternal gratitude goes to my beloved wife, Selma S. Cernea, MD, for her serenity, patience and support.

Claudio R. Cernea, São Paulo

Cernea CR, Dias FL, Fliss D, Lima RA, Myers EN, Wei WI (eds): Pearls and Pitfalls in Head and Neck Surgery. Basel, Karger, 2008, pp 2–3

1.1 How to Avoid Injury of Inferior Laryngeal Nerve

Jacob Moalem, Orlo H. Clark

University of California, Division of Endocrine Surgery, San Francisco, Calif., USA

PEARLS

- Detailed knowledge of the inferior laryngeal nerve (ILN)'s anatomic relationships and variations is imperative to safely perform thyroidectomy or parathyroidectomy.
- Avoid mass ligature and stay as close as possible to the thyroid gland at all times.
- Definitively identify the ILN prior to sacrificing branches of the inferior thyroid artery (ITA).
- Maintain meticulous hemostasis and a clean dissecting field at all times for excellent visualization.
- Fully evaluate the thyroid gland and adjacent lymph nodes for suspicious nodules prior to performing thyroidectomy or parathyroidectomy to eliminate the potential for reoperation.
- Consider a 'you touch it – you buy it' policy: soften the indications for thyroid lobectomy any time a lobe is exposed for another reason.
- Perform preoperative direct laryngoscopy on all patients with dysphonia or risk factors for unilateral vocal cord dysfunction at baseline.

PITFALLS

- Injury to the ILN is up to 5-fold higher in reoperative surgery. This risk is even higher when operating for malignancy as opposed to benign conditions.
- The most common site where the ILN is injured is near the ligament of Berry. Injury may occur because of excessive traction, cautery, a branched ILN, or misplaced hemostatic sutures.

Introduction

The terms 'inferior' and 'recurrent' laryngeal nerve have been used interchangeably to describe a branch of the thoracic vagus that loops around the subclavian artery (on the right) or aortic arch (on the left), and then ascends to terminally arborize [1]. The ILN carries sensory, motor and parasympathetic fibers, and divides into an internal branch (sensory to the vocal cords and subglottis) and external branch (motor to the intrinsic muscles of the larynx except cricothyroid). In as many as 70% of cases, this branching is extralaryngeal, predisposing a branch of the nerve to injury. In the vast majority of these cases, this bifurcation occurs more than 1.0 cm from the cricoid cartilage [2, 3].

ILN dysfunction is among the most common, feared and litigious complications of cervical explorations, and is associated with temporary or permanent vocal cord dysfunction. When bilateral injury occurs, the morbidity is even more dramatic, often requiring tracheostomy.

Practical Tips

❶ Most authors assert that routine identification of the ILN, as opposed to its avoidance, is the method of choice to reduce the chance of injury [4].
❷ In the modern surgical literature, the ILN has never been reported to enter the fascia of the thyroid gland. However, the nerve can be surrounded or displaced by a thyroid nodule or by an invasive thyroid cancer.

3 Many surgeons use relationships with the ITA, tracheoesophageal groove, and ligament of Berry as anatomical landmarks to identify the nerve. However:

• While the majority of ILNs lie posterior to the ITA, approximately 1/3 have been identified either anterior to, or interdigitating with, its branches (12–32.5 and 6.5–27%, respectively) [3, 5].

• In approximately 2/3 of the cases the ILN lies within the tracheoesophageal groove. However, in approximately 1/3 of the cases the nerve is lateral to the trachea, and in approximately 1% the nerve is anterior to the trachea [3].

• Autopsy studies demonstrate that the ILN is usually located dorsolaterally to the ligament of Berry, at a mean distance of 3 mm [6]. There are reports, however, where the nerve passes posteromedially to, or through, the ligament of Berry [7].

4 A particularly feared variant is the nonrecurrent ILN (NRILN). Known to occur in 0.3–1.6% of cases, NRILN is virtually always encountered on the right side where it is associated with (and may be predicted by [8]) an anomalous origin of the brachiocephalic artery. Of note, an NRILN may be associated with the superior thyroid artery (type A) or with the ITA (type B) [8]. In either case, its course is much more oblique (or even transverse) than expected. There are two reports of left-sided NRILN, both in association with a right-sided aortic arch [9].

5 The use of loupes with 2.5–3.5× magnification helps to optimize visualization and minimize risk of injury to the ILN.

6 Although increasingly employed, there is no convincing evidence that routine use of intraoperative ILN monitoring or stimulation results in lower rates of nerve injury [10].

7 Recovery of function is possible in cases where postoperative palsy occurs despite intraoperative identification and preservation of the ILN. In this group, vocal cord recovery is described in as many as 94.6% of patients at a mean of 31 days [4].

Conclusion

As is widely reported, consistently safe thyroidectomy is feasible, but relies upon a meticulous surgical technique. Surgeon experience, intimate familiarity with the anatomy of the ILN, magnification, and constant vigilance all minimize the risk of highly morbid complications.

References

1 Mirilas P, Skandalakis JE: Benign anatomical mistakes: the correct anatomical term for the recurrent laryngeal nerve. Am Surg 2002;68:95–97.
2 Nemiroff PM, Katz AD: Extralaryngeal divisions of the recurrent laryngeal nerve. Surgical and clinical significance. Am J Surg 1982;144:466–469.
3 Ardito G, Revelli L, D'Alatri L, et al: Revisited anatomy of the recurrent laryngeal nerves. Am J Surg 2004;187:249–253.
4 Chiang FY, Wang LF, Huang YF, et al: Recurrent laryngeal nerve palsy after thyroidectomy with routine identification of the recurrent laryngeal nerve. Surgery 2005;137:342–347.
5 Steinberg JL, Khane GJ, Fernandes CM, et al: Anatomy of the recurrent laryngeal nerve: a redescription. J Laryngol Otol 1986; 100:919–927.
6 Sasou S, Nakamura S, Kurihara H: Suspensory ligament of Berry: its relationship to recurrent laryngeal nerve and anatomic examination of 24 autopsies. Head Neck 1998;20:695–698.
7 Yalcin B, Ozan H: Detailed investigation of the relationship between the inferior laryngeal nerve including laryngeal branches and ligament of Berry. J Am Coll Surg 2006;202:291–296.
8 Toniato A, Mazzarotto R, Piotto A, et al: Identification of the nonrecurrent laryngeal nerve during thyroid surgery: 20-year experience. World J Surg 2004;28:659–661.
9 Henry JF, Audiffret J, Denizot A, et al: The nonrecurrent inferior laryngeal nerve: review of 33 cases, including two on the left side. Surgery 1988;104:977–984.
10 Dralle H, Sekulla C, Haerting J, et al: Risk factors of paralysis and functional outcome after recurrent laryngeal nerve monitoring in thyroid surgery. Surgery 2004;136:1310–1322.

Cernea CR, Dias FL, Fliss D, Lima RA, Myers EN, Wei WI (eds): Pearls and Pitfalls in Head and Neck Surgery. Basel, Karger, 2008, pp 4–5

1.2 How to Avoid Injury of the External Branch of Superior Laryngeal Nerve

Claudio R. Cernea, Alberto R. Ferraz

Department of Head and Neck Surgery, University of São Paulo Medical School, São Paulo, Brazil

Pearls

- Keep in mind that the external branch of superior laryngeal nerve (EBSLN) may be found in the operative field of a thyroidectomy in 15–20% of the cases.
- Avoid mass ligatures of the superior thyroid pole vessels.
- Use nerve monitoring or, at least, a nerve stimulator, especially when performing a thyroidectomy in a voice professional.

Pitfalls

- Risk of EBSLN injury is much higher in large goiters.
- Excessive burning with the Bovie near the cricothyroid muscle (CTM) can cause the same functional impact on voice performance.

Introduction

The EBSLN is the main motor supply to the CTM. The contraction of this muscle stretches the vocal fold, especially during the production of high frequency sounds [1]. Therefore, EBSLN paralysis leads to an important impairment of voice performance, mainly among women and voice professionals.

This nerve crosses the superior thyroid vessels, usually more than 1 cm above the upper border of the superior thyroid pole, before reaching the CTM, in a region defined as the sternothyroid triangle [2]. However, in 15–20% of the instances, it may cross the vessels closer or even inferiorly to the border. This is the type 2b nerve [3], and in this instance the nerve is more vulnerable to inadvertent injury during a thyroidectomy [4]. Moreover, if the thyroid gland is markedly enlarged, the superior thyroid pole is elevated, increasing the likelihood of a type 2b nerve and, consequently, the risk of its injury as well [5]. In half of the cases who presented this complication after thyroidectomy, it was permanent [4], and no effective treatment has been reported so far. Therefore, prevention of damage to the EBSLN during thyroidectomy is strongly advised.

Practical Tips

Although it is probably not necessary to actively search for the EBSLN during a routine thyroidectomy in the majority of the cases, it is important to keep in mind some situations that could increase the risk of its injury and to be prepared to prevent it:

1. According to some authors, type 2b EBSLN is more prevalent among patients with short stature [6] and with large thyroid growth [5, 6].
2. Ask your anesthesiologist not to paralyze your patient.
3. Consider using some kind of nerve monitoring or, at least, a simple disposable nerve stimulator. If a nerve monitoring system is employed, the potential noted after EBSLN stimulation, despite being much smaller than the recurrent nerve record, is very typical. In addition, the contraction

of the CTM, in response to a simple 0.5-mA stimulus on the EBSLN is very easily demonstrated in the surgical field. These measures are mandatory when operating on a voice professional or within a reoperative field.

4 Always keep in mind that there is a 15–20% chance to find a type 2b nerve. Therefore, any anatomical structure resembling a small nerve going towards the CTM should be carefully preserved.

5 Magnification is advisable. Wide-angled surgical loupes, with 2.5–3.5× magnifying lenses, help to identify the EBSLN.

6 Sectioning the sternothyroid muscle markedly improves the visualization of the superior thyroid pole with no negative impact on voice performance [7].

7 Try to avoid mass ligatures of the superior thyroid pedicle. Instead, identify and ligate separately the branches of the superior thyroid vessels. If a harmonic scalpel or a sealing device is used, be sure not to include the EBSLN in the instrument.

8 The anatomical classification of the EBSLN was created based upon a conventional thyroidectomy field. However, when performing a video-assisted thyroidectomy, remember that the EBSLN is greatly approximated to the superior thyroid pole, because no hyperextension of the neck is exerted. On the other hand, the great magnification offered by the endoscope helps to identify and preserve the nerve in virtually all patients, as long as the surgeon is aware of this different positioning.

Conclusion

In this chapter, the reader is introduced to a frequently overlooked complication of thyroidectomy, the injury of the EBSLN. The resulting paralysis of CTM is often permanent. It is important to realize that 15–20% of the nerves may be found during a thyroidectomy, and the surgeon must be able to identify them, preferably with nerve monitoring or with a nerve stimulator, in order to keep their integrity when dissecting the superior thyroid pole.

References

1 Kark AE, Kissin MW, Auerbach R, et al: Voice changes after thyroidectomy: role of the external laryngeal nerve. Br Med J (Clin Res Ed) 1984;289:1412–1415.

2 Moosman DA, DeWeese MS: The external laryngeal nerve as related to thyroidectomy. Surg Gynecol Obstet 1968;127:1011–1016.

3 Cernea CR, Ferraz AR, Nishio S, et al: Surgical anatomy of the external branch of the superior laryngeal nerve. Head Neck 1992;14:380–383.

4 Cernea CR, Ferraz AR, Furlani J, et al: Identification of the external branch of the superior laryngeal nerve during thyroidectomy. Am J Surg 1992;164:634–639.

5 Cernea CR, Nishio S, Hojaij FC: Identification of the external branch of the superior laryngeal nerve (EBSLN) in large goiters. Am J Otolaryngol 1995;16:307–311.

6 Furlan JC, Cordeiro AC, Brandao LG: Study of some 'intrinsic risk factors' that can enhance an iatrogenic injury of the external branch of the superior laryngeal nerve. Otolaryngol Head Neck Surg 2003;128:396–400.

7 Cernea CR, Ferraz AR, Cordeiro AC: Surgical anatomy of the superior laryngeal nerve; in Randolph GW (ed): Surgery of the Thyroid and Parathyroid Glands. Philadelphia, Saunders-Elsevier, 2003, pp 293–299.

Cernea CR, Dias FL, Fliss D, Lima RA, Myers EN, Wei WI (eds): Pearls and Pitfalls in Head and Neck Surgery. Basel, Karger, 2008, pp 6–7

1.3 Recurrent Laryngeal Nerve Monitoring in Thyroid and Parathyroid Surgery: Technique for the NIM 2 System

David J. Lesnik[a], Lenine Garcia Brandao[b], Gregory W. Randolph[a]

[a] Massachusetts Eye and Ear Infirmary, Thyroid Surgical Division, Harvard Medical School, Boston, Mass., USA;
[b] Head and Neck Surgery, Hospital das Clínicas, University of São Paulo Medical School, São Paulo, Brazil

PEARLS

- The recurrent laryngeal nerve (RLN) monitoring will aid in identification and protection of the RLN during thyroid and parathyroid surgery especially in difficult or revision cases.
- The nerve monitor may be used to localize the RLN prior to visual identification expediting surgery and minimizing nerve dissection.
- Monitoring may be used to prognosticate postoperative function and impact the decision to perform bilateral surgery.
- When using the NIM 2 system, attention to detail and confirmation of tube position preoperatively is essential.

PITFALLS

- The monitor is not a substitute for careful surgical technique and meticulous hemostasis.
- True negative RLN stimulation cannot be trusted until definitive RLN identification and positive stimulation are achieved.
- No structure in the lateral thyroid region should be clamped, ligated, or cut until the RLN is identified both visually and electrically.

Introduction

Injury to the RLN is a significant risk associated with thyroid and parathyroid surgery. While permanent deficit is rare, this postoperative complication may lead to appreciable difficulties with speech and swallowing. Numerous studies have determined that routine identification of the RLN is associated with lower rates of injury. Therefore, RLN monitoring represents a useful technical development that may greatly aid the surgeon in identifying and protecting the RLN during surgery, especially in difficult cases, e.g. large or toxic goiter, malignancy, or reoperative cases.

RLN monitoring has three functions: (1) to facilitate neural identification, (2) to aid in neural dissection and (3) to prognosticate regarding postoperative neural function. Monitoring may reduce the incidence of nerve injury and yet, it is not used universally. Herein we describe our preferred method of RLN identification and monitoring and offer some tips for success.

NIM 2 Nerve Monitoring

In our experience the NIM 2 system (Xomed NIM 2, Jacksonville, Fla., USA) is the state of the art in RLN monitoring. The NIM 2 system employs a specially designed endotracheal (ET) tube (NIM 2 EMG ET tube) equipped with bilateral surface electrodes that are in contact with the medial aspect of the true vocal folds. A sterile, handheld stimulator probe is connected to a monitor and this is used to deliver the adjustable stimulus (0.5–2 mA) to the RLN. This allows passive and evoked monitoring of the thyroarytenoid muscles from monitor to the surgeon during thyroid or parathyroid surgery.

An added benefit to using the NIM 2 system is often in initial nerve localization before definite visual identification. The blunt-tipped stimulus probe may be used at higher intensity (e.g. 2 mA) to probe the soft tissue of the RLN triangle starting at a more superficial level proceeding more deeply. This technique often expedites identification of the proximal portion of the RLN without more extensive dissection.

Practical Tips for the NIM 2 System [from 1]

1. Succinylcholine or other short-acting paralytic agents allow full relaxation for good ET tube position with quick return of EMG activity.
2. Care must be taken to position the surface electrodes at the level of the glottis and the ET tube cuff in the subglottis.
3. Position patient prior to securing ET tube.
4. Check for:

   a) Respiratory variation in baseline EMG tracing; this is universal and confirms good tube position.

   b) Impedance of less than 5 kΩ with impedance imbalance of less than 1 kΩ.
5. Monitor settings:

   a) Event threshold (EMG response): 100 μV.

   b) Stimulator probe: 1 mA.
6. Surgical field notes:

   a) Test stimulator on strap muscle to confirm twitch and that current is received on Xomed monitor.

   b) Visually identify RLN and confirm true positive before accepting any stimulation as negative.

Conclusions

Nerve monitoring may assist the surgeon with more rapid and confident identification of the RLN during thyroid and parathyroid surgery. It will also facilitate dissection along the RLN, which is especially useful in certain cases such as a distally branching RLN.

If used properly, nerve monitoring may help the surgeon prevent postoperative RLN dysfunction.

References

1 Randolph GW: Surgical anatomy of the recurrent laryngeal nerve; in Randolph GW (ed): Surgery of the Thyroid and Parathyroid Glands. Philadelphia, Saunders-Elsevier, 2003, pp 316–320.

2 Brandão JSN, Brandão LG, Cavalheiro BG, Sondermann A, Vitols I: Intraoperative monitoring of inferior laringeal nerve during thyroidectomies and neck dissections. XIX Congresso Brasileiro de Cirurgia de Cabeça e Pescoço, Curitiba, 2003.

3 Horn D, Rötzscher VM: Intraoperative electromyogram monitoring of the recurrent laryngeal nerve: experience with an intralaryngeal surface electrode. Langenbecks Arch Surg 1999;384:392–395.

4 Sasaki CT, Mitra S: Recurrent laryngeal nerve monitoring by cricopharyngeus contraction. Laryngoscope 2001;111:738–739.

5 Riddell V: Thyroidectomy: prevention of bilateral recurrent laryngeal nerve palsy: results of identification of the nerve in over 23 consecutive years (1946–1969) with description of an additional safety measure. Br J Surg 1970;57:1–11.

6 Satoh I: Evoked electromyographic test applied for recurrent laryngeal nerve paralysis. Laryngoscope 1978;88:2022–2031.

7 Premachandra DJ, Radcliffe GJ, Stearns MP: Intraoperative identification of the recurrent laryngeal nerve and demonstration of its function. Laryngoscope 1990;100:94–96.

8 Thomusch O, Dralle H: Advantages of intraoperative neuromonitoring in thyroid gland operations (in German). Dtsch Med Wochenschr 2000;125:774.

Cernea CR, Dias FL, Fliss D, Lima RA, Myers EN, Wei WI (eds): Pearls and Pitfalls in Head and Neck Surgery. Basel, Karger, 2008, pp 8–9

1.4 How to Preserve the Parathyroid Glands during Thyroid Surgery

Ashok R. Shaha, Vergilius José F. de Araújo Filho

Head and Neck Service, Memorial Sloan-Kettering Cancer Center, Cornell University Medical Center, New York, N.Y., USA

PEARLS

- Incidence of temporary hypoparathyroidism is 25–30%, while the incidence of permanent hypoparathyroidism is 2–3% and depends upon certain technical modifications, such as neck dissection, paratracheal lymph node dissection (level VI), large and substernal goiters, or Hashimoto's thyroiditis.
- Parathyroid blood supply from the inferior thyroid artery, and occasionally from the superior thyroid artery or directly from the thyroid vessels. Preserve parathyroids with blood supply.
- Devascularized parathyroid should be autotransplanted in the neck muscle. Parathyroid glands may mimic lymph nodes, thyroid tissue, or fat.

PITFALLS

- Symptoms of hypoparathyroidism may be subtle. However, the symptoms may become serious, especially with the development of tetany.
- Severe hypocalcemia may occur even 2–3 days after the initial surgery.
- Intravenous calcium supplement may have cardiac toxicity if given rapidly, and may irritate the skin if infiltrated.
- Large doses of oral calcium and vitamin D may lead to iatrogenic hypercalcemia.

Introduction

Since Ivor Sandstrom described parathyroid glands in humans, there has been considerable interest in their function and preservation, particularly during total thyroidectomy [1]. One of the serious complications of total thyroidectomy is temporary (25–30%) or permanent hypoparathyroidism (2–3%). The morbidity from permanent hypoparathyroidism is considerable, with a lifetime requirement of calcium and vitamin D. These small, elusive glands are crucial to sustain good health in patients undergoing total thyroidectomy. Serial calcium levels are helpful and the trending of calcium levels between 8 and 23 h is helpful. Parathormone assay has also been helpful regarding safe discharge of the patients.

Surgical Technique

1. Recognize normal and abnormal locations of parathyroids. They may occasionally be undescended, located between the trachea and the esophagus, in the superior mediastinum, or inside the thyroid gland.
2. The branches of the inferior thyroid artery should be ligated close to the thyroid capsule, so that the minute branches supplying the parathyroid glands can be preserved [2, 3].
3. Avoid surface hematoma or retraction injury of the parathyroid glands. Use electrocautery judiciously. Anterior parathyroids on the surface of the thyroid, receiving their blood supply directly

from the thyroid gland, may be very difficult to preserve in situ and may require autotransplantation. Intense care should be taken to identify and preserve the parathyroid glands in patients undergoing total thyroidectomy with neck dissection, surgery for large and substernal goiters, and Hashimoto's thyroiditis. Patients undergoing total laryngopharyngectomy and total thyroidectomy are at highest risk for permanent hypoparathyroidism [4].

Parathyroid Autotransplantation

During surgery, if the parathyroid gland appears to be devascularized by change of color or separation from the surrounding soft tissue, it should be autotransplanted after confirming with a small piece on frozen section that it is parathyroid gland. Confirm the presence of parathyroid tissue to avoid autotransplantation of a metastatic thyroid carcinoma. The parathyroid gland should be minced into small pieces and autotransplanted, preferably in the contralateral sternomastoid muscle. There is no need to autotransplant the parathyroid gland in the forearm. Generally 60–70% of the autotransplanted parathyroid glands will function within 6–12 weeks.

Management of Temporary and Permanent Hypoparathyroidism

The patient should be observed closely postoperatively. Check serial calcium levels 8 and 23 h postsurgery. Ionized calcium is a much better parameter. If the patient is asymptomatic, calcium replacement is generally not suggested. However, if calcium levels are below 7.5 mg/dl, calcium supplementation should be considered, as the patients may develop serious signs and symptoms of hypocalcemia. Patients should be checked for Chvostek's and Trousseau's signs [5, 6]. If the patient has severe symptoms, intravenous calcium gluconate is recommended. Subsequent maintenance calcium supplementation is recommended with calcium and vitamin D. Generally, vitamin D takes approximately 48 h for biochemical effects. Such patients will require increased dosage of calcium supplementation, approximately 500 mg of elemental calcium, 4–6 times/day. It is important to check the calcium levels 48–72 h after this intensive supplementation to avoid iatrogenic hypercalcemia. A parathormone assay may be helpful.

Conclusion

An understanding of the anatomy of normal parathyroid glands, their variations, blood supply and preservation during total thyroidectomy is crucial to avoid hypoparathyroidism. Every attempt should be made to preserve the parathyroid glands and their blood supply, or autotransplant if necessary. The patients should be observed closely for hypoparathyroidism, and treated expeditiously to avoid severe symptoms of hypocalcemia.

References

1 Halsted WS, Evans HM: The parathyroid glandules: their blood supply and their preservation in operations on the thyroid gland. Ann Surg 1907;46:489–507.
2 Shaha AR, Jaffe BM: Parathyroid preservation during thyroid surgery. Am J Otol 1988;19:113–117.
3 Araujo Filho VJF, Silva Filho GB, Brandao LG, Santos LRM, Ferraz AR: The importance of the ligation of the inferior thyroid artery in parathyroid function after subtotal thyroidectomy. Clinics 2000;55:113–120.
4 Alveryd A: Parathyroid glands in thyroid surgery. Acta Chir Scand Suppl 1968;389:1–120.
5 Roh JL, Park CI: Routine oral calcium and vitamin D supplements for prevention of hypocalcemia after total thyroidectomy. Am J Surg 2006;192:675–678.
6 Chia SH, Weisman RA, Tieu D, Kelly C, Dillmann WH, Orloff LA: Prospective study of perioperative factors predicting hypocalcemia after thyroid and parathyroid surgery. Arch Otolaryngol Head Neck Surg 2006;132:41–45.

Cernea CR, Dias FL, Fliss D, Lima RA, Myers EN, Wei WI (eds): Pearls and Pitfalls in Head and Neck Surgery. Basel, Karger, 2008, pp 10–11

1.5 Completion Thyroidectomy

Eveline Slotema, Jean-François Henry

Department of Endocrine Surgery, University Hospital Marseille, Marseille, France

PEARLS

- Minimizing the need for reoperative surgery is the most effective way to decrease operative risks.
- Consider each parathyroid gland (PT) as if it were the last one left, even in unilateral resection.

PITFALLS

- Avoid reoperations in previously dissected planes by neither performing subtotal lobectomies nor enucleations.
- Contralateral lobe assessment by palpation is old-fashioned and inferior to ultrasonic assessment.

Introduction

Completion thyroidectomy (CT) is a unilateral reoperation on a previously unoperated thyroid lobe (TL) to avoid the risk of recurrence on the contralateral lobe. The incidence of bilateral thyroid carcinoma reported in the literature ranges from 30 to 88% [1, 2]. No initial tumor feature reliably predicts the presence of tumor on the second side [3], except multifocality. CT is recommended for all patients with differentiated cancer (>10 mm) who have significant residual thyroid tissue remaining in the neck (^{131}I uptake >5% over 24 h) [2]. The use of postoperative radioiodine therapy decreases recurrence rate and distant metastasis, improving survival when compared with unilateral thyroid lobectomy [4]. Finally, CT permits tumor surveillance by thyroglobulin measurements.

To avoid CT, try to obtain a correct diagnosis before or during initial surgery with fine needle aspiration cytology (FNA), preoperative ultrasound and frozen section (FS). Nevertheless, neither FNA nor FS are absolutely reliable in the diagnosis of cancer, especially in follicular and oncocytic lesions [5]. Hence, for neoplasms >4 cm in diameter with these FNA results, prophylactic total thyroidectomy may be considered [2].

Practical Tips to Facilitate CT

To avoid reoperations in previously dissected planes, total unilateral lobectomies, always including isthmus and Lallouette's pyramid, are preferred to subtotal resections. Assessing lymph nodes during initial operation is important.

The recurrent and superior laryngeal nerves and both PTs should be preserved at the original operation. The inferior thyroid artery (TA) should therefore not be ligated. A devascularized gland should be autotransplanted. Consider each PT as if it were the last one left, even in unilateral resection.

Intraoperative assessment of contralateral lobe via palpation is useless. Ultrasonography is much more accurate. Do not dissect between the sternothyroid muscle (STM) and the thyroid gland. If palpation is deemed necessary, it should be done between STM and sternohyoid muscles (SHM) to prevent adhesions along the thyroid capsula [6].

Practical Tips to Perform CT

The timing of CT can substantially contribute to surgical difficulty. Within 1 week, no dense adhesions occur. Therefore, reoperation should be performed no later than 5 days postoperatively or postponed for at least 3 months [7]. Psychologically, it is in the patient's best interest to reoperate as soon as possible.

Direct laryngoscopy should be performed in all cases before CT, because 30–40% of unilateral recurrent laryngeal nerve (RLN) paralysis is asymptomatic [6]. Transient palsy can be a temporary contraindication for reoperation. In patients with definitive RLN palsy the indication of CT must be discussed considering the risk of bilateral RLN palsy and the need for tracheostomy. In such cases electromyographic monitoring of the RLN is strongly advised, if not in all reoperative thyroid surgery [8].

Preferably, the original scar is incised for access to the thyroid. Strap muscles are dissected in the midline and retracted laterally, if they did not adhere to the TL as a result of former proper surgery. This is the ideal situation. In moderate adhesions, access is gained between the SHM and STM. If there is dense fibrosis, a posterolateral approach by Henry and Sebag [9] may be used.

Direct RLN visualization is mandatory. In case of adhesions, the RLN is to be identified in a previously undissected area and then followed into the dissected area. The nerve may be identified inferiorly, below the inferior TA, in the tracheoesophageal groove, and then followed upwards, or superiorly, after division of the superior TA, with subsequent lateral and downward traction of the superior thyroid pole, identified at its entry point. Then, it may be followed downwards.

A meticulous review of previous operative notes and pathology for possible symmetry of parathyroids can be useful. To autotransplant devascularized PT the operative specimen should be examined carefully before passing it on for pathological analysis.

Conclusion

When a unilateral thyroid lobectomy is indicated, the surgeon and cytopathologist should be careful to avoid or at least to facilitate possible CT. This implies obtaining a correct diagnosis at initial surgery, performing nothing but a total lobectomy with preservation of both PTs and RLN, and avoiding any dissection into the contralateral side. Therefore, when indicated, CT is simply a unilateral operation on a previously undissected TL and a procedure that can be performed safely.

References

1 Clark OH: Total thyroidectomy: the treatment of choice for patients with differentiated thyroid cancer. Ann Surg 1982;196:361–370.
2 Pasieka JL, Thompson NW, McLeod MK, Burney RE, Macha M: The incidence of bilateral well-differentiated thyroid cancer found at completion thyroidectomy. World J Surg 1992;16:711–716.
3 DeGroot LJ, Kaplan EL: Second operations for 'completion' of thyroidectomy in treatment of differentiated thyroid cancer. Surgery 1991;110:936–939.
4 Hamming JF, Van de Velde CJ, Goslings BM, Schelfhout LJ, Fleuren GJ, Hermans J, Zwaveling A: Prognosis and morbidity after total thyroidectomy for papillary, follicular and medullary thyroid cancer. Eur J Cancer Clin Oncol 1989;25:1317–1323.
5 Raber W, Kaserer K, Niederle B, Vierhapper H: Risk factors for malignancy of thyroid nodules initially identified as follicular neoplasia by fine-needle aspiration: results of a prospective study of one hundred twenty patients. Thyroid 2000;10:709–712.
6 Pasieka JL: Reoperative thyroid surgery; in Randolph GW (ed): Surgery of the Thyroid and Parathyroid Glands. Philadephia, Saunders, 2003, pp 385–391.
7 Tan MP, Agarwal G, Reeve TS, Barraclough BH, Delbridge LW: Impact of timing on completion thyroidectomy for thyroid cancer. Br J Surg 2002;89:802–804.
8 Timmermann W, Dralle H, Hamelmann W, Thomusch O, Sekulla C, Meyer T, Timm S, Thiede A. Does intraoperative nerve monitoring reduce the rate of recurrent nerve palsies during thyroid surgery? Zentralbl Chir 2002;127:395–399.
9 Henry JF, Sebag F: Lateral endoscopic approach for thyroid and parathyroid surgery. Ann Chir 2006;131:51–56.

Cernea CR, Dias FL, Fliss D, Lima RA, Myers EN, Wei WI (eds): Pearls and Pitfalls in Head and Neck Surgery. Basel, Karger, 2008, pp 12–13

1.6 Surgery for Intrathoracic Goiters

Ashok R. Shaha[a], James L. Netterville[b], Nadir Ahmad[b]

[a] Cornell University Medical College, Memorial Sloan-Kettering Cancer Center, New York, N.Y., and
[b] Department of Otolaryngology-Head and Neck Surgery, Vanderbilt University Medical Center, Nashville, Tenn., USA

PEARLS

- Total thyroidectomy (TT) is the optimal management.
- Symptoms related to pressure effects are the main indication for surgery, but potential malignancy is also a concern.
- Cervical approach is usually sufficient to manage large intrathoracic goiters (IG) and sternal split (SS) is rarely indicated.
- Large incision, transection of the strap muscles, and ligation of the inferior thyroid vessels are recommended.
- Preoperative CT scan determines both location and extension of the goiter and its relationship to surrounding structures, especially the recurrent laryngeal nerve (RLN).
- Despite significant tracheal deviation and compression, tracheomalacia is very rare.

PITFALLS

- Intraoperative bleeding may be a major concern.
- Risk of RLN injury is much higher though it is usually located in the normal anatomic position.
- Parathyroid glands (PG) may be quite difficult to identify.
- Aggressive, rather than gentle blunt finger dissection is dangerous.
- Approximately 10% of these patients may present with acute airway issues.

Introduction

Intrathoracic or substernal goiter (SG) is defined as a goiter with 50% or more of its mass in the mediastinum (MS) [1]. Its incidence ranges between 2 and 19% of patients undergoing thyroidectomy [1–3]. IG should always be considered in the differential diagnosis of both neck and anterior mediastinal masses.

The origin of IG is commonly an extension of the cervical thyroid gland into the MS, rather than an abnormal growth of a mediastinal-based gland. The cervical source of blood supply to IG attests to its cervical origin in most cases. The majority of IG are benign and can remain asymptomatic for many years. Symptoms typically arise from tracheoesophageal compression.

IGs often extend into the anterosuperior MS, keeping the RLN in its normal configuration. However, IG involving the posterior MS (1–2%) displace the nerve anteriorly. Preoperative imaging with CT scan is important.

Complications inherent to thyroidectomy are more common after IG operations, but still low in experienced hands. Tracheomalacia secondary to long-term compression is surprisingly rare [1]. However, other reports state that it can occur, suggesting to keep a patient intubated for 24–48 h, with controlled extubation [2, 3].

Practical Tips

❶ Nontraumatic intubation with No. 6 or 7 tube is a must. A majority of these patients can be easily intubated since the larynx is generally in its normal position.

❷ The endotracheal tube should be well below the vocal cords, as there is a frequent tendency for the tube to slide back.

❸ The patient should be totally paralyzed during surgery for full relaxation.

❹ A wide skin excision and transection of the strap muscles is recommended for better exposure.

❺ The dissection in the neck should begin with ligation of the middle thyroid vein, ligation of the superior thyroid vessels, and dissection along the lateral border of the thyroid. The area between the anterior border of the trachea and the lateral border of the thyroid should be exposed under vision.

❻ There are several inferior thyroid veins which should be ligated carefully. This procedure can lead to unwarranted bleeding which may be extremely difficult to control. Hemoclips, bipolar electrocautery or Ligasure may assist in this portion of the surgical procedure.

❼ The RLN is better identified after retrieving the thyroid gland from the substernal region. Rarely, a retrograde technique of dissecting the RLN may be necessary, where the nerve is identified near the ligament of Berry and dissected retrograde using a toboggan technique.

❽ PGs are difficult to identify, and if devascularized may occasionally require autotransplantation in the sternomastoid muscle.

❾ SS is seldom necessary, and can involve partial (manubriectomy) or clamshell thoracotomy. A full SS is essential if the thyroid is adherent to the surrounding structures or there is suspicion of malignancy.

❿ Most of the patients can be extubated in the operating room; however, if there is any concern, the tube should remain in place for 24 h.

⓫ Suction drain is recommended.

⓬ Technical variations, such as retrieving the SG with spoons, or morcellation, have been described, but are not used [2, 3].

Conclusions

SGs form 2–19% of all goiters. The main surgical indication is compression. Approximately 10% of SGs may harbor malignancy. The vast majority can be retrieved through the neck. TT is usually indicated. The surgeon should be familiar with intraoperative manipulation of large SGs and technical variations to retrieve the goiter from the neck. The major complication is hemorrhage in the superior MS.

References

1 Netterville JL, Coleman SC, Smith JC, et al: Management of substernal goiter. Laryngoscope 1998;108:1611–1617.
2 Newman E, Shaha AR: Substernal goiter. J Surg Oncol 1995;60: 207–212.
3 Singh B, Lucente FE, Shaha AR: Substernal goiter: a clinical review. Am J Otolaryngol 1994;15:409–416.
4 Shaha AR: Surgery for benign thyroid disease causing tracheoesophageal compression. Otolaryngol Clin North Am 1990;23: 391–401.
5 Shaha A, Alfonso A, Jaffe BM: Acute airway distress due to thyroid pathology. Surgery 1987;102:1068–1074.
6 Shaha AR, Burnett C, Alfonso A, Jaffe BM: Goiters and airway problems. Am J Surg 1989;158:378–381.
7 Katlic MR, Wang C, Grillo HC: Substernal goiter. Ann Thorac Surg 1985;39:391–399.

Cernea CR, Dias FL, Fliss D, Lima RA, Myers EN, Wei WI (eds): Pearls and Pitfalls in Head and Neck Surgery. Basel, Karger, 2008, pp 14–15

1.7 How to Decide the Extent of Thyroidectomy for Benign Diseases

Jeremy L. Freeman

Mount Sinai Hospital, University of Toronto, Toronto, Ont., Canada

PEARLS

- Hyperthyroidism is best treated with total thyroidectomy.
- Compressive and cosmetic problems are best treated with total thyroidectomy.
- Low-risk nodular disease is best treated with subtotal thyroidectomy with the option to total depending on intraoperative pathology.
- High-risk nodular disease is best treated with total thyroidectomy.

PITFALLS

- Lack of knowledge of risk factors results in inadequate surgery in the high-risk patient or too aggressive surgery (total thyroidectomy) in the low-risk patient.

Introduction

Diseases of the thyroid can be divided into functional and structural. Functional problems include hypo- and hyperthyroid states. Hypothyroidism generally is managed with administration of thyroid hormone. Hyperthyroid states can be treated with a surgical resection primarily or secondarily in cases refractory to management with medication and/or radioactive iodine. Hyperthyroid surgical cases are best managed by total thyroidectomy to ensure eradication of all diseased tissue mitigating against persistence [1].

Structural problems of the thyroid can be divided into those cases treated for cosmetic reasons, compressive symptoms or risk of cancer.

Patients with cosmetically unsightly goiters or compression of foodway and/or airway are best managed by total thyroidectomy. Usually those large thyroids entering the mediastinum can be retrieved through a neck approach but those goiters that have grown deeply into the mediastinum (i.e. to the level of the carina) may have to be managed surgically through a sternal split [2].

Although controversial, we feel that cancer cases are best managed with total thyroidectomy although there is a school of thought that less than total thyroidectomy is appropriate for low-risk cancer cases such as small nodules in younger individuals [3]. The literature suggests that outcomes (survival/recurrence) are enhanced by total thyroidectomy [4].

The problems in decision-making arise in patients presenting with thyroid nodular disease without a definite preoperative diagnosis. Patients presenting with thyroid nodular disease should have a comprehensive history and physical examination, a fine needle aspirate biopsy and ultrasonic examination of the neck. Patients can then be classified into low- and high-risk disease based on risk factors (table 1) [5]. Low-risk patients have few risk factors usually of minor import whereas higher-risk patients have several risk factors or one or two significant ones. Patients with no definite tissue diagnosis of cancer with nodular dis-

Table 1. Risk factors

Patient risk factors	Tumor risk factors	Imaging risk factors
Age (very young or very old)	Rapid size increase	Metastatic nodes[1]
Place of birth (e.g. Belarus)[1]	Lymphadenopathy[1]	Stippled calcification[1]
Ethnicity (e.g. Filipino)[1]	Vocal cord paresis[1]	Invasive primary lesion[1]
Radiation exposure[1]	Dysphagia	
Familial syndrome (e.g. Cowden syndrome)[1]	Firm/fixed nodule	
Family history of thyroid cancer	Suspicious/atypical/positive cytology[1]	
Elevated serum calcitonin[1]	Size >4 cm	

[1] Denotes major risk factor.

ease in a low-risk category may be treated with partial thyroidectomy with the option to proceed to total thyroidectomy depending on intraoperative pathology. Sometimes intraoperative pathology is not available or conclusive at which time definitive cancers diagnosed subsequently may be managed with completion thyroidectomy. This approach mitigates against total thyroidectomy for benign disease and thus reduces the risk of complication and the need for subsequent supplementation with thyroid hormone.

A further decision-making challenge is the patient with a putative solitary nodule which is benign who undergoes surgery and during the procedure, on palpation of the opposite lobe, is found to have more nodules of significant size which are of indeterminate pathology. It is prudent to proceed with removal of the opposite lobe in these cases to deal with possible undetected malignancy and/or to avoid diagnostic dilemmas in the future given nodular disease in the opposite lobe of an operated thyroid field. Palpation should be done over the strap muscles in order to avoid unnecessary fibrosis rendering future surgery more technically difficult.

It is wise to remove the pyramidal lobe with any surgery be it subtotal or total thyroidectomy to avoid leaving hard-to-find thyroid tissue in the event that the patient would require a completion procedure in the future. In addition, if the disease turns out to be malignant, as much thyroid tissue as possible would have been removed to allow maximum effect of radioactive iodine administration.

An elevated serum calcitonin in a patient with thyroid nodular disease necessitates a total thyroidectomy with appropriate neck dissection for probable medullary thyroid cancer [6].

Conclusion

Hyperthyroidism treated surgically is best treated by total thyroidectomy.

Structural problems including unsightly cosmetic goiters, compressive symptoms and cancer are treated with total thyroidectomy.

Nodular lesions with benign or indeterminate cytopathology are then viewed from the perspective of risk stratification and extent of thyroidectomy is based on whether patients fall into low- or high-risk categories.

References

1 Barakate MS, Agarwal G, Reeve TS, et al: Total thyroidectomy is now the preferred option for the surgical management of Graves' disease. ANZ J Surg 2002;72:321–324.
2 de Perrot M, Fadel E, Mercier O, et al: Surgical management of mediastinal goiters: when is a sternotomy required? Thorac Cardiovasc Surg 2007;55:39–43.
3 Shah JP, Loree TR, Dharkar D, et al: Lobectomy versus total thyroidectomy for differentiated carcinoma of the thyroid: a matched-pair analysis. Am J Surg 1993;166:331–335.
4 Mazzaferri EL, Massoll N: Management of papillary and follicular (differentiated) thyroid cancer: new paradigms using recombinant human thyrotropin. Endocr Relat Cancer 2002;9:227–247.
5 Cooper DS, Doherty GM, Haugen BR, et al: Management guidelines for patients with thyroid nodules and differentiated thyroid cancer. Thyroid 2006;16:109–142.
6 Clark JR, Fridman TR, Odell MJ, et al: Prognostic variables and calcitonin in medullary thyroid cancer. Laryngoscope 2005;115: 1445–1450.

Cernea CR, Dias FL, Fliss D, Lima RA, Myers EN, Wei WI (eds): Pearls and Pitfalls in Head and Neck Surgery. Basel, Karger, 2008, pp 16–17

1.8 Minimally Invasive Video-Assisted Thyroidectomy

Erivelto M. Volpi, Gabrielle Matterazzi, Fernando L. Dias, Paolo Miccoli

Head and Neck Surgery Department, School of Medicine, University of São Paulo, São Paulo, Brazil

PEARLS

- A careful preoperative selection of the patients is the only guarantee of a low complication rate.
- Minimally invasive, video-assisted thyroidectomy (MIVAT) allows an excellent endoscopic visualization of nerves and parathyroid glands (PG) and a good control of major vessels.
- When using Harmonic Scalpel® (HS), keep the tip far from the nerves (more than 5 mm) and, if necessary, do not hesitate to use a clip.
- Do not prolong the endoscopic dissection too much. Once the nerves and PGs are identified and dissected, extract the lobe and continue resection under direct vision.
- Better postoperative course and cosmetic outcome are major benefits of MIVAT.

PITFALLS

- Unexpected thyroiditis or the presence of metastatic lymph nodes in the central compartment are the most frequent reasons for conversion.
- At the beginning, operative time and complication rate might be higher.
- Improper use of HS can jeopardize tracheal surface (avoid neck hyperextension).

Introduction

MIVAT was developed at the University of Pisa by Paolo Miccoli [1, 2]. When a new surgical procedure, like MIVAT, is introduced, especially if the operative technique employs innovative instruments and is based on peculiar surgical steps, there will be a natural learning curve for the surgeons. At the beginning, operative time and complication rate may rise, but after an adequate period of training, results can be compared with conventional operation.

Practical Tips

A careful selection of the patients results in a low complication rate and a good outcome. Only a minority of the cases are eligible for an MIVAT [3–5].

1 MIVAT is performed by a unique central incision of 1.5 cm, 2 cm above the sternal notch.

2 The operative space is maintained by external retraction; no gas insufflation is utilized. Subcutaneous fat and platysma are carefully dissected to avoid any minimum bleeding. The midline is divided longitudinally as much as possible (3–4 cm).

3 A 30° 5-mm endoscope is inserted through the skin incision. Under endoscopic vision the dissection of the thyrotracheal groove is completed by using small (2 mm in diameter) instruments: atraumatic spatulas, spatula-shaped aspirator,

ear-nose-throat forceps and scissors. Hemostasis is achieved by HS and small (3 mm) vascular clips.

4 Section of the upper pedicle is performed endoscopically as the first step. The orientation of the endoscope is of paramount importance. It must now be held on a line almost parallel to the neurovascular trunk, with the 30° rotated upward, looking at the roof of the operative space, thus offering the best view of the field. After visualizing the external branch of the superior laryngeal nerve (EBSLN), the branches of the superior thyroid pedicle will be selectively and safely sectioned.

5 In most cases the EBSLN can be much more easily identified near the upper pedicle than during the standard procedure. Also PGs are easily visualized by endoscopic magnification and their manipulation by spatulas is more delicate.

6 The inferior laryngeal nerve (ILN) can also be simply identified during MIVAT thanks to the magnification of the endoscope. During this phase of the operation, the endoscope must be held in an orthogonal position with the thyroid lobe and neurovascular trunk, with the 30° directed downward. Look for the ILN near the posterior lobe of the thyroid (Zuckerkandl tuberculum). In conventional surgery the ILN is generally identified at its emergence from the thoracic outlet; during MIVAT, this area can be difficult to visualize; the nerve can be found near the middle part of the thyroid gland.

7 Always remember to keep the inactive blade of the HS oriented to avoid jeopardizing the nerve, which is very sensitive to heat transmission. A minimal distance (5 mm) between the inactive blade and the nerve must be kept.

Conclusion

In selected cases, MIVAT offers the same results as conventional thyroidectomy, with best cosmetic outcome, less postoperative pain and best postoperative recovery.

References

1 Miccoli P, Berti P, Conte M, Bendinelli C, Marcocci C: Minimally invasive surgery for small thyroid nodules: preliminary report. J Endocrinol Invest 1999;22:849–851.

2 Terris DJ: Minimally invasive thyroidectomy: an emerging standard of care. Minerva Chir 2007;62:327–333.

3 Miccoli P, Berti P, Frustaci GL, Ambrosini CE, Materazzi G: Video-assisted thyroidectomy: indications and results. Langenbecks Arch Surg 2006;391:68–71.

4 Miccoli P, Berti P, Materazzi G, Minuto M, Barellini L: Minimally invasive video-assisted thyroidectomy: five years of experience. J Am Coll Surg 2004;199:243–248.

5 Shimizu K, Akira S, Jasmi AY, Kitamura Y, Kitagawa W, Akasu H, Tanaka S: Video-assisted neck surgery: endoscopic resection of thyroid tumors with a very minimal neck wound. J Am Coll Surg 1999;188:697–703.

Cernea CR, Dias FL, Fliss D, Lima RA, Myers EN, Wei WI (eds): Pearls and Pitfalls in Head and Neck Surgery. Basel, Karger, 2008, pp 18–19

1.9 Video-Assisted Parathyroidectomy

William B. Inabnet

Columbia University, New York, N.Y., USA

PEARLS

- Prior to making the initial incision, place a clear dressing over the skin to prevent abrasions or heat injury to the skin surface.
- Use an angled 30 or 45° endoscope.
- Never grasp the adenoma in order to avoid violation of the parathyroid capsule.
- For high superior parathyroid adenomas, a lateral 'backdoor' approach can be used to gain access to the parathyroid basin by developing the space between the carotid artery and the lateral border of the strap muscles [1].
- For parathyroid adenomas located in the superior mediastinum, insert a table-mounted sternal retractor to elevate the sternum to increase the working space [2].

PITFALLS

- Video-assisted parathyroidectomy requires multiple assistants with a knowledge of video-assisted techniques.
- Since the surgical field is a small space, the tip of the camera may get smudged by touching surrounding tissue leading to impaired visualization and the need for frequent cleaning of the endoscope.
- The dissection of the adenoma can seem unnatural as the working space requires different ergonomics than with conventional or focused open parathyroidectomy.

Introduction

Video-assisted endocrine neck surgery has gained a strong foothold in the surgical armamentarium of parathyroid surgeons. Advantages over conventional parathyroid surgery and other minimally invasive techniques include improved illumination of the operative field, access to deep and ectopic locations, and uniform visualization of the operation by all members of the operative team.

Surgical Technique and Practical Tips

(1) Before proceeding with parathyroidectomy, the diagnosis of primary hyperparathyroidism (PHPT) must be firmly established. Elevated total and/or ionized calcium and intact parathyroid hormone (PTH) levels support a diagnosis of PHPT. Twenty-four hour urine calcium levels may be normal or elevated. Video-assisted parathyroidectomy is not recommended for patients with risk factors for multigland disease, such as patients with multiple endocrine neoplasia or familial hyperparathyroidism, as these cases may be more complex and have a higher incidence of parathyroid hyperplasia.

(2) Preoperative localization plays an important role for patient selection, especially early in the surgeon's experience. Patients with a solitary parathyroid adenoma visualized on ultrasonography and/or sestamibi scanning are ideally situated for a video-assisted approach. Once the surgeon has increased experience with video-assisted parathyroidectomy, bilateral neck exploration

may be permissible in patients with PHPT and negative imaging [3]. Be aware that the incidence of multigland disease is higher in patients with negative sestamibi scans [1]. Video-assisted parathyroidectomy should not be performed in patients with parathyroid adenomas that appear to be greater than 5 g on preoperative ultrasonography, as the large size of the adenoma may interfere with intraoperative visualization.

3 Video-assisted parathyroidectomy can be performed under either local anesthesia with conscious sedation or general anesthesia [4]. When local anesthesia is used, a combined deep and superficial cervical block is recommended using a solution of 0.5% lidocaine and 0.25% bupivacaine.

4 A small 1.5- to 2-cm incision is made 2–3 finger breadths above the sternal notch. The strap muscles are separated at the midline without raising myocutaneous flaps. Narrow retractors are inserted laterally and medially and an angled endoscope is inserted directly through the small incision [5].

5 Using flat spatulated instruments, the thyroid lobe is mobilized until the targeted parathyroid gland is visualized. A small hook cautery may be useful as well as a small aspirator. After identifying the recurrent laryngeal nerve, the vascular pedicle of the adenoma is isolated, clipped and divided. A gentle lateral retraction of the adenoma may facilitate visualization of the vascular pedicle.

6 Intraoperative PTH (IOPTH) monitoring is recommended in all cases. Levels are drawn at baseline and 0, 5 and 10 min following parathyroid excision [6]. The extent of neck exploration is determined by a combination of intraoperative findings and IOPTH levels. If IOPTH levels decrease by greater than 50% of the highest preexcision value, the operation is concluded without exploring the other quadrants of the neck. If IOPTH monitoring is not available or is being used selectively due to cost constraints, video-assisted 4-gland exploration can be performed with excellent results [3].

7 Skin closure is in layers and the patient may be discharged to home the same day of surgery.

Conclusions

Video-assisted parathyroidectomy permits focused parathyroid exploration through the smallest possible incision with excellent visualization.

References

1 Sebag F, Hubbard JG, Maweja S, et al: Negative preoperative localization studies are highly predictive of multiglandular disease in sporadic primary hyperparathyroidism. Surgery 2003; 134:1038–1042.

2 Inabnet WB, Chu CA: Transcervical endoscopic-assisted mediastinal parathyroidectomy with intraoperative parathyroid hormone monitoring. Surg Endosc 2003;17:1678.

3 Miccoli P, Berti P, Materazzi G, et al: Endoscopic bilateral neck exploration versus quick intraoperative parathormone assay (qPTHa) during endoscopic parathyroidectomy: a prospective randomized trial. Surg Endosc 2007, E-pub ahead of print.

4 Miccoli P, Barellini L, Monchik JM, et al: Randomized clinical trial comparing regional and general anaesthesia in minimally invasive video-assisted parathyroidectomy. Br J Surg 2005;92: 814–818.

5 Barczynski M, Cichon S, Konturek A, et al: Minimally invasive video-assisted parathyroidectomy versus open minimally invasive parathyroidectomy for a solitary parathyroid adenoma: a prospective, randomized, blinded trial. World J Surg 2006;30: 721–731.

6 Lee JA, Inabnet WB 3rd: The surgeon's armamentarium to the surgical treatment of primary hyperparathyroidism. J Surg Oncol 2005;89:130–135.

Cernea CR, Dias FL, Fliss D, Lima RA, Myers EN, Wei WI (eds): Pearls and Pitfalls in Head and Neck Surgery. Basel, Karger, 2008, pp 20–21

1.10 Limited Parathyroidectomy

Keith S. Heller

New York University School of Medicine, New York, N.Y., USA

Pearls

- Preoperative imaging can localize the adenoma in 90% of cases.
- Focused minimally invasive parathyroidectomy (FMIP) can be performed under local/regional anesthesia as an outpatient.
- Position the patient with the head turned away from the side of the adenoma.
- Make the incision slightly off center, positioned higher or lower in the neck based on the position of the adenoma determined by imaging.
- Go through or lateral to the strap muscles, not through the midline.

Pitfalls

- Imaging frequently fails to detect multiple gland involvement.
- Pneumothorax can occur in parathyroidectomies (PTX) performed under local anesthesia.
- The recurrent laryngeal nerve (RLN) can be very close to adenomas on the undersurface of the thyroid.
- Intraoperative PTH 'spike' due to manipulation of the adenoma can be misleading.

Introduction

FMIP can be performed because 85% of cases of primary hyperparathyroidism are due to a solitary adenoma. Imaging studies can predict the location of solitary adenomas in up to 90% of cases. Patients with multigland disease can only be identified in 50% of cases [1, 2]. For this reason, the removal of all hyperfunctioning parathyroid (PT) tissue needs to be confirmed by intraoperative PTH measurement. Focused PTX can be accomplished by several different surgical approaches. I use conventional surgical techniques and instruments working through an incision about 2.5 cm in length.

Practical Tips

(1) *Intraoperative PTH Measurement.* It is preferable that the assay be performed in the operating room suite rather than in the central chemistry laboratory to minimize delay. Blood samples are obtained from a peripheral intravenous catheter when possible or from an intra-arterial catheter, but never directly from the jugular vein. A baseline sample is drawn when the patient is first brought into the operating room, before the neck is manipulated to avoid an inappropriately elevated baseline PTH due to massaging the adenoma. Additional samples are drawn when the adenoma is removed and at 5-min intervals thereafter. Occasionally, there is a marked spike in the PTH level at the time the adenoma is removed. Failure to recognize this spike could result in the errone-

ous conclusion that additional hyperfunctioning PT tissue is present if the 5-min sample is the same as the baseline. Adequacy of PTX is assured when the PTH value falls more than 50% from the baseline value and into the normal range. A 50% decrease that plateaus at a level above normal is indicative of another abnormal PT and should prompt a conventional bilateral exploration.

2 *Anesthesia.* My preference is to use local/regional anesthesia. Contraindications include obesity, sleep apnea syndrome, and significant gastroesophageal reflux. The technique described by LoGerfo and Kim [3] is used. Intravenous sedation using propofol minimizes patient anxiety. Transient (several hours) vocal cord paralysis resulting from inadvertent vagus nerve block can occur. Pneumothorax occurs in 1% of patients after PTX under local/regional anesthesia due to negative intrathoracic pressure in spontaneous breathing.

3 *Surgery.* The patient is positioned supine with the head extended and turned away from the side of the adenoma. A horizontal incision measuring 2–4 cm, slightly lateral to the midline, is planned. The location of the incision is based on preoperative imaging. Skin flaps are elevated. The fibers of the strap muscle are separated longitudinally. If the adenoma is in an inferior PT located inferior to the thyroid, the muscles are separated in the midline or close to it. If the adenoma is in the retroesophageal location, the muscles are separated more laterally and dissection is continued just medial to the carotid sheath. The retroesophageal space can then be explored without having to mobilize the thyroid. To expose PT lying anywhere behind the thyroid, the carotid sheath is retracted laterally and the thyroid medially. It is occasionally necessary to divide the middle thyroid vein. Although the RLN may be near adenomas lying in the tracheal-esophageal groove, I do not routinely identify the nerve. Blunt dissection is employed and tissues are spread rather than divided. The adenoma is within a thin layer of fascia. Dissection under this layer will free the PT from its surrounding tissues and leave it hanging on its vascular pedicle, which then can be clipped. The nerve can cross directly over the PT. It can be easily recognized and bluntly dissected away from the adenoma.

4 *Postoperative Care.* Patients are discharged after 3 h of observation on oral calcium supplements (1,000 mg/day).

References

1 Johnson NA, Tublin ME, Ogilvie JB: Parathyroid imaging: technique and role in the preoperative evaluation of primary hyperparathyroidism. AJR Am J Roentgenol 2007;188:1706–1715.
2 Bergson EJ, Sznyter LA, Dubner S, Palestro CJ, Heller KS: Sestamibi scans and intraoperative parathyroid hormone measurement in the treatment of primary hyperparathyroidism. Arch Otolaryngol Head Neck Surg 2004;130:87–91.
3 LoGerfo P, Kim LJ: Technique for regional anesthesia: thyroidectomy and parathyroidectomy. Oper Tech Gen Surg 1999;1:95–102.

Cernea CR, Dias FL, Fliss D, Lima RA, Myers EN, Wei WI (eds): Pearls and Pitfalls in Head and Neck Surgery. Basel, Karger, 2008, pp 22–23

1.11 Practical Tips for the Surgical Management of Secondary Hyperparathyroidism

Fábio Luiz de Menezes Montenegro[a], Rodrigo Oliveira Santos[b], Anói Castro Cordeiro[a]

[a] Department of Head and Neck Surgery, University of São Paulo Medical School and
[b] Department of Otolaryngology-Head and Neck Surgery, Federal University of São Paulo, São Paulo, Brazil

PEARLS

- Ultrasound (US) may be helpful to disclose associated thyroid disorders or intrathyroidal parathyroids.
- Intraoperative parathyroid hormone (PTH) monitoring may indicate a supernumerary hyperfunctioning gland.
- Implant of cryopreserved parathyroid tissue may revert postoperative hypoparathyroidism.

PITFALLS

- Not all patients with chronic kidney disease (CKD) and elevation of PTH levels are candidates for parathyroidectomy (PTX).
- There is a high risk of hypocalcemia after PTX due to the hungry bone syndrome.
- Decrease of renal graft function after PTX may occur in some cases with tertiary hyperparathyroidism (3HPT).
- Autotransplantation of nodular areas increases the chance of recurrence.

Introduction

Parathyroid hyperfunction due to a previous metabolic derangement is characterized as secondary hyperparathyroidism (2HPT). The commonest cause is CKD.

As renal function decreases, PTH increases. A mild elevation of the PTH level is necessary for an adequate bone metabolism in patients with CKD. However, prolonged stimulation of parathyroid cells may induce parathyroid autonomy, i.e. loss of physiological response. Excessive secretion of PTH is often associated with deleterious effects.

In the past, bone complications of osteitis fibrosa with fractures and pain were the major concern. At present, it is well recognized that other mineral metabolism conditions are also important as regards morbidity and mortality of renal patients. Hyperphosphatemia and vascular calcifications are associated with an increased risk of cardiovascular events [1].

The denomination of 3HPT is usually employed in patients with hyperparathyroidism after successful kidney transplantation. In the text below, 2HPT will refer to patients with CKD on dialysis and 3HPT will be restricted to renal transplant cases.

Practical Tips

(1) Indication of PTX: Under specific conditions, PTX will significantly improve quality of life and prolong survival. Contrariwise, worsening is expected if PTX is performed in patients with disturbances and complaints not related to hyperparathyroidism. In 2HPT, the Guidelines of the National Kidney Foundation (K/DOQI) establish

that PTX is indicated in patients with persistent serum levels of PTH higher than 800 pg/ml (88.0 pmol/l) which are associated with hypercalcemia and/or hyperphosphatemia that are refractory to medical therapy [2]. In 3HPT, increased PTH and persistent hypercalcemia after kidney transplantation suggest that PTX is required.

2 Preoperative imaging: Even though all hyperfunctioning parathyroid tissue must be inspected and the sensitivity of imaging studies is variable, preoperative US and technetium-sestamibi (MIBI) scanning may represent a helpful tool in intraoperative decision making. US may identify associated thyroid disease as papillary thyroid carcinoma [3]. Although not frequent, intrathyroidal parathyroid glands can be suggested by ultrasonography [4]. Rarely does the MIBI scan detect all hyperfunctioning parathyroid glands, but it may provide information about ectopic glands (mediastinal, high cervical, retropharyngeal).

3 Preoperative care: Comorbidities are common and they must be evaluated before surgery. Dialysis is performed the day before the operation, and a lower heparin dose is advised.

4 Intraoperative care: Nephrotoxic drugs and hypotension must be avoided in patients with 3HPT. If feasible, intraoperative PTH should be employed. Reduction of 80% of basal levels after 10–20 min seems to indicate an adequate excision [5]. A failure to achieve this level is indicative of a supernumerary hyperfunctioning parathyroid.

5 Extent of the surgery: There is no consensus in the literature about the best approach to 2HPT and 3HPT. Subtotal PTX and total PTX with immediate heterotopic autotransplantation are reported with good results. Forearm and presternal autotransplantation are acceptable techniques. Areas of nodular hyperplasia should be avoided for autotransplantation, as they carry an increased risk of graft-dependent recurrence. The risk of malignant tissue transplantation is rare as parathyroid carcinoma is rather infrequent in both 2HPT and 3HPT [6, 7].

6 Postoperative care: Right after surgery for 2HPT, a continuous infusion of calcium in a small volume of saline or dextrose is started. Usually, 900 mg of elemental calcium of calcium gluconate are diluted in 200–250 ml. The concentrated solution can cause chemical phlebitis if it is infused into a peripheral vein. As soon as possible, oral calcium and calcitriol are added in large daily doses (4.0–7.0 g of calcium salts and 2–4 μg of calcitriol) [8]. Hypoparathyroidism may be reverted by autotransplantation of cryopreserved tissue [9]. In 3HPT, hypocalcemia is less pronounced and lower doses of calcium and calcitriol are required. Renal function should be evaluated closely. There is evidence that acute PTH reduction affects renal function [10].

References

1 Moe SM, Drüeke T, Lameire N, Eknoyan G: Chronic kidney disease-mineral-bone disorder: a new paradigm. Adv Chronic Kidney Dis 2007;14:3–12.
2 National Kidney Foundation: Clinical practice guidelines for bone metabolism and disease in chronic kidney disease. Am J Kidney Dis 2003;42(suppl 3):s1–s201. http://www.kidney.org/professionals/kdoqi/guidelines_bone/index.htm.
3 Montenegro FLM, Smith RB, Castro IV, Tavares MR, Cordeiro AC, Ferraz AR: Association of papillary thyroid carcinoma and hyperparathyroidism. Rev Col Bras Cir 2005;32:115–119.
4 Montenegro FLM, Tavares MR, Cordeiro AC, Ferraz AR, Ianhez LE, Buchpiguel CA: Intrathyroidal supernumerary parathyroid gland in hyperparathyroidism after renal transplantation. Nephrol Dial Transplant 2007;22:293–295.
5 Ohe MN, Santos RO, Kunii IS, Abrahao M, Cervantes O, Carvalho AB, Lazaretti-Castro M, Vieira JG: Usefulness of intraoperative PTH measurement in primary and secondary hyperparathyroidism: experience with 109 patients. Arq Bras Endocrinol Metab 2006;50:869–875.
6 Cordeiro AC, Montenegro FLM, Kulcsar MAV, Dellanegra LA, Tavares MR, Michaluart P, Ferraz AF: Parathyroid carcinoma. Am J Surg 1998;175:52–55.
7 Montenegro FLM, Tavares MR, Durazzo MD, Cernea CR, Cordeiro AC, Ferraz AR: Clinical suspicion and parathyroid carcinoma management. Sao Paulo Med J 2006;124:42–44.
8 Cozzolino M, Gallieni M, Corsi C, Bastagli A, Brancaccio D: Management of calcium refilling post-parathyroidectomy in end-stage renal disease. J Nephrol 2004;17:3–8.
9 Montenegro FLM, Custódio MR, Arap SS, Reis LM, Sonohara S, Castro IV, Jorgetti V, Cordeiro AC, Ferraz AR: Successful implant of long-term cryopreserved parathyroid glands after total parathyroidectomy. Head Neck 2007;29:296–300.
10 Schwarz A, Rustien G, Merkel S, Radermacher J, Haller H: Decreased renal transplant function after parathyroidectomy. Nephrol Dial Transplant 2007;22:584–591.

Cernea CR, Dias FL, Fliss D, Lima RA, Myers EN, Wei WI (eds): Pearls and Pitfalls in Head and Neck Surgery. Basel, Karger, 2008, pp 24–25

1.12 Reoperative Parathyroidectomy

Alfred Simental

Otolaryngology Head Neck Surgery, Loma Linda University, Loma Linda, Calif., USA

PEARLS

- Confirm initial diagnosis.
- Maximize localization techniques.
- Read previous operative and pathology reports.
- Work in previously undissected field first where scarring is least and probability of finding affected gland is highest.
- Develop an organized dissection pattern and understand ectopic locations.
- Remove concomitant thyroid pathology.

PITFALLS

- Risk of failing to recognize improper diagnosis.
- Risk of permanent hypocalcemia and vocal cord paralysis is greatly increased in reoperative surgery.
- Risk of removing normal parathyroid glands.
- Risk of pharyngoesophageal injury.

Introduction

Hyperparathyroidism (HPT) can be surgically cured on initial exploration in greater than 90% of cases, and in experienced hands greater than 95%. However, uncontrolled HPT in patients with unsuccessful explorations may result in severe osteoporosis, fatigue, depression, nephrolithiasis, renal failure, hypertension, and increased cardiovascular risk. This necessitates consideration for reexploration and surgical correction of the hyperparathyroid state, especially in younger patients.

Reexploration for HPT is complicated by previous scarring, higher incidence of tumors in ectopic locations, multigland hyperplasia, and may be associated with recurrence of parathyroid carcinoma. Ectopic parathyroid locations include thymus, thyroid, carotid sheath, retroesophageal, superior mediastinum, tracheoesophageal groove, submandibular, and posterior mediastinum [1, 2].

Patients and physicians should understand that reoperative surgery has inherently increased risks. Reoperation in a scarred field increases the risk of injury to the recurrent laryngeal and superior laryngeal nerves, resulting in subsequent dysphonia. In addition, the incidence of either postoperative hypoparathyroidism or persistent HPT is increased and may approach 10% [3]. Localization studies may aid in identifying ectopic and hyperfunctioning glands, while reducing the morbidity of reexploration [4].

Practical Tips

(1) Before embarking on a rigorous reoperative surgery, the initial diagnosis of HPT should be confirmed taking care to rule out medications, dietary contributions, or any secondary reason to have hypercalcemia, especially benign familial hypocalciuric hypercalcemia. The patient should be evaluated by an endocrinologist who can con-

firm the diagnosis and determine whether medical management may be effective. Reexploration should be delayed at least 6–9 months to allow inflammation to subside and increase the efficacy of repeat imaging studies.

2 The previous operative and pathological reports should be reviewed to determine previous sites of exploration, pathological confirmation of removed tissues, and other intraoperative findings. In situations of unilateral exploration, the unexplored side is utilized unless localization studies suggest that the initial side is active.

3 Imaging studies should be repeated and should include sestamibi imaging to look for new or ectopic activity [5]. Ultrasound examination should determine the presence of thyroid nodules and paratracheal masses, which may represent enlarged parathyroid glands. Computed tomography (CT) or MRI may also be considered to evaluate the mediastinal and retroesophageal regions that may not be visualized by ultrasound [6]. Selective venous sampling by interventional radiology may help determine laterality and possibly venous outflow location of the most active gland [7].

4 Intraoperative parathyroid hormone monitoring should be employed to determine adequacy of resection, beginning with a preincision 'defined baseline level' [8]. Postresection intraoperative PTH levels drawn at 10 min should be at least reduced by 50% unless the level is within the normal range. A draw at 15 min should continue to reveal a drop of 25–30% as an additional half-life has occurred.

5 Reoperative strategy should routinely begin by exposing the carotid artery, then working from lateral to medial towards the cricoid cartilage. The recurrent laryngeal nerve should be identified early, either just inferior to the cricoid cartilage or lower in the lateral paratracheal region where scarring is minimal. Once the carotid and recurrent nerve are dissected, exploration of the paratracheal region, retropharyngeal, retrothyroid, and superior mediastinum should be systematically undertaken. Any intrathyroidal lesions should prompt thyroidectomy as these may represent intrathyroidal parathyroid glands, especially in the face of unsuccessful exploration. Early exploration of the superior mediastinum with resection of thymus should be considered after the routine areas have been explored.

Conclusion

Reoperative surgery for HPT is associated with an increased incidence of complications including vocal fold paralysis, permanent hypoparathyroidism, and persistent hypercalcemia. The use of nuclear medicine imaging, ultrasound and high resolution CT/MRI may aid in surgical planning. However, knowledge of potential ectopic locations and a well-planned surgical approach from lateral to medial are critical in ensuring adequate resection, which may be verified by intraoperative parathyroid hormone monitoring.

References

1 Phitayakorn R, McHenry CR: Incidence and location of ectopic abnormal parathyroid glands. Am J Surg 2006;191:418–423.
2 Shen W, Duren M, Morita E, et al: Reoperation for persistent or recurrent primary hyperparathyroidism. Arch Surg 1996;131: 861–869.
3 Allendorf J, Digorgi M, Spanknebel K, et al: 1112 consecutive bilateral neck explorations for primary hyperparathyroidism. World J Surg 2007, E-pub ahead of print.
4 Rodriguez JM, Tezelman S, Siperstein AE, et al: Localization procedures in patients with persistent or recurrent hyperparathyroidism. Arch Surg 1994;129:870–875.
5 Chen CC, Skarulis MC, Fraker DL, et al: Technetium-99m-sestamibi imaging before reoperation for primary hyperparathyroidism. J Nucl Med 1995;36:2186–2191.
6 Rodgers SE, Hunter GJ, Hamberg LM, et al: Improved preoperative planning for directed parathyroidectomy with 4-dimensional computed tomography. Surgery 2006;140:932–940.
7 Ogilvie CM, Brown PL, Matson M, et al: Selective parathyroid venous sampling in patients with complicated hyperparathyroidism. Eur J Endocrinol 2006;155:813–821.
8 Riss P, Kaczirek K, Heinz G, et al: A 'defined baseline' in PTH monitoring increases surgical success in patients with multiple gland disease. Surgery 2007;142:398–404.

Cernea CR, Dias FL, Fliss D, Lima RA, Myers EN, Wei WI (eds): Pearls and Pitfalls in Head and Neck Surgery. Basel, Karger, 2008, pp 26–27

1.13 Paratracheal Neck Dissection: Surgical Tips

A. Khafif[a], L.P. Kowalski[b], Dan M. Fliss[a]

[a] Department of Otolaryngology-Head and Neck Surgery, Tel Aviv Sourasky Medical Center (affiliated to the Sackler Faculty of Medicine), Tel Aviv University, Tel Aviv, Israel;
[b] Department of Head and Neck Surgery and Otorhinolaryngology, Hospital A.C. Camargo, São Paulo, Brazil

Pearls

- Gentle endotracheal intubation by experienced anesthesiologist.
- Divide the sternothyroid muscle if necessary to get a good exposure.
- Identify the recurrent laryngeal nerve (RLN) through its entire course in all patients.
- Left RLN is more vertical and dissection of this side may necessitate retraction of the RLN using a nerve hook.
- Identify and preserve well-vascularized parathyroid glands.
- Implants of parathyroid glands may be necessary if they are ischemic by the end of the dissection.
- Do not coagulate near the nerve.
- Treat hypocalcemia aggressively.

Pitfalls

- Risk of hypocalcemia is much higher in reoperations and when a neck dissection is performed simultaneously.
- Nerve monitoring can be used, especially in reoperations, but identification of the RLN is always mandatory.

Introduction

Therapeutic paratracheal neck dissection (PTND) is common practice for the treatment of positive nodes at levels VI–VII originating from well-differentiated and medullary thyroid carcinoma. The high rate of recurrence following 'berry picking', presumably due to subclinical involvement of lymph nodes, has led to routine performance of a formal unilateral or bilateral PTND in patients with clinically positive nodes in the paratracheal region [1,2]. It has also been indicated as an elective procedure for patients with positive jugular chain adenopathy [3], especially in high-risk patients with well-differentiated thyroid carcinoma (older male patients with aggressive tumors) and certainly for patients with medullary carcinoma. Dissection of this region does not necessarily carry an increased risk of RLN injury [3, 4]; however, the rates of postoperative hypocalcemia can be as high as 25% [5].

Practical Tips for PTND

1. Intubation should be done by an experienced anesthesiologist, preferably with a soft endotracheal tube to avoid injury to the vocal cords.
2. PTND starts with dissection of the carotid artery and internal jugular vein through their entire course into the mediastinum. Remember, the RLN passes underneath the artery and is thus safe at this point.

③ The RLN has to be identified in all patients through its entire course in the paratracheal region from the upper mediastinum to the cricothyroid membrane. Remember that nerve monitoring is not a substitute for proper identification of the nerve.
④ Exposure of the left RLN may necessitate complete sharp dissection of the nerve through its circumference and retraction using a nerve hook, to facilitate removal of the specimen underneath the nerve towards the trachea. At times, the specimen may be separated to avoid injury to the RLN during retraction.
⑤ For better exposure of the paratracheal region, the sternothyroid muscle can be divided, preferably at its uppermost attachment to the thyroid cartilage.
⑥ If the parathyroid glands are devascularized during dissection, they should be resected and reimplanted in the sternocleidomastoid muscle.
⑦ While dissecting the upper mediastinum, care must be taken to avoid injury to the subclavian or innominate arteries. These vessels serve as the lowermost limit of our dissection.
⑧ Remember, the right common carotid artery may have a somewhat oblique course inferiorly and may cross the trachea towards the innominate artery. Care is taken not to injure this vessel at this last step of the dissection.
⑨ Postoperatively, hypocalcemia is more common in reoperations, and oral supplementation of calcium should be considered even prior to the development of hypocalcemia in these patients. Aggressive supplementation may help with early hospital discharge.

At times, edema of the ipsilateral side of the larynx may be anticipated and treated with a short course of corticosteroids.

Conclusions

PTND may be a complicated maneuver and care must be taken during the procedure to minimize the morbidity. When performed properly the morbidity is relatively low [3] even in reoperations [4].

References

1 Watkinson JC, Franklyn JA, Olliff JF: Detection and surgical treatment of cervical lymph nodes in differentiated thyroid cancer. Thyroid 2006;16:187–194.
2 Shaha AR: Management of the neck in thyroid cancer. Otol Clin North Am 1998;31:823–831.
3 Khafif A, Ben Yosef R, Abergel A, Kesler A, Landsberg R, Fliss DM: Elective paratracheal neck dissection for lateral metastases from papillary carcinoma of the thyroid: is it indicated? Head Neck 2007, E-pub ahead of print.
4 Kim MK, Mandel SH, Baloch Z, Livolsi VA, Langer JE, Didonato L, Fish S, Webber RS: Morbidity following central compartment reoperation for recurrent or persistent thyroid cancer. Arch Otolaryngol Head Neck Surg 2004;130:1214–1216.
5 Filho JG, Kowalski LP: Postoperative complications of thyroidectomy for differentiated thyroid carcinoma. Am J Otolaryngol 2004;25:225–230.

Cernea CR, Dias FL, Fliss D, Lima RA, Myers EN, Wei WI (eds): Pearls and Pitfalls in Head and Neck Surgery. Basel, Karger, 2008, pp 28–29

1.14 Management of Lymph Nodes in Medullary Thyroid Cancer

Marcos R. Tavares

Department of Head and Neck Surgery, University of São Paulo Medical School, São Paulo, Brazil

Pearls

- Lymph node metastasis is frequent in medullary thyroid cancer (MTC) (±70%).
- Preoperative thyroid and lymph node evaluation by ultrasound and computed tomography is very useful.
- Parathyroid glands are better identified during thyroidectomy.
- Elective dissection of the lateral compartment of the neck may be postponed until a second time.
- Reoperation is indicated if serum calcitonin is elevated after adequate initial treatment and after confirmation of the disease in the neck by fine needle aspiration cytology, without distant metastasis.
- Dissection of the level I is unnecessary.

Pitfalls

- Inadequate clinical and pathological evaluation of the neck.
- Insufficient dissection of the central compartment of the neck.
- Assumption of cure without a negative stimulated calcitonin test.
- Parathyroid function is more frequently impaired after dissection of the central neck.
- RET test not performed in patients with MTC and first degree relatives of those with a positive test.
- Dissection of the lateral neck without localization of persistent or recurrent disease.

Introduction

MTC occurs in sporadic or familial clinical settings and corresponds to 5% of thyroid carcinomas and as much as 63% of them present initially with lymph node metastasis [1]. Complete surgical resection is critical for cure because cervical reoperation for persistent or recurrent disease benefits only select patients [2]. Total thyroidectomy and neck dissection are mandatory when metastases are clinically evident, and it is accepted by consensus that dissection of the central compartment of the neck is the minimal adequate initial treatment, even when neck metastases are not identified [3]. Dissection of the central compartment of the neck is risky for the parathyroid glands and laryngeal recurrent nerves, and must be performed by an experienced head and neck surgeon.

Practical Tips

1. Dissection of the central neck must be performed in virtually all patients to avoid damage done by reoperation in this anatomical site. The only exception that might be considered is in a patient with low-risk RET mutation at the age of 5 years or below and with negative stimulated calcitonin test.
2. All tissue between the carotid arteries laterally and between the hyoid bone and the brachiocephalic venous trunk is to be removed.
3. Parathyroid glands are better identified at the time of the thyroidectomy. It is recommended to remove and to transplant them, since parathyroid

adenoma occurs in about 50% of the patients with familial disease [3] and it is hard to preserve its function with an aggressive dissection of the central neck.

4 Dissection of the lateral neck must be performed for positive neck and may be modified; it is unnecessary to include the submandibular echelon in the specimen. Elective dissection of the lateral compartment may be postponed as a second staged procedure.

5 Reoperation is indicated if calcitonin does not reach a low level. Dissection of the lateral neck (levels II–V) is performed only after detection of the disease by fine needle aspiration or a positive MIBI test, as long as distant metastases are ruled out. The most efficient imaging workup for depicting MTC tumor sites includes a neck US, chest CT, liver MRI, bone scintigraphy and axial skeleton MRI. FDG-PET scan appears to be less sensitive with low prognostic value [4].

References

1 Moley JF, DeBenedetti MK: Patterns of nodal metastases in palpable medullary thyroid carcinoma. Recommendations for extent of node dissection. Ann Surg 1999;229:880–888.

2 You YN, Lakhani V, Wells SA Jr, Moley JF: Medullary thyroid cancer. Surg Oncol Clin N Am 2006;15:639–660.

3 Brandi ML, Gagel RF, Angeli A, Bilezikian PB, Bordi C, Conte-Devolx B, Flachetti A, Giheri RG, Libroia A, Lips CJM, Lombardi C, Mannelli M, Pacini F, Ponder BAJ, Raue F, Skojeseid GT, Tamburrano G, Thakker RV, Thompson PT, Tonelli F, Wells S Jr, Marx S: Guidelines for diagnosis and therapy of MEN type 1 and type 2. J Clin Endocrinol Metab 2001;86:5568–5571.

4 Giraudet AL, Vanel D, Leboulleux S, Aupérin A, Dromain C, Chami L, Tovo NN, Lumbroso J, Lassau N, Bonniaud G, Hartl D, Travagli JP, Baudin E, Schlumberger M: Imaging medullary thyroid carcinoma with persistent elevated calcitonin levels. J Clin Endocrinol Metab 2007;92:4185–4190.

Cernea CR, Dias FL, Fliss D, Lima RA, Myers EN, Wei WI (eds): Pearls and Pitfalls in Head and Neck Surgery. Basel, Karger, 2008, pp 30–31

1.15 How to Manage a Well-Differentiated Carcinoma with Recurrent Nerve Invasion

Patrick Sheahan, Jatin P. Shah

Department of Head and Neck Surgery, Memorial Sloan-Kettering Cancer Center, New York, N.Y., USA

PEARLS

- In patients who have a preoperative vocal cord paralysis (VCP) secondary to tumor involvement of the recurrent laryngeal nerve (RLN), resection of the RLN should be performed.
- With functioning vocal cords (VCs), every effort should be made to preserve the RLN, not leaving gross tumor behind.
- When there is RLN invasion, the minimum operation should be a total thyroidectomy (TT), to use postoperative radioiodine treatment.
- In cases of bilateral RLN invasion, at least one RLN should be preserved.
- When an invaded RLN is found, explore the contralateral side, to ensure the integrity of the contralateral RLN, prior to considering sacrifice of the involved RLN.

PITFALL

- Gross disease should never be left behind, as this leads to a high local failure rate, often with transformation to a more aggressive histology.

Introduction

The reported incidence of extrathyroid extension of well-differentiated thyroid cancer (WDTC) varies from 1 to 15% [1]. After the strap muscles, the RLN is the next most commonly invaded structure by WDTC [2]. Complete surgical resection of all gross disease is the cornerstone therapy; however, resection of the RLN may lead to significant long-term sequelae. Thus, the management of the RLN invaded by WDTC is a contentious area.

RLN invasion usually occurs either in the region of Berry's ligament or in the tracheoesophageal groove from tumor in metastatic paratracheal lymph nodes [2]. Male sex, older age, and aggressive histological subtypes of papillary carcinoma are associated with increased risk of RLN invasion [3, 4].

Practical Tips

1. RLN invasion may or may not lead to VCP. Preoperative indirect or flexible laryngoscopy is mandatory in patients with suspected thyroid cancer.
2. The presence of RLN invasion implies extrathyroid spread of tumor, and upstages the tumor to T4 [1]. However, in contrast to invasion of the larynx, trachea, or esophagus [3], this does not necessarily portend a poor prognosis [2].
3. WDTC with extrathyroid extension is best treated with complete resection of all gross disease. Margins of only a few millimeters are generally adequate.
4. Removal of all gross tumor leaving behind microscopic disease does not necessarily lead to an increased failure rate, as long as postoperative treatment with radioiodine or external beam radiotherapy is administered.

5 Patients with preoperative VCP rarely regain VC movement. Thus, there is little benefit in preserving the RLN in them.

6 In patients with normal VC function preoperatively, RLN resection per se does not necessarily lead to improved local control or survival [5–7]. Therefore, every effort should be made to preserve the functioning RLN.

7 When the RLN is sacrificed, an adequate three-dimensional resection should be performed to secure clear margins.

8 The surgeon should endeavor to preserve the nerve on at least one side, if feasible. Prior to sacrificing an invaded nerve, integrity of contralateral RLN should be ensured. The immediate effect of bilateral RLN sacrifice or injury is stridor, which usually necessitates re-intubation. Tracheostomy should be performed as soon as feasible.

9 Postoperative adjuvant treatment with radioiodine or external beam radiotherapy (in cases with poorly differentiated histology, massive extrathyroid extension, or older age) or both improves local control and survival. Hence, TT is the minimum operation.

10 Symptoms of unilateral VCP (breathy voice and/or aspiration of thin liquids) are variable and may initially fluctuate. As most patients will experience spontaneous improvement, surgical medialization should be delayed for several months.

11 Immediate RLN reconstruction by either direct repair or cable grafting has been advocated by some [8]. Despite not leading to any return in VC movement, it may improve voice by preventing muscle atrophy [8, 9].

Conclusion

The management of the RLN invaded by WDTC is an important issue. As a general rule, a paralyzed nerve should be resected, whereas every effort should be made to preserve a functioning nerve. However, preservation should only be attempted without leaving gross tumor behind. In all cases, TT facilitates postoperative adjunctive treatment with radioiodine.

References

1 Morton RP, Ahmad Z: Thyroid cancer invasion of neck structures: epidemiology, evaluation, staging and management. Curr Opin Otolaryngol Head Neck Surg 2007;15:89–94.
2 McCaffrey TV, Bergstralh EJ, Hay ID: Locally invasive papillary thyroid carcinoma: 1940–1990. Head Neck 1994;16:165–172.
3 Shaha A: Implications of prognostic factors and risk groups in the management of differentiated thyroid cancer. Laryngoscope 2004;114:393–402.
4 Kebebew E, Clark OH: Locally advanced differentiated thyroid cancer. Surg Oncol 2003;12:91–99.
5 Chan WF, Lo CY, Lam KY, Wan KY: Recurrent laryngeal nerve palsy in well-differentiated thyroid carcinoma: clinicopathological features and outcome study. World J Surg 2004:1093–1098.
6 Nishida T, Nakao K, Hamaji M, Kamiike W, Kurozumi K, Matsuda H: Preservation of recurrent laryngeal nerve invaded by differentiated thyroid cancer. Ann Surg 1997;226:85–91.
7 Falk SA, McCaffrey TV: Management of the recurrent laryngeal nerve in suspected and proven thyroid cancer. Otolaryngol Head Neck Surg 1995;113:42–48.
8 Yumoto E, Sanuki T, Kumai Y: Immediate recurrent laryngeal nerve reconstruction and vocal outcome. Laryngoscope 2006; 116:1657–1661.
9 Chou FF, Su CY, Jeng SF, Hsu KL, Lu KY: Neurorrhaphy of the recurrent laryngeal nerve. J Am Coll Surg 2003;197:52–57.

Cernea CR, Dias FL, Fliss D, Lima RA, Myers EN, Wei WI (eds): Pearls and Pitfalls in Head and Neck Surgery. Basel, Karger, 2008, pp 32–33

1.16 Management of Invasive Thyroid Cancer

Thomas V. McCaffrey

Department of Otolaryngology, Head and Neck Surgery, University of South Florida, Tampa, Fla., USA

PEARLS

- Hoarseness, airway obstruction and particularly hemoptysis are signs of upper aerodigestive tract (UADT) invasion by thyroid cancer.
- Laryngeal function can often be preserved by partial laryngectomy procedures even if invasion has occurred.
- Postoperative external beam radiation therapy (EBRT) may control unresectable invasive thyroid cancer (ITC) and preserve laryngeal function.

PITFALLS

- Inadequate resection of ITC will result in severe morbidities of airway obstruction, hemoptysis and dysphagia.
- Overestimating the need for radical resection may lead to the loss of salvageable laryngeal function.

Introduction

Well-differentiated carcinoma of the thyroid (WDTC) is a generally curable disease with a mortality rate quoted as between 11 and 17%. When WDTC extends beyond the thyroid capsule and produces invasion of the UADT structures, it is the cause of considerable increased morbidity and increased mortality.

In a review by McConahey et al. [1], cause of death from WDTC was related to untreatable local disease in 36% of cases and metastatic disease in 39% of cases. Control of ITC is therefore an important clinical problem, and it would be expected that successful treatment of ITC would include survival and reduced morbidity. ITC can produce symptoms as a result of paralysis of one or both recurrent laryngeal nerves (LN) resulting in hoarseness or airway obstruction, direct invasion of the trachea or larynx with the potential of airway obstruction and bleeding, invasion of the esophagus resulting in bleeding and dysphagia. Treatment goals for ITC include the prevention of hemorrhage and air obstruction, preservation of the function of the UADT, prevention of local/regional recurrence, and optimally long-term survival.

Practical Tips

Surgical Techniques

Larynx. Invasion can occur by direct extension and erosion of the laryngeal cartilage or by invasion around the posterior and inferior aspects of the thyroid cartilage into the paraglottic space. Often, it is unilateral, permitting conservative operations (e.g., partial vertical laryngectomy, PVL). If the mucosa is not directly involved, removal of the thyroid cartilage without entering the airway is also possible. LN invasion presents special problems. If paralysis has occurred, LN is resected with the tumor. Rehabilitation by thyroplasty offers an excellent result. However, in some cases, perineural invasion occurs without paralysis of the nerve. Although some controversy exists, peeling of tumor from the nerve preserving its function does not appear to result in reduced survival.

Trachea. Invasion may be relatively superficial with erosion or invasion of the cartilage rings without mucosal involvement, or it may be deep with intraluminal extension (IE). When IE occurs, full-thickness resection (FTR) of the trachea is the optimal treatment, occasionally as a window resection if the invasion is localized. The defect can be repaired with a myofacial flap from the sternocleidomastoid or other adjacent muscles. If the invasion is circumferential, tracheal resection is indicated, eventually extended up to include part of the cricoid, if necessary.

Pharynx/Esophagus. Because of the loose submucosal layer, tumor may involve the muscle coat without invasion through the underlying mucosa. This usually permits stripping of the muscle with preservation of the mucosa. If limited mucosal invasion does occur, resection with primary repair is possible. Extensive esophageal invasion may require laryngopharyngectomy and reconstruction with a jejunal or cutaneous free flap.

Shave Resection (SR) versus FTR. Some controversy still remains on the appropriate resection of minimally invasive tumors. Advocates for FTR of the airway state that, although the tumor may appear to be superficially invasive, usually extension into the submucosal plane occurs and that leaving a tumor behind results in higher recurrence rate [2]. Proponents of SR argue that there is no evidence to indicate survival improvement by FTR and that adding postoperative EBRT results in a similar disease-free survival [3]. Presently, the final word is not yet established. Certainly, in elderly patients or those who have other morbidities which may limit their survival, a less invasive, less traumatic procedure may be of benefit. Younger patients, in whom eradication of disease could extend survival, would benefit from more aggressive resections. This still remains an individual surgical decision.

EBRT has become more widely used in treating ITC. There are no controlled trials, although anecdotal results indicate that it may be helpful in selected cases [4].

Conclusion

WDTC invading the UADT and LN causes significant morbidity/mortality. Successful treatment is possible while preserving function. PVL, tracheal resections, SR and EBRT eliminate morbidity, preserve function, reduce local recurrence and may improve survival.

References

1 McConahey WM, Woolner LB, van Heerden JA, Taylor WF: Papillary thyroid cancer treated at the Mayo Clinic, 1946–1970: initial manifestations, pathological findings, therapy, and outcome. Mayo Clin Proc 1986;61:978–996.

2 Grillo HC, Suen HC, Mathisen DJ, Wain JC: Resectional management of thyroid cancer invading the airway. Ann Thorac Surg 1992;54:3–9.

3 Lipton RJ, McCaffrey TV, van Heerden: Surgical treatment of invasion of the upper aerodigestive tract by well-differentiated thyroid carcinoma. Am J Surg 1987;154:363–367.

4 Brierley JD, Tsang RW: External beam radiation therapy in the treatment of differentiated thyroid cancer. Semin Surg Oncol 1999;16:42–49.

Cernea CR, Dias FL, Fliss D, Lima RA, Myers EN, Wei WI (eds): Pearls and Pitfalls in Head and Neck Surgery. Basel, Karger, 2008, pp 34–35

2.1 Preoperative Workup of the Neck in Head and Neck Squamous Cell Carcinoma

Michiel van den Brekel, Frans J.M. Hilgers

Netherlands Cancer Institute – Antoni van Leeuwenhoek Hospital and Academic Medical Center, University of Amsterdam, Amsterdam, The Netherlands

Pearls

- Imaging is crucial in evaluating the extent of metastatic disease and can play a pivotal role in treatment planning.
- Imaging, especially PET-CT and US-FNAC, can detect occult metastases if larger than 5–6 mm.
- Only an invasive technique further improves detection of occult metastases: a sentinel node biopsy.
- Prediction of the metastatic potential of a tumor might soon be available in the form of gene expression profiling.

Pitfalls

- The majority of occult metastases cannot be detected using the current imaging techniques.
- Not treating the neck electively with either surgery or radiotherapy is only warranted in tumors with a moderate to low risk of occult metastases and when adequate imaging follow-up is ensured.
- As the pathology of neck dissection specimens is not very accurate either, a negative pathology report does not guarantee that no metastases are present.

Introduction

Pretreatment workup of the neck is important to decide on indication and extent of the treatment. An important use of pretreatment imaging is the assessment of the extent of neck disease or the infiltration into crucial structures, in order to determine operability. Tumors with encasement of the carotid artery over more than 270° are rarely operable. Other important issues for prognostication are: assessment of necrosis, tumor volume, extranodal spread, involvement of levels IV and V, retropharyngeal lymph nodes or paratracheal lymph nodes.

Although for individual patients it is an advantage when occult metastases are detected with CT or MRI, the unreliable criteria to assess small nonpalpable metastases make these techniques unreliable for the detection of metastases smaller than 8–9 mm. The advent of PET and PET-CT has certainly increased the sensitivity and specificity, but metastases smaller than 5 mm are seldom detected [1]. As US-FNAC is an ideal technique both for initial assessment and follow-up, it has been widely studied for the assessment of the N0 neck [2]. However, the reported sensitivity of US-guided FNAC in the N0 neck varies from 42 to 73%. In a routine setting we recently found that the sensitivity of US-FNAC in small (T1) oral carcinomas treated with transoral excision and a 'wait and see' strategy for the neck was significantly lower (18%) than in patients who had an elective neck dissection for T2–3 oral carcinomas (27%) or T2–3 oropharyngeal carcinomas (50%).

Sentinel node biopsy is reported to be a very sensitive technique. The major disadvantage, of course, is that the sentinel node procedure implicates a surgical procedure that has to be followed by a completion neck dissection when the SN is tumor positive.

Practical Tips

❶ As no currently available imaging technique can reliably detect small metastases, in treatment planning one should consider the risk of occult metastases and either treat the neck electively or use a very stringent follow-up protocol, including imaging, at regular intervals.

❷ As a 'wait and see' policy for the N0 neck leads to delayed detection of neck metastases in 15–40% of the patients (depending on the accuracy of imaging and patient population), these patients are treated at a later stage, either implicating more extensive treatment or a poorer prognosis. A very strict follow-up using US-FNAC leads to a similar prognosis.

❸ To obtain well-interpretable images, CT and MRI should be done with intravenous contrast agents and thin slices (3–4 mm) or spiral CT.

❹ Ultrasound is only trustworthy if performed by a skilled ultrasonographer, either the surgeon or the radiologist. The same holds true for the interpretation of the cytology.

❺ Although the levels I–III are at risk in most head and neck carcinomas, special attention should be given to retropharyngeal and paratracheal nodes. Any node larger than 5–6 mm in these areas is suspicious.

Conclusion

Although in the last decades imaging has tremendously increased our ability to stage tumors and optimize treatment planning, we are still unable to detect small metastases that frequently occur in early-stage head and neck cancers. Recent advances in the prediction of neck metastases using gene expression profiling or detection using sentinel node biopsy might help us solve this problem in the future. Imaging does have a place in evaluating tumor extent, assessing operability and determining optimal treatment.

References

1 Brouwer J, De Bree R, Comans EF, Castelijns JA, Hoekstra OS, Leemans CR: Positron emission tomography using [18F] fluorodeoxyglucose (FDG-PET) in the clinically negative neck: is it likely to be superior? Eur Arch Otorhinolaryngol 2004;261:479–483.

2 van den Brekel MW, Castelijns JA: What the clinician wants to know: surgical perspective and ultrasound for lymph node imaging of the neck. Cancer Imaging 2005;5(suppl):S41–S49.

Cernea CR, Dias FL, Fliss D, Lima RA, Myers EN, Wei WI (eds): Pearls and Pitfalls in Head and Neck Surgery. Basel, Karger, 2008, pp 36–37

2.2 N0 Neck in Oral Cancer: Wait and Watch

Yoav P. Talmi

Department of Otorhinolaryngology – Head and Neck Surgery, Chaim Sheba Medical Center, Tel Hashomer, and Department of Otorhinolaryngology, Tel Aviv University Sackler School of Medicine, Tel Aviv, Israel

PEARLS

Wait and Watch Policy

- Avoid performing surgery not indicated in the majority of patients.
- Avoid complications of surgery and irradiation.
- Keep the option of surgery and/or radiation for recurrences/second primaries.
- Reduce cost.

Active Neck Treatment

- Complications and sequelae of selective neck dissection (ND) are minimal.
- Delayed neck presentation may be rapid and in a more advanced stage.
- More extended ND procedures indicated when treating delayed neck recurrences.
- Incidence of neck recurrence is significantly reduced when treated simultaneously.
- Chances of cure are significantly elevated.

Introduction

Cervical metastases are the worst prognostic indicator apart from distant metastases in patients with cancer of the head and neck, decreasing survival by approximately 50%.

The incidence of occult nodes was reported in the range of 21–45% of oral cavity cases. It is recommended that when the probability of occult cervical lymph node metastasis is more than 20%, the neck should be electively treated either by surgery or radiotherapy. Both, however, are associated with adverse effects.

The argument in favor of observation is that with elective treatment, the majority of patients receive an intervention that is necessary only in 25–30%. While morbidity of elective ND is usually minimal, a neck intervention in the future may be hampered by former surgery. Radiation treatment is not without consequences either, i.e. local effects or induction of second primaries, and we may also deny the patients the opportunity of such interventions in the future.

The assumption that the N0 neck can be readily observed and treated when the patient develops early regional N1 metastatic disease has often been proven erroneous. Forty-nine percent of patients who underwent salvage neck surgery after a close 'watch and wait' policy were found to have advanced neck disease (N2b) [1].

In a group of 137 patients [2] with T1/T2, N0 tongue cancer, patients that required ND when becoming N+ had a significantly greater number of positive nodes, a higher incidence of extracapsular spread, and decreased survival compared to patients undergoing simultaneous ND.

In a group [3] where elective ND and 'watchful waiting' in stage I/II oral tongue squamous cell cancer (SCC) was compared, the regional recurrence rate was 47% (23% mortality) in N0 patients who had no ND. Elective ND significantly reduced the regional recurrence rate to 9% (3% mortality).

In a group of 233 patients with stage I/II oral cavity SCC treated by brachytherapy [4], 47% underwent elective ND and 53% were only followed and underwent ND in case of relapses. In the first group, salvage treatment was successful in 47% of cases and it was successful in 62% of the second group. Ten-year survival, however, was 37 and 31%, respectively.

Increased patient morbidity associated with salvage surgery was due to the need for more radical forms of ND in established neck disease and the need for postoperative radiotherapy [5].

A significant decrease in survival in high-risk patients was reported [6]. Among the cases that had metastases at follow-up, 50% were not even candidates for salvage treatment. Kligerman et al. [7] stipulated that ND remains mandatory in the early stage of oral SCC because of better survival rates compared to resection alone and the poor salvage rate. This was noted in particular in patients with tumor thickness >4 mm.

In a group of 156 similar patients [8] elective ND increased survival to 55% compared with 33% with observation. Wei et al. [9] reviewed the accepted approaches to the N0 neck summarizing the issues at hand.

An approach of close ultrasound follow-up with FNA cytology has been suggested and may be of value in watch and wait cases. Sentinel node biopsy in selected cases may also change our approach to a more conservative one. A negative sentinel node biopsy may obviate the need to perform ND whereas if the sampled node or nodes are positive, there is no question regarding the need for ND.

Conclusion

It is my view that a selective ND should be performed in the majority of the N0 necks, which is supported by the literature cited. However, in cases where a sentinel node biopsy was negative, a careful watch and wait approach may be justified. Also, in superficial T1 lesions with a depth ranging to no more than 4–6 mm, or anterior tongue small lesions, a watch and wait policy may be reasonable.

References

1 Andersen PE, Cambronero E, Shaha AR, Shah JP: The extent of neck disease after regional failure during observation of the N0 neck. Am J Surg 1996;172:689–691.

2 Haddadin KJ, Soutar DS, Oliver RJ, Webster MH, Robertson AG, MacDonald DG: Improved survival for patients with clinically T1/T2, N0 tongue tumors undergoing a prophylactic neck dissection. Head Neck 1999;21:517–525.

3 Yuen AP, Wei WI, Wong YM, Tang KC: Elective neck dissection versus observation in the treatment of early oral tongue carcinoma. Head Neck 1997;19:583–588.

4 Piedbois P, Mazeron JJ, Haddad E, Coste A, Martin M, Levy C, et al: Stage I–II squamous cell carcinoma of the oral cavity treated by iridium-192: is elective neck dissection indicated? Radiother Oncol 1991;21:100–106.

5 Shasha D, Harrison LB: Elective irradiation of the N0 neck in squamous cell carcinoma of the upper aerodigestive tract. Otolaryngol Clin North Am 1998;31:803–813.

6 Kowalski LP, Bagietto R, Lara JR, Santos RL, Silva JF Jr, Magrin J: Prognostic significance of the distribution of neck node metastasis from oral carcinoma. Head Neck 2000;22:207–214.

7 Kligerman J, Lima RA, Soares JR, Prado L, Dias FL, Freitas EQ, et al: Supraomohyoid neck dissection in the treatment of T1/T2 squamous cell carcinoma of oral cavity. Am J Surg 1994;168:391–394.

8 Lydiatt DD, Robbins KT, Byers RM, Wolf PF: Treatment of stage I and II oral tongue cancer. Head Neck 1993;15:308–312.

9 Wei WI, Ferlito A, Rinaldo A, Gourin CG, Lowry J, Ho WK, et al: Management of the N0 neck – reference or preference. Oral Oncol 2006;42:115–122.

Cernea CR, Dias FL, Fliss D, Lima RA, Myers EN, Wei WI (eds): Pearls and Pitfalls in Head and Neck Surgery. Basel, Karger, 2008, pp 38–39

2.3 N0 Neck in Oral Cancer: Elective Neck Dissection

Fernando L. Dias, Roberto A. Lima

Head and Neck Surgery Department, Brazilian National Cancer Institute and Postgraduation School of Medicine, Catholic University of Rio de Janeiro, Rio de Janeiro, Brazil

Pearls

- Consider elective supraomohyoid neck dissection in early oral tongue and floor of mouth squamous cell carcinoma (SCC).
- Consider extending supraomohyoid neck dissection to level IV in SCC of the posterior 1/3 of the tongue.
- Identification of the posterior belly of the digastric muscle will ease the dissection of level IIa–b.

Pitfalls

- Avoid traction of nerve XI while dissecting level IIb.
- Avoid dissection of level II before identification of nerve XI.

Introduction

Lymph node metastasis (LNM) from oral cavity (OC) SCC occurs in a predictable and sequential fashion. For primary tumors of the OC the first echelon lymph node at highest risk for early dissemination includes levels I, II and III [1–5].

Poor salvage rates for regional recurrence ranging from 11 to 40%, despite the use of aggressive therapy, emphasize the role of elective treatment of the neck in OC SCC [6].

Practical Tips

Tumors more than 1 cm away from the midline present a low risk of bilateral/contralateral LNM (7%). Tumors crossing the midline by less than 1 cm have a risk increased to 16%, which reaches 46% in those patients where the crossing is more than 1 cm.

The depth of invasion and thickness, the characteristics of the tumor-normal tissue boundary (i.e., well-demarcated vs. diffuse invasion at the boundary), lymphatic or vascular space invasion, perineural invasion, and the degree of inflammatory (lymphoplasmacytic) response are considered predictive factors for LNM as well as its diameter and grade [6].

(1) The incision is placed in an upper neck skin crease extending from the posterior border of the sternocleidomastoid muscle towards the hyoid bone up to the midline (at least two finger breadths below the angle of the mandible).

(2) Nerves at risk during supraomohyoid neck dissection are marginal mandibular branch of the facial nerve (MBFN), lingual nerve, hypoglossal nerve, spinal accessory nerve, cutaneous and muscular branches of the cervical plexus, and great auricular nerve. They should be carefully identified and preserved [4, 7].

(3) Start dissecting the anterior border of the sternomastoid muscle from its intersection with the omohyoid muscle (posterior belly) up to the mastoid tip. This maneuver will ease the identifica-

tion of the posterior belly of the digastric muscle and, consequently, the dissection of the apex of the posterior triangle.

4 Nerve XI usually runs parallel and deep to the great auricular nerve. Avoid traction on nerve XI while dissecting level IIb.

5 There is a close relationship between the MBFN and the facial vessels. A surgical maneuver attributed to Hayes Martin, i.e. keeping the cranial stumps of facial vessels retracted upward during the dissection of the submandibular triangle, helps to protect the nerve. The use of nerve monitoring and magnification can be of help [7].

6 Only after the identification of the MBFN is exposure of the prevascular facial LN (level Ib) accomplished.

7 A brisk hemorrhage is expected during dissection along the lower border of the body of the mandible up to the attachment of the anterior belly of the digastric muscle [4].

8 Adequate exposure of the undersurface of the floor of the mouth is achieved with gentle traction of the submandibular gland downward and medial retraction of the lateral border of the mylohyoid muscle. Such exposure allows precise identification of the hypoglossal and lingual nerves as well as its secretomotor fibers to the submandibular gland and the Wharton's duct. Once the lingual nerve is clearly identified, the secretomotor fibers to the submandibular gland can be safely divided between clamps and ligated.

9 In N0 neck, levels IV and V LN are generally not at risk of harboring micrometastasis. The exception to this observation are SCC of the posterior 1/3 lateral border of the tongue in which level IV may be at risk of occult LNM [4, 5].

10 To facilitate accurate description of the excised LN, it is important to apply numerical tags to the LN depicting each level.

Conclusion

The limitations for the identification of occult cervical metastases and the negative impact of recurrent disease in the neck are important issues in the management of OC SCC [1–3]. Elective treatment of the neck must be strongly considered in OC, even in early stages when the primary tumor is located at the tongue and/or floor of the mouth.

References

1 Shah JP, Candela FC, Poddar AK: The patterns of cervical lymph node metastases from squamous carcinoma of the oral cavity. Cancer 1990;66:109–113.

2 Dias FL, Kligerman J, Matos de Sá G, et al: Elective neck dissection versus observation in stage I squamous cell carcinomas of the tongue and floor of the mouth. Otolaryngol Head Neck Surg 2001;125:23–29.

3 Laubenbacher C, Saumweber D, Wagner-Manslau C, et al: Comparison of fluorine-18-fluorodeoxyglucose PET, MRI and endoscopy for staging head and neck squamous carcinomas. J Nucl Med 1995;36:1747–1757.

4 Shah JP, Patel SG: Cervical lymph nodes; in Shah JP, Patel SG (eds): Head and Neck Surgery and Oncology, ed 3. Edinburgh, Mosby, 2003, pp 353–394.

5 Dias FL, Lima RA, Kligerman J, et al: Relevance of skip metastases for squamous cell carcinoma of the oral tongue and floor of the mouth. Otolaryngol Head Neck Surg 2006;136:460–465.

6 Dias FL, Lima RA: Cancer of the floor of the mouth. Oper Tech Otolaryngol Head Neck Surg 2005;16:10–17.

7 Dias FL, Lima RA, Cernea CR: Management of tumors of the submandibular and sublingual glands; in Myers EN, Ferris RL (eds): Salivary Gland Disorders. Berlin, Springer, 2007, pp 339–376.

Cernea CR, Dias FL, Fliss D, Lima RA, Myers EN, Wei WI (eds): Pearls and Pitfalls in Head and Neck Surgery. Basel, Karger, 2008, pp 40–41

2.4 Sentinel Node Biopsy in the Management of the N0 Oral Cancer

Francisco Civantos

Department of Otolaryngology, Head and Neck Surgery, Sylvester Cancer Center, University of Miami, Miami, Fla., USA

PEARLS

- Select early lesions without extremely deep invasion.
- Use preoperative contrasted CT or MRI to detect grossly involved lymph nodes (LN).
- Accurate radiotracer injection requires a comfortable patient.
- Inject closely into normal tissue around the lesion.
- Manage background activity from the primary site.
- Tag identified nerves.
- Exhaustive step sectioning and immunohistochemistry.
- Close follow-up.

PITFALLS

- Counsel patients regarding potential reexploration.
- Avoid large lesions as an excessive number of nodes will result.
- Use of the gamma probe is not intuitive.
- Do not inject local anesthetic directly into the primary tumor.
- Avoid blue dye for mucosal lesions.
- Avoid paralysis.

Introduction

Traditional 'watchful waiting' minimized morbidity in the majority of patients [1]. However, recent opinion favors neck dissection (ND) in patients at risk for cervical metastases [2, 3].

Sentinel lymph node biopsy (SLNB) could consign this debate to history, as accrued experience demonstrates that micrometastases can be accurately detected with this less invasive technique. More than 60 single institution trials, two international conference consensus documents, a meta-analysis, and a rigorous cooperative group validation trial have evaluated this technique for oral cancer [4–6]. The negative predictive value of SLNB approximates 95%; step sectioning and immunohistochemistry prove essential and lead to significant upstaging, and unexpected patterns of drainage can occur [7].

Practical Tips

① *Patient Selection.* Select T1 and smaller T2 lesions. Rule out nonpalpable gross disease through strictly interpreted imaging. SLNB will detect micrometastases, but not nonfunctional, grossly involved nodes.

② *Radionuclide Injection and Imaging of the Primary Tumor.* Avoid direct injection of the tumor with local anesthetic as it affects radionuclide uptake. Narrow injection circumferentially encompasses the lesion with an additional injection in the center of the lesion. Use 500 mCi on the morning of surgery, or a slightly higher dose the night before. We prefer unfiltered 99Tc sulfur colloid. The optional radiologic imaging can provide an anatomic guide and improve preoperative counseling.

③ *Removal of the Primary Tumor.* We resect the primary tumor transorally first to reduce background activity.

④ *Gamma Probe-Guided SLNB.* The incision must be consistent with possible ND. Small flaps are elevated. Palpate the open neck to detect unanticipated gross disease.

Initial readings are taken of the precordium, back table, and primary resection bed, to assess background. The probe is gradually passed over the neck while assessing the auditory input. Avoid rapid or unsteady movement which leads to falsely higher readings. The probe is moved radially across each hot spot, indicating the direction in which to proceed. Angling the probe indicates depth. Using a fine hemostat, the surgeon bluntly dissects towards the sentinel node (SN). Bipolar cautery is used to divide tissues. Avoid paralysis and unipolar electrocautery. Tag identified nerves with permanent suture to facilitate identification if reexploration is necessary.

The SN is excised and ex vivo readings are taken. Repeat readings of the lymphatic bed seeking additional SN. Any LN exhibiting 10% or more of the radioactivity of the most radioactive node will be harvested. Greater than six highly radioactive nodes represent technical failure and call for SN dissection (SND). Rarely, a hot node occurs in a completely separate anatomic region (i.e. submental vs. level II) that does not reach 10% of the radioactivity of the hottest node but is significantly radioactive above background. It may represent drainage from a different portion of the tumor and should be harvested.

To assess level I nodes with floor of mouth tumors, the surgeon may dissect below the marginal mandibular nerve towards the mylohyoid muscle, mobilizing the nodes away from the oral cavity. The gamma probe is introduced into the tunnel created and directed inferiorly.

⑤ *Rigorous Histopathologic Assessment of the SN.* Fine sectioning and immunohistochemistry should be performed. Accelerate pathologic evaluation to permit early reexploration prior to onset of inflammation.

Conclusions

Though less morbid than radical dissections, SND has measurable morbidity [8–10]. Morbidity is much less with SLNB [7].

At issue is our limited ability to immediately evaluate SN. For a minority of patients we must reexplore a recently operated wound.

SLNB has an increasing role for early oral cancers. We encourage surgeons to gain experience with cutaneous malignancies, early oral cancers, and gamma probe-guided ND for more invasive cancers.

References

1 Spiro RH, Strong EW: Epidermoid carcinoma of the mobile tongue. Treatment by partial glossectomy alone. Am J Surg 1971; 122:707–710.

2 Shah JP, Andersen PE: Evolving role of modifications in neck dissection for oral squamous carcinoma. Br J Oral Maxillofac Surg 1995;33:3–8.

3 Kligerman J, Lima RA, Soares JR, et al: Supraomohyoid neck dissection in the treatment of T1/T2 squamous cell carcinoma of oral cavity. Am J Surg 1994;168:391–392.

4 Ross GL, Soutar DS, Gordon MacDonald D, Shoaib T, Camilleri I, Roberton AG, Sorensen JA, Thomsen J, Grupe P, Alvarez J, Barbier L, Santamaria J, Poli T, Massarelli O, Sesenna E, Kovacs AF, Grunwald F, Barzan L, Sulfaro S, Alberti F: Sentinel node biopsy in head and neck cancer: preliminary results of a multicenter trial. Ann Surg Oncol 2004;11:690–696.

5 Paleri V, Rees G, Arullendran P, Shoaib T, Krishman S: Sentinel node biopsy in squamous cell cancer of the oral cavity and oral pharynx: a diagnostic meta-analysis. Head Neck 2005;27:739–747.

6 Civantos FJ, Moffat FL, Goodwin WJ: Lymphatic mapping and sentinel lymphadenectomy for 106 head and neck lesions: contrasts between oral cavity and cutaneous malignancy. Laryngoscope 2006;112(suppl 109):1–15.

7 Civantos FJ, Zitsch R, Schuller D, Agrawal A, Smith R, Nason R, Petruzelli G, Gourin C, Yarbrough W, Ridge JD, Myers J: Sentinel node biopsy for oral cancer: a multi-center validation trial (abstract). Arch Otolaryngol Head Neck Surg 2006;132:8.

8 Chepeha DB, Taylor RJ, Chepeha JC, et al: Functional assessment using Constant's Shoulder Scale after modified radical and selective neck dissection. Head Neck 2002;24:432–436.

9 Kuntz AL, Weymuller EA Jr: Impact of neck dissection on quality of life. Laryngoscope 1999;109:1334–1338.

10 Rogers SN, Ferlito A, Pelliteri PK, Shaha AR, Rinaldo A: Quality of life following neck dissections. Acta Otolaryngol 2004;124: 231–236.

Cernea CR, Dias FL, Fliss D, Lima RA, Myers EN, Wei WI (eds): Pearls and Pitfalls in Head and Neck Surgery. Basel, Karger, 2008, pp 42–43

2.5 Selective Neck Dissection in the Treatment of the N+ Neck in Cancers of the Oral Cavity

Jesus E. Medina, Greg Krempl

Department of Otorhinolaryngology, University of Oklahoma Health Sciences Center, Oklahoma City, Okla., USA

PEARLS

- Patients with cancer of the oral cavity (COC) rarely have isolated lymph node metastasis (LNM) in levels IV or V.
- A selective neck dissection (SND) is an appropriate operation for the management of selected patients with an N+ neck.
- Postoperative radiation (PORDT) is usually indicated with an SND in such cases.

PITFALL

- Lack of appropriate informed consent may hinder the surgeon's ability to extend the operation when necessary to remove all the disease encountered in the neck.

Introduction

An SND consists of the en bloc removal of the lymph node groups that are most likely to harbor metastases depending upon the location of the primary tumor. The goal of such operation is to remove the nodes at risk while preserving function and minimizing morbidity. A selective dissection of the nodes of levels I, II and III/IV (supraomohyoid neck dissection) is currently the preferred operation for the initial management of the neck in patients with COC who have no clinical evidence of LNM, but in whom the risk of subclinical metastases is reasonably high. In the presence of palpable LNM, a radical or modified radical neck dissection is the preferred operation. SNDs are being used with increasing frequency in selected N+ patients, either alone or in combination with PORDT [1–10].

Since the use of these operations in the treatment of the N+ neck is still controversial, we reviewed our experience and attempt to outline the appropriate role of SND in the management of the N+ neck in patients with cancers of the oral cavity.

Practical Tips

1 At least levels I, II and III must be included. In a cohort of 164 patients with oral cancer, who had a single clinically positive node (N1 or N2a), Kowalski and Carvalho [8] found no isolated LNM in levels IV or V. Furthermore, in patients with clinically N1 neck disease involving levels I or II, these nodes were histopathologically negative (pN0) in 57.4% of the cases.

2 In other reports the prevalence of metastases in level IV in clinically N+ cases is 17%, suggesting that it is a safer practice to include level IV whenever an SND is done for an N+ neck in patients with COC.

3 The prevalence of LNM in level V is so low in such patients (0.5% in cN0 and 3% in cN+) that dissection of this region of the neck is rarely necessary.

4 PORDT is beneficial in terms of locoregional control of tumor in pN+ patients, particularly in cases with adverse prognostic factors such as multiple metastatic lymph nodes or extracapsular spread [8]. Furthermore, when SND is used in combination with PORDT, survival and recurrence results are comparable to those obtained with comprehensive neck dissections [7].

Results

We analyzed our results in a cohort of 22 consecutive patients with COC who had limited pN+ (13 pN1, 1 pN2a and 8 pN2) confined to levels I and II, and underwent an SND. The primary tumor was in the oral tongue in 7 patients, the lower lip in 6, the floor of the mouth in 4, the alveolar ridge in 2, the retromolar trigone in 2, and the buccal mucosa in 1 patient. In the majority of patients (72.7%) the dissection included levels I–III (11/50%) or levels I–IV (5/22.7%). Six patients had received radiation to the neck previously and 8 patients received PORDT. With a mean follow-up of 28 months, a recurrence in the neck occurred in 3 patients (13.6%), all of whom had received PORDT. In a previous review we encountered a similar neck recurrence rate of 12.5% in 53 patients with pathological N+ disease undergoing SND and radiotherapy. Ambrosch et al. [6] reported a recurrence in the dissected neck in 6.6% of patients with pN+ necks. More recently, the same group reported their results with therapeutic SND. The 3-year regional recurrence rate was 4.9% among pN1 cases and 12.1% among pN2 cases [8].

Conclusion

This review and other investigations reported in the literature suggest that SND has a role in the management of patients with COC who have clinically positive LNM in level I or II, particularly when appropriately combined with PORDT.

2

References

1 Byers RM, Wolf PF, Ballantyne AJ: Rationale for elective modified neck dissection. Head Neck Surg 1988;10:160–167.
2 Traynor SJ, Cohen JI, Gray J, et al: Selective neck dissection and the management of the node-positive neck. Am J Surg 1996;172: 654–657.
3 Davidson J, Khan Y, Gilbert R, et al: Is selective neck dissection sufficient treatment for the N0/Np+ neck? J Otolaryngol 1997;26: 229–231.
4 Pellitteri PK, Robbins KT, Neuman T: Expanded application of selective neck dissection with regard to nodal status. Head Neck 1997;19:260–265.
5 Muzaffar K: Therapeutic selective neck dissection: a 25-year review. Laryngoscope 2003;113:1460–1465.
6 Ambrosch P, Kron M, Pradier O, et al: Efficacy of selective neck dissection: a review of 503 cases of elective and therapeutic treatment of the neck in squamous cell carcinoma of the upper aerodigestive tract. Otolaryngol Head Neck Surg 2001;124:180–187.
7 Andersen PE, Warren F, Spiro J, et al: Results of selective neck dissection in management of the node-positive neck. Arch Otolaryngol Head Neck Surg 2002;128:1180–1184.
8 Kowalski LP, Carvalho AL: Feasibility of supraomohyoid neck dissection in N1 and N2a oral cancer patients. Head Neck 2002; 24:921–924.
9 Shah JP: Patterns of cervical lymph node metastasis from squamous carcinomas of the upper aerodigestive tract. Am J Surg 1990;160:405–409.
10 Medina JE, Byers RM: Supraomohyoid neck dissection: rationale, indications, and surgical technique. Head Neck 1989;11:111–122.

Cernea CR, Dias FL, Fliss D, Lima RA, Myers EN, Wei WI (eds): Pearls and Pitfalls in Head and Neck Surgery. Basel, Karger, 2008, pp 44–45

2.6 How to Manage the XI Nerve in Neck Dissections

Lance E. Oxford, John C. O'Brien, Jr.

Sammons Cancer Center, Baylor University Medical Center, Dallas, Tex., USA

Pearls

- Where there are nodes in the posterior triangle, there you will find the spinal accessory nerve (SAN).
- Raise the posterior triangle skin flap carefully. Dissect over the veins and nerves.
- Preserve the innervation to the levator scapulae and the cervical nerve root contributions to the SAN that may provide innervation to the trapezius.

Pitfalls

- The SAN is more superficial than you think.
- Avoid traction and the use of electrocautery around the SAN.
- The potential for postoperative irradiation does not justify inadequate surgery.

Introduction

The head and neck surgeon should be able to identify the SAN in multiple locations throughout its course. Primary tumors, nodal metastases and prior chemoradiotherapy may distort the neck anatomy, which can dictate the initial approach to the identification of the SAN.

Careful elevation of the posterior skin flaps is crucial to prevent injury. Dorsal to the free edge of the platysma, the SAN may be injured if thick skin flaps are elevated. Dissect over the nerves and veins that are found during the dissection.

The SAN travels from the jugular foramen to enter the upper one third of the sternocleidomastoid (SCM). The transverse process of the atlas (C1 vertebra) is a good landmark [1]. The internal jugular vein passes anterior to this prominence; the SAN is lateral to the vein. The SAN passes through the SCM giving off muscular branches. It exits posteriorly, approximately 1 cm superior to Erb's point [2]. The SAN travels posteroinferiorly through the posterior triangle neck to enter deep to the free edge of the trapezius approximately 2–5 cm superior to the clavicle. The supraclavicular nerves are superficial and the SAN deep to the trapezius.

The SAN is identified as it enters the SCM by dissecting the fascia off of the medial aspect of the superior SCM. Vascular landmarks have been reported to help localize the SAN [3, 4]. In the lower neck, the SAN is identified by dissecting the fascia along the anterior edge of the trapezius, approximately two finger breadths superior to the clavicle. There are multiple terminal branches of the SAN that must be preserved. The SAN can be traced proximally. With gentle traction on the SAN with vessel loops, the contributions of the cervical nerve roots to the nerve can be identified by the fixation points where the fibers enter.

A nerve stimulator can be utilized to confirm the SAN. Some authors recommend SAN monitoring similar to that which is done for the recurrent laryngeal and facial nerves [5].

Practical Tips

Identification of the SAN is a standard component in a neck dissection:

1. Surface landmarks such as the junction of the superior and middle thirds of the SCM estimate the location of the SAN; however, surface landmarks are not always reliable [5].
2. If the SAN is sacrificed, the sural nerve may be used to reconstruct it. A cervical sensory nerve may also be used as a donor; however, the nerve should be widely clear of nodal disease often making the great auricular nerve a poor candidate. Margins of the SAN should be evaluated with frozen section prior to grafting.
3. In postirradiation patients who are treated with surgery, the surgeon must be more aggressive in resection of recurrent nodal disease. This often results in sacrifice of the SAN.
4. Avoid excessive traction and the use of the electrocautery near the SAN.
5. Preserve the cervical nerve root contributions to the accessory nerve. The C3 nerve roots to the levator scapulae help support the shoulder and preserve function.

Conclusion

Preservation of SAN can be done safely in properly selected patients. The ability to choose patients with the appropriate indications, knowledge of anatomy, and careful dissection can result in excellent results from an oncologic and functional endpoint. There is no SAN worth the life of a patient.

References

1 Sheen TS, Chung TT, Snyderman CH: Transverse process of the atlas (C1) – an important surgical landmark of the upper neck. Head Neck 1997;19:37–40.

2 Eisele DW, Weymuller EA, Price JC: Spinal accessory nerve preservation during neck dissection. Laryngoscope 1991;101:433–435.

3 Rafferty MA, Goldstein DP, Brown DH, Irish JC: The sternomastoid branch of the occipital artery: a surgical landmark for the spinal accessory nerve in selective neck dissections. Otolaryngol Head Neck Surg 2005;133:874–876.

4 Chaukar DA, Pai A, D'Cruz AK: A technique to identify and preserve the spinal accessory nerve during neck dissection. J Laryngol Otol 2006;120:494–496.

5 Witt R, Gillis G, Pratt R Jr: Spinal accessory nerve monitoring with clinical outcomes measures. Ear Nose Throat J 2006;85:540–544.

6 Symes A, Ellis H: Variations in the surface anatomy of the spinal accessory nerve in the posterior triangle. Surg Radiol Anat 2005;27:404–408.

Cernea CR, Dias FL, Fliss D, Lima RA, Myers EN, Wei WI (eds): Pearls and Pitfalls in Head and Neck Surgery. Basel, Karger, 2008, pp 46–47

2.7 Preservation of the Marginal Mandibular Nerve in Neck Surgery

K. Thomas Robbins

Otolaryngology – Head and Neck Surgery, SimmonsCooper Cancer Institute, Southern Illinois University School of Medicine, Springfield, Ill., USA

PEARLS

- Proper draping of the patient with exposure of the surface anatomy of the neck and lower face helps to maintain proper orientation.
- Carefully monitor the placement of retractors by your assistant in order to avoid direct compression of the ramus.
- Preoperative counseling of patients is important to inform them of the slight risk of developing paresis of the lower facial mimetic muscles.

PITFALLS

- Paralysis of the patient will preclude the effective use of a nerve stimulator.
- Beware of patients with ptosis of the submandibular gland because the marginal branch of the facial nerve may lie lower than usual.
- Always locate the ramus mandibularis when dissecting the perifacial and buccinator lymph nodes.

Introduction

Surgery performed in the upper neck carries the risk of injury to the marginal mandibular nerve (MMN) resulting in a cosmetic deformity caused by interruption of nerve fibers to the depressor anguli oris and the depressor labii inferioris. However, division of the platysma muscle and in some cases the cervical branch of the facial nerve can result in pseudoparalysis of the MMN that usually recovers spontaneously [1]. The reported rate of mandibular nerve injury varies from 0 to 20% following submandibular gland removal [2]. Following neck dissection involving level I, temporary apraxia was found in 29% of patients and persistent paralysis in 16% [3]. Temporary dysfunction usually resolves in 3–6 months.

Practical Tips

Two or more rami of the mandibular branch of the facial nerve can be found in the region of the angle of the mandible always crossing the superficial surface of the anterior facial vein [4]. In the region immediately posterior to the junction of the facial artery and the mandible, the nerve lies above the inferior border of the mandible in 81% of specimens, and 1 cm or less below the inferior border of the mandible in 19% [4]. Anterior to the facial artery and mandible junction, all branches of the MMN lie above the inferior border of the mandible. However, in elderly patients with ptosis of the neck structures, the nerve could lie as low as 3–4 cm below this point [5].

Incisions made in the upper neck must be made for optimal exposure of the surgical bed. However, the planning of the incisions must take into account the location of the MMN. A safe rule is to make the incision parallel to the pathway of the nerve located 3 cm inferior to the lower border of the mandible. The neck flaps should be lifted in the plane, immediately below the platysma muscle.

The traditional maneuver designed to protect the MMN was to identify the anterior facial vein, ligate it and lift it superiorly. In recent years I have abandoned this 'indirect technique' for one that I would term 'the direct approach'. I prefer to identify the nerve by careful separation of the tissue overlying the angle of the mandible until the small whitish nerve branch is visualized. This can be facilitated with a nerve stimulator to help localize the exact pathway of the nerve [6]. Next, it is important to skeletonize the nerve for a short distance (2–3 cm) in order to determine its direction and to facilitate transposing it away from the surgical bed if necessary. Alternatively, retrograde dissection of the cervical branch upwards will usually help to identify the MMN since both nerves arise from a common trunk [7].

References

1 Tulley P, Webb A, Chana JS, Tan T, Hudson D, Grobbelaar AO, Harrison DH: Paralysis of the marginal mandibular branch of the facial nerve: treatment options. Br J Plast Surg 2000;53:378–385.

2 Hald J, Andreassen UK: Submandibular gland excision: short- and long-term complications. ORL J Otorhinolaryngol Relat Spec 1994;56:87–91.

3 Nasan RW, Binahmed A, Torchia MG, Thliversis J: Clinical observations of the anatomy and function of the marginal mandibular nerve. Int J Oral Maxillofac 2007;36:712–715.

4 Dingman RO, Grabb WC: Surgical anatomy of the mandibular ramus of the facial nerve based on the dissection of 100 facial halves. Plast Reconstr Surg 1962;29:266–272.

5 Baker DC, Conley J: Avoiding facial nerve injuries in rhytidectomy. Plast Reconstr Surg 1979;64:781–795.

6 Sadoughi B, Hans S, de Monès E, Brasnu DF: Preservation of the marginal mandibular branch of the facial nerve using a plexus block nerve stimulator. Laryngoscope 2006;116:1713–1716.

7 Mohd S, Zaidi S: A simple nerve dissecting technique for identification of marginal mandibular nerve in radical neck dissection. J Surg Oncol 2007;96:71–72.

Cernea CR, Dias FL, Fliss D, Lima RA, Myers EN, Wei WI (eds): Pearls and Pitfalls in Head and Neck Surgery. Basel, Karger, 2008, pp 48–49

2.8 Bilateral Neck Dissections: Practical Tips

Jonas T. Johnson

Department of Otolaryngology, University of Pittsburgh School of Medicine, Pittsburgh, Pa., USA

PEARLS

- The side with less disease should be dissected first to assure preservation of at least 1 internal jugular vein (IJV).
- The incision employed should reflect the need for exposure and resection of the primary tumor as applicable.
- Bilateral neck dissection (BND) can be accomplished simultaneously in the vast majority of patients.
- Reconstruction of one IJV should be considered if the tumor burden requires bilateral resection of both IJVs.

PITFALLS

- Bilateral occlusion of both IJVs will be associated with extensive, prolonged edema of the face and neck.
- Bilateral simultaneous occlusion of both IJVs may be associated with dangerous increase in intracranial pressure and even blindness and death.

Introduction

Surgical care of cervical metastatic disease remains a mainstay in the treatment of patients with cancer involving structures of the head and neck. All primary tumors, irrespective of laterality, may on occasion be associated with contralateral metastases. Many head and neck sites including anterior floor of mouth, tongue base, supraglottic larynx, and pharynx are commonly associated with a significant risk for bilateral cervical metastases.

These considerations mandate that head and neck surgeons be prepared to offer patients simultaneous treatment to both sides of the neck under circumstances which are commonly encountered.

Practical Tips

Modified selective BND can be safely accomplished in a single session for the majority of patients. BND results in approximately 90 min of extra surgery and less than 1 unit of blood loss. It should not be expected to extend the hospital stay [1].

The particular incision employed to expose the neck for BND should be chosen according to the needs of the particular patient. There is no universally accepted approach. I recommend that an incision be chosen which allows adequate exposure for both necks as well as resection of the primary tumor. For patients with cancer involving the thyroid gland or larynx, a superiorly based apron flap seems most convenient. When working on a primary in the oral cavity (OC), it may be appropriate to use a shorter apron, allowing a tracheotomy to be placed through a separate incision if needed. A short apron flap may be used to deglove the mandible if the surgeon prefers this exposure for OC resection. In some cases, two separate utility incisions may be used.

I prefer to operate upon the side with the least tumor burden first. This is especially important if the surgeon plans to resect the IJV on the contralateral side. In so doing, it is possible for the surgical team to reassure themselves that one IJV has been preserved before the contralateral vein is sacrificed intentionally. If the IJV is inadvertently injured or sacrificed, the surgical team can then decide to either resect and reconstruct the contralateral side or stage the second ND.

Bilateral simultaneous resection of both IJVs results in almost certain severe facial edema with potential for obstruction of the airway, swallowing, and the Eustachian tubes. Tracheotomy is always required. Increased intracranial pressure, blindness, and even death may be encountered in some patients under these circumstances [2]. Accordingly, radical BND with occlusion of both IJVs should not be accomplished in a single session. Blindness is, fortunately, very rarely encountered following BND. The pathophysiologic cause is controversial and is perhaps variable according to the patient's particular situation. Blindness may be due to hypotension secondary to excessive blood loss. Another potential mechanism for blindness is anterior ischemic optic neuropathy. This is characterized by pale edematous optic nerves with increased intraocular pressure. Unfortunately, staging radical BND may not completely obviate the risk [2].

Radical BND can be safety accomplished in most circumstances when staged 6 weeks apart. Alternatively, a number of reconstructive methods are available which would allow repair of a single IJV electively. This would allow BND to proceed simultaneously.

Patients undergoing BND may benefit from perioperative prophylactic antibiotic administration even when the wound is not contaminated by exposure to the OC or pharynx [3].

Conclusion

BND is frequently indicated in patients treated for cancer of the structures of the head and neck. This can be safely accomplished in most patients who require modified or selective ND. When excessive tumor burden is present bilaterally, consideration should be given to reconstruction of a single JV or staging the procedure 6 weeks apart.

References

1 Weber PC, Johnson JT, Myers EN: Impact of bilateral neck dissection on recovery following supraglottic laryngectomy. Arch Otolaryngol Head Neck Surg 1993;119:61–64.
2 Worrell L, Rowe M, Petti G: Amaurosis: a complication of bilateral radical neck dissection. Am J Otolaryngol 2002;23:56–59.
3 Seven H, Sayin I, Turgut S: Antibiotic prophylaxis in clean neck dissections. J Laryngol Otol 2004;118:213–216.

Cernea CR, Dias FL, Fliss D, Lima RA, Myers EN, Wei WI (eds): Pearls and Pitfalls in Head and Neck Surgery. Basel, Karger, 2008, pp 50–51

2.9a How to Manage Retropharyngeal Lymph Nodes 1. Transoral Approach

James Cohen[a], Randal S. Weber[b]

[a] Department of Otolaryngology/Head and Neck Surgery, Oregon Health Sciences University, PV-01, Portland, Oreg., and
[b] Department of Head and Neck Surgery, Unit 441, University of Texas M.D. Anderson Cancer Center, Houston, Tex., USA

PEARLS

- Tumor histology (thyroid vs. squamous cell carcinoma) and nodal configuration by imaging (CT, MRI) determine the likelihood of extracapsular extension, which in turn determines whether the transoral or transcervical approach to excision should be used.
- Identification of the internal carotid artery (ICA) and superior sympathetic trunk is essential to safe removal of this nodal group.

PITFALLS

- Nodes that are not palpable transorally are very difficult to excise with the transoral approach.
- Adequate illumination, loupe magnification and meticulous hemostasis are essential for safe transoral removal.

Introduction

Retropharyngeal lymph node (RPLN) metastasis by thyroid cancer has been suggested to occur either by retrograde spread from the lymphatic pathways of the jugular chain and paratracheal nodes or through the superior thyroid pole [1, 2]. The proximity of the RPLN to the posterior oropharyngeal mucosa and the generally well-circumscribed, noninvasive nature of thyroid cancer metastases, which usually lack macroscopic extracapsular spread (as compared to the extracapsular spread usually seen with squamous cell metastasis to this location), make a direct transoral approach to their removal technically feasible and oncologically sound.

Practical Tips

1. CT and MRI are the principle means of detecting disease within the RPLN as they are usually asymptomatic. Nodes being considered for transoral removal should be well circumscribed without radiographic evidence of extracapsular spread. Nodes that are greater than 1 cm in size, particularly if asymmetrically enlarged, or those with central lucency should be considered suspicious for disease [3, 4]. Where doubt exists transoral FNA is possible, in the clinic for larger nodes that are palpable, or in the operating room with ultrasound guidance if needed.
2. Surgical excision should only be considered for those nodes that are clinically palpable transorally after the patient is appropriately positioned in the operating room with the head slightly extended on the neck and a Crowe-Davis or similar tongue-retracting mouth gag inserted. Otherwise they can be extremely difficult to locate surgically since the lateral RPLN sit in the groove lateral to the prominence of the central portion of the vertebral body and tend to be pushed later-

ally into this groove by palpation or retracted laterally with the carotid artery at the time of surgical exposure.

3 Exposure of the nodes is best achieved by vertically incising the mucosa of the posterior pharyngeal wall and the constrictor muscles just posterior to the posterior tonsillar from the level of the inferior tonsillar pole to just above the level of the soft palate [5]. The ICA is then located by palpating its pulse lateral to the nodes and the buccopharyngeal fascia overlying the nodes is incised just medial to the artery. The nodes are separated from the undersurface of the fascia by sharp and blunt dissection and excised. The superior sympathetic ganglion can be mistaken for an RPLN if care is not taken to ensure that the mass is not continuous with a nerve inferiorly. Beginning the nodal dissection inferiorly ensures that the node will not be mistaken for the superior sympathetic ganglion.

4 Meticulously hemostasis is critical to prevent a retropharyngeal hematoma and is facilitated throughout the dissection by the use of monopolar and bipolar cautery combined with loupe magnification and a headlight for best visualization. The incision is closed with interrupted chromic sutures as a single layer incorporating fascia, muscle, and mucosa in each bite. No more than 3–4 sutures are required. If hemostasis is questionable, the superior aspect of the incision that lies in the nasopharynx behind the soft palate is left open to prevent formation of a hematoma.

5 Antibiotics are administered preoperatively. The patient is allowed to eat a regular diet in the immediate postoperative period and is discharged on the same day or the next morning.

Conclusions

The RPLN represent a nodal group at risk for metastatic spread from cancers of the head and neck region. Detection of metastasis occurs almost entirely by imaging (CT or MRI). With appropriate patient selection based on histology, nodal size and configuration, metastatic disease can be safely excised from this location with a minimum of patient morbidity.

References

1 Robbins KT, Woodson GE: Thyroid carcinoma presenting as a parapharyngeal mass. Head Neck Surg 1985;7:434–436.
2 Dileo MD, Baker KB, Deschler DG, Hayden RE: Metastatic papillary thyroid carcinoma presenting as a retropharyngeal mass. Am J Otol 1998;19:404–406.
3 Morrissey DD, Talbot JM, Cohen JI, Wax MK, Anderson PE: Accuracy of computed tomography in determining the presence or absence of metastatic retropharyngeal adenopathy. Arch Otolaryngol Head Neck Surg 2000;126:1478–1481.
4 Davis WL, Harnsberger HR, Smoker WRK, Watanabe AS: Retropharyngeal space: evaluation of normal anatomy and diseases with CT and MR imaging. Radiology 1990;174:50–64.
5 Le TD, Cohen JI: Transoral approach to removal of the retropharyngeal lymph nodes in well differentiated thyroid cancer. Laryngoscope 2007;117:1155–1158.

2

Cernea CR, Dias FL, Fliss D, Lima RA, Myers EN, Wei WI (eds): Pearls and Pitfalls in Head and Neck Surgery. Basel, Karger, 2008, pp 52–53

2.9b How to Manage Retropharyngeal Lymph Nodes 2. Transcervical Approach

Randal S. Weber

Department of Head and Neck Surgery, Unit 441, University of Texas M.D. Anderson Cancer Center, Houston, Tex., USA

PEARLS

- The transcervical approach is used for metastasis to the retropharyngeal lymph nodes (RPLN) from primary tumors of the pharynx and thyroid or lymph nodes that display extracapsular spread where a transoral approach would be hazardous.
- Identification of the internal carotid artery (ICA) and superior sympathetic trunk is essential for safe removal of this nodal group.
- Take down the digastric and styloid muscles, follow the ICA to the skull base and resect the areolar tissue and lymph nodes medially to the ICA.

PITFALLS

- Adequate illumination, loupe magnification and meticulous hemostasis are essential for the transcervical retropharyngeal lymph node dissection (TRPLND).
- Inform the patient about first bite syndrome, Horner's syndrome and the possibility of dysphagia.

Introduction

RPLN lie within the retropharynx and have a medial and lateral group. The lateral RPLN that occur near the base of skull are of greatest clinical significance. They lie adjacent to the ICA and the sympathetic chain. For squamous cell carcinoma arising from the pharyngeal walls the incidence of RPLN metastasis is 44% [1, 2]. In the absence of pathologic involvement the RPLN are not usually visible on CT or MRI. In the setting of malignant disease of the upper aerodigestive tract or thyroid, RPLN that are visible should be considered to harbor metastatic disease.

TRPLND is not frequently performed today because many cancers of the pharynx are treated with primary radiotherapy with or without chemotherapy and the RPLN lie within the radiation field. This procedure is reserved for patients with RPLN metastasis from tumors of the upper aerodigestive tract or thyroid who will undergo primary surgical resection and have radiographically positive lymph nodes in the retropharynx. At times patients with metastatic thyroid cancer who have RPLN metastasis display bulky nodal disease or evidence of extracapsular spread that would make a transoral resection hazardous. The latter group should undergo TRPLND.

Practical Tips

1. CT and MRI are the imaging modalities for detecting RPLN.
2. Most often TRPLND is performed through an external approach for squamous cell carcinoma of the pharyngeal walls [3]. The external approach is facilitated in patients undergoing laryngopharyngectomy or composite resection. The need for

an isolated RPLND without resection of the primary tumor for squamous cell carcinoma is infrequent.

3 Key to TRPLND is to first perform a lateral neck dissection including all levels of the neck at risk for occult or apparent metastasis. The primary tumor should be resected as indicated prior to the TRPLND. The lateral neck and the TRPLND do not need to be done in continuity.

4 First complete the lateral neck dissection. Identify the ICA and place a vascular loop around the vessel for control. Skeletonize the internal jugular vein, ligate the common facial vein and the internal jugular vein branches in the upper neck. Completely dissect the XIIth nerve and ligate any of the external carotid artery branches that prevent superior dissection of the ICA.

5 Divide the posterior belly of the digastric muscle and the styloid musculature. Follow the internal carotid to the skull base and reflect the fibrofatty tissue medially. Search for the IXth nerve at or near the tip of the styloid process and preserve it if at all possible.

6 To facilitate superior dissection medial to the mandible, divide the stylomandibular ligament. This will allow distraction of the mandible anteriorly by placing a bone hook or retractor on the angle.

7 Dissect the fibroareolar tissue from the superior constrictor and the prevertebral fascia to the midline. This will include the RPLN within this tissue compartment.

Conclusions

The RPLN represent a nodal group at risk for metastatic spread from cancers of the head and neck region. Detection of metastasis occurs almost entirely by imaging (CT or MRI). Selection of the TRPLND depends upon the primary tumor site and the presence or absence of extracapsular spread. With appropriate patient selection based on histology, nodal size and configuration, metastatic disease can be safely excised from this location with a minimum of patient morbidity.

References

1 Ballantyne AJ: Principles of surgical management of cancer of the pharyngeal walls. Cancer 1967;20:663–667.

2 Saito H, Sato T, Yamashita Y, Amagasa T: Topographical analysis of lymphatic pathways from the meso- and hypopharynx based on minute cadaveric dissections: possible application to neck dissection in pharyngeal cancer surgery. Surg Radiol Anat 2002; 24:38–49.

3 Hasegawa Y, Matsuura H: Retropharyngeal node dissection in cancer of the oropharynx and hypopharynx. Head Neck 1994;16: 173–180.

2

Cernea CR, Dias FL, Fliss D, Lima RA, Myers EN, Wei WI (eds): Pearls and Pitfalls in Head and Neck Surgery. Basel, Karger, 2008, pp 54–55

2.10 Management of the Node-Positive Neck in Patients Undergoing Chemoradiotherapy

Rod P. Rezaee, Pierre Lavertu

Department of Otolaryngology – Head and Neck Surgery, University Hospitals Case Medical Center, Ireland Cancer Center, Cleveland, Ohio, USA

PEARLS

- Obtain appropriate posttreatment imaging to augment the physical exam for accurate assessment.
- The role of neck dissection (ND) continues to evolve and must be individualized based on the patient, institutional resources available, and physician factors.
- Selective ND may be utilized in the posttreatment setting [1].

PITFALLS

- Suboptimal timing of posttreatment imaging (CT/PET) leads to treatment dilemmas.
- Neck management schemes remain controversial in the patient undergoing chemoradiotherapy.
- Viability of positive posttreatment neck specimen has been questioned [2].

It is of paramount importance to have an appreciation for the prognostic significance of the presence, persistence or recurrence of nodal disease in the head and neck cancer patient (HNCP). As such, a sound management scheme for addressing and treating the nodal basins at risk is critical to maximizing the potential for successful patient outcomes.

The introduction of intensity-modulated radiation therapy has enhanced the ability to deliver curative doses to the disease fields while reducing patient morbidity. Organ preservation protocols using chemotherapy with modern radiation have raised a discussion of the evolving need, role and timing of ND in the patient undergoing chemoradiotherapy [3]. Management schemes for these patients include planned ND based on initial patient staging or ND based on response to treatment.

Little controversy exists when considering ND in the N1 patient. The role of ND should be reserved for those with less than complete clinical response (CR) or those requiring surgical salvage for persistence or recurrence at the primary site.

Controversy surrounds the management scheme for the patient initially staged with N2–N3 disease. Planned ND continues to be advocated by some, regardless of response to treatment [4]. Rationale is based on the concept that it can be difficult to diagnose neck recurrence and that when found, the disease is often unresectable, precluding successful salvage neck surgery (SNS) [5]. Furthermore, when subsequently looking at potential factors to determine pathologic complete response (pCR), the same authors failed to identify reliable clinical predictors. Thus, recommendation for ND for all N2–N3 necks regardless of response to treatment was made [6]. In patients with N2–N3 disease treated with chemoradiotherapy, regional control was significantly inferior at 5 years in 49 patients not treated with

ND compared to the 100 that did undergo dissection (82.0 vs. 93.9%, respectively, p = 0.028). This, however, was based on positive pathologic findings. The viability of these cells has been questioned, thus clouding their significance. Additionally, SNS was rarely successful, thus supporting planned ND in the N2–N3 neck [7].

Observation exists as an alternative to planned ND and is based on patient response to treatment. Clinical exam alone is not a reliable indicator of pCR and should be combined with imaging studies when making a decision for neck surgery. While combined PET/CT is emerging as the imaging modality of choice, a variety of acceptable imaging techniques exists.

Liauw et al. [8] used CT scan 4 weeks posttreatment to indicate ND. They defined radiographic complete response (rCR) using strict criteria of nodal size <1.5 cm with no focal abnormality and with negative predictive value (NPV) of 94%. They recommended observation of all patients with rCR, regardless of initial N stage. These patients showed no significant decrease in 5-year survival rate compared with those with negative posttreatment ND (97 vs. 98%, respectively).

The use of PET or PET/CT has been shown to be an effective method. Studies have concluded that PET imaging has a low false-negative rate and thus a high NPV of 97% and positive predictive value (PPV) approaching 70%. Problems with high false-positive rates generally are due to the timing of the scan and the continued inflammatory effects of treatment. To allow these effects to dissipate, it is recommended that PET or PET-CT be obtained at least 8–12 weeks posttreatment [9]. If the PET scan is positive at 8–12 weeks, then ND is indicated. If negative, then the patient may safely be observed [10].

Control of nodal disease is a critically important aspect of treatment of the HNCP. It is essential to consider key concepts when making treatment decisions. Planned ND for N2–N3 disease remains a viable option for these patients. Advances in treatment and imaging have created a subset of patients that now may be just observed.

References

1 Robbins KT, Shannon K, Viera F: Is there a role for selective neck dissection after chemoradiotherapy for head and neck cancer? J Am Coll Surg 2004;199:913–916.

2 Strasser MD, Gleich LL, Miller MA, et al: Management implications of evaluating the N2 and N3 neck after organ preservation therapy. Laryngoscope 1999;109:1776–1780.

3 Pellitteri PK, Ferlito A, Rinaldo A, et al: Planned neck dissection following chemoradiotherapy for advanced head and neck cancer: is it necessary for all? Head Neck 2006;28:166–175.

4 Sewall GK, Palazzi-Churas KL, Richards GM, et al: Planned postradiotherapy neck dissection: rationale and clinical outcomes. Laryngoscope 2007;117:121–128.

5 Lavertu P, Adelstein DJ, Saxton JP, et al: Management of the neck in a randomized trial comparing concurrent chemotherapy and radiotherapy alone in respectable stage III and IV squamous cell head and neck cancer. Head Neck 1997;19:559–566.

6 McHam SA, Adelstein DJ, Rybicki LA, et al: Who merits a neck dissection after definitive chemoradiotherapy for N2–N3 squamous cell head and neck cancer? Head Neck 2003;10:791–798.

7 Adelstein DJ, Saxton JP, Rybicki LA, et al: Multiagent concurrent chemoradiotherapy for locoregionally advanced squamous cell head and neck cancer: mature results from a single institution. J Clin Oncol 2006;24:1064–1071.

8 Liauw SL, Mancuso AA, Amdur RJ, et al: Postradiotherapy neck dissection for lymph node-positive head and neck cancer: the use of computed tomography to manage the neck. J Clin Oncol 2006;24:1421–1427.

9 Nayak VN, Walvekar RR, Andrade RS, et al: Deferring planned neck dissection following chemoradiotherapy for stage IV head and neck cancer: the utility of PET-CT. Laryngoscope 2007;117:1–6.

10 Porceddu SV, Jarmolowski E, Hicks RJ, et al: Utility of positron emission tomography for the detection of disease in residual neck nodes after chemoradiotherapy in head and neck cancer. Head Neck 2005;27:175–181.

Cernea CR, Dias FL, Fliss D, Lima RA, Myers EN, Wei WI (eds): Pearls and Pitfalls in Head and Neck Surgery. Basel, Karger, 2008, pp 56–57

2.11 How to Avoid Injury to Thoracic Duct during Surgical Resection of Left Level IV Lymph Nodes

Gary L. Clayman

Department of Head and Neck Surgery, The University of Texas M.D. Anderson Cancer Center, Houston, Tex., USA

Pearls

- The thoracic duct (TD) is usually not a single ductal structure. It is usually a series of arborized vessels containing chylous and lymphatic drainage. Meticulous surgery in the inferior level III through inferior-most level IV lymphatics is required with vascular ligatures on all retained deep structures. Although the TD is located within the left neck, similar chylous and lymphatic structures are located within the right level IV lymphatics.
- Loupe magnification improves visualization and control of these lymph and chylous-containing vessels.

Pitfalls

- TD injury is most common in metastatic thyroid cancer cases with metastases located in the posterior carotid/vertebral junction areas. Blunt dissection of metastatic disease within inferior level IV lymphatics may cause injury to the TD and difficulty in obtaining proximal control of this structure.
- Drain placement overlying the TD may increase the risk for delayed chylous drainage.

Introduction

The TD is an endothelial lined vascular structure transporting chylous material from the left TD into the inferior portion of the internal jugular vein (IJV). Although generally named a single vascular structure, the TD is frequently an arborized series of chylous vessels intermingled with lymphatic drainage structures. The immediate proximity of this deeply penetrating structure to the phrenic nerve (PN) must be appreciated to adequately control this vessel as well as maintain PN function.

The complex and beautiful anatomy of level IV within the left neck must be appreciated. The anatomic variations of location of the subclavian vein (SV), PN, IJV, branches of the TD, common carotid artery, and vertebral system must be appreciated. Generally speaking, the identification of the transverse cervical artery (TCA) and vein is usually the superior-most recognition of the potential distal entry of the TD into the IJV. Nevertheless, this is only an approximation.

Probably most important, although the TD does not in fact exist within the right neck, similar chylous structures can be present and lead to chylous leakage. Meticulous attention in the left as well as right level IV and deep lymphatic structures must be strongly advised.

Practical Tips

1 Meticulous surgical technique is the best method of which I am aware in preventing chylous leakage. In general, I utilize 3.5 loupe magnification for modified neck dissections (MND).

2 As the left MND is performed, which is dissecting the level IV lymphatics (and similarly executed on the right side as well), the sternocleidomastoic muscle is skeletonized along its entire length to the sternal notch. As the ventral surface of the muscle is also skeletonized, the transition to the dissection of the anterior component of the inferior level V lymphatics is also included in most comprehensive dissections of this area.

3 The transverse cervical vessels are usually encountered in level IV and visible through the fascia overlying the deep scalene musculature (except in obese individuals). The anterior surface of the IJV is dissected with careful attention to its lateral border. It is critically important that the dissection be performed on the vein adventitia.

4 For thyroid malignancies, the lymphatics of the medial aspect of level IV, overlying the PN and extending even more medially to the posterior carotid sheath and vertebral vessel, must be included. This is where the TD vessels are placed at greatest risk. To avoid damage or leakage from these vessels, a lateral to medial approach with ligation of all fibrous and fatty/lymphatic structures in the infraclavicular area is undertaken. The SV is dissected to be the inferior aspect of the dissection. From lateral to medial, the clamping and cutting is completed inferiorly along the dissection which has already been accomplished by identifying the lateral border of the IJV. Once the inferior aspect is completed, the posterior medial dissection of the carotid/vertebral area needs to be performed. Again, meticulous clamping and tying is undertaken to at least the level of the TCA takeoff. This clamping and tying is performed even if the surgeon does not visualize ductal structures in the vicinity. The PN, vagus nerve, and carotid and vertebral arteries must be carefully dissected and preserved.

5 Following completion of dissection the area must be dry during Valsalva. No suction drains should directly contact the area of the chylous vessels. To prevent suction drain trauma, a small piece of gelfoam or similar barrier can be utilized in the posterior carotid sheath area.

Cernea CR, Dias FL, Fliss D, Lima RA, Myers EN, Wei WI (eds): Pearls and Pitfalls in Head and Neck Surgery. Basel, Karger, 2008, pp 58–59

2.12 What Are the New Concepts in Functional Modified Neck Dissection?

Bhuvanesh Singh

Laboratory of Epithelial Cancer Biology, Head and Neck Service, Memorial Sloan-Kettering Cancer Center, New York, N.Y., USA

PEARLS

- Neck nodal metastasis from nonnasopharyngeal head and neck squamous cell carcinomas (HNSCC) involves level V of the neck in fewer than 5% of cases. The vast majority (>90%) of incidences of level V metastasis involves the infra-accessory nerve lymphatics (primarily level Vb).
- Adjuvant therapy (either radiation or chemoradiation) is required in most cases with metastasis to the regional lymphatics.
- All nodal basins at risk can be adequately addressed with removal of levels I–IV and Vb lymphatics.

PITFALLS

- Even with anatomic preservation of the accessory nerve, functional deficit can still occur consequently to devascularization and stretch injury during modified neck dissections.
- All nodal levels must be examined intraoperatively prior to proceeding with a functional modified neck dissection (fMND).

Introduction

As our understanding of the patterns of nodal metastasis has emerged, we have progressively modified neck dissections to address the nodal basins at risk for metastasis from HNSCC [1]. As a consequence, radical neck dissections (RND) are rarely performed, physicians opting instead for selective or modified dissections based on the location of the primary tumor and the extent of nodal metastasis [2–6]. While modifications to the classical RND have not improved overall survival, they have reduced sequelae resulting from classical RND including winging of the scapula and resultant chronic pain. Although less morbid than RND, modified neck dissections are not without significant sequelae, uniformly resulting in sensory losses due to sacrifice of cutaneous nerves, as well as functional loss due to devascularization and/or stretch injury consequent to dissection of the accessory nerve.

Understanding the patterns of level V neck metastasis allows us to consider further modifications of neck dissection that do not compromise tumor control while allowing enhanced sensory and motor preservation. Overall, level V metastasis is very rare, occurring in fewer than 5% of all cases of HNSCC. Published data and our own experience suggest that the vast majority of level V metastasis occurs in level Vb, or more precisely, in the infra-accessory lymphatic chain [1, 2]. Accordingly, we now routinely perform a fMND on patients with HNSCC, removing lymphatic-bearing tissue in levels I–IV and Vb, while preserving the accessory nerve without devascularization injury, sternocleidomastoid muscle (SCM), internal jugular vein, as well as the sensory spinal rootlets and the ansa cervicalis. The fMND tumor outcomes are not compromised, while functional outcomes are optimized.

Practical Tips

1. Surgical access is achieved through a single horizontal incision that approximates a skin crease. If level I lymphatics are to be removed, the incision is extended beyond the midline to allow easier access to this region. Flaps are elevated in a routine manner.
2. The fascia investing the SCM is elevated off in a circumferential manner, thereby allowing access to the level V lymphatics in a plane deep to the muscle. The accessory nerve is elevated in the flap. Care must be taken not to injure the accessory nerve as it exits the SCM in level V.
3. All nodal basins are carefully examined to assure the absence of detectable metastasis to level Va.
4. The lymph node-bearing tissue can be dissected in level V starting from the trapezius muscle.
5. As the dissection proceeds anteriorly, the spinal sensory rootlets are identified and preserved, while meticulously removing all node-bearing tissue.
6. The spinal contribution to the ansa is identified and preserved, as is the descending hypoglossi.
7. Node-bearing tissue is removed in levels I–IV as performed in the supraomohyoid neck dissection.

Conclusions

Modifications in neck dissection have allowed improvements in functional outcome without compromising tumor outcomes. Given the patterns of metastasis to level V from HNSCC, fMND can be performed to include nodal basins at highest risk for metastasis (levels I–IV and Vb) resulting in improved functional outcomes without compromising tumor control. The fMND is also applicable to papillary thyroid carcinomas.

2

References

1 Shah JP: Patterns of cervical lymph node metastasis from squamous carcinomas of the upper aerodigestive tract. Am J Surg 1990;160:405–409.

2 Davidson BJ, Kulkarny V, Delacure MD, Shah JP: Posterior triangle metastases of squamous cell carcinoma of the upper aerodigestive tract. Am J Surg 1993;166:395–398.

3 Byers RM: Neck dissection: concepts, controversies, and technique. Semin Surg Oncol 1991;7:9–13.

4 End results of a prospective trial on elective lateral neck dissection vs type III modified radical neck dissection in the management of supraglottic and transglottic carcinomas. Brazilian Head and Neck Cancer Study Group. Head Neck 1999;21:694–702.

5 Ferlito A, Rinaldo A, Silver CE, et al: Elective and therapeutic selective neck dissection. Oral Oncol 2006;42:14–25.

6 Martins EP, Filho JG, Agra IM, et al: Preservation of the internal jugular vein in the radical treatment of node-positive neck – is it safe? Ann Surg Oncol 2007;15:364–370.

Cernea CR, Dias FL, Fliss D, Lima RA, Myers EN, Wei WI (eds): Pearls and Pitfalls in Head and Neck Surgery. Basel, Karger, 2008, pp 60–61

3.1 How to Reconstruct Small Tongue and Floor of Mouth Defects

Remco de Bree, C. René Leemans

Department of Otolaryngology-Head and Neck Surgery, VU University Medical Center (VUmc), Amsterdam, The Netherlands

PEARLS

- In the planning of surgical treatment of tumors in the oral cavity, reconstructive options also have to be considered.
- Reconstructive objectives include adequate wound healing, optimal residual function, and restoration of sensation.
- To restore function, even small defects may need flap reconstruction.

PITFALLS

- Primary closure or secondary healing harbors the risk of tethering the tongue.
- Inadequate reconstruction may have a severe impact on swallowing and speech and thus on quality of life.

Introduction

Resection of early tongue and floor of mouth cancers results in defects of soft tissues, sometimes in combination with jaw bone. Reconstructive objectives include adequate wound healing, optimal residual function, and restoration of sensation. Because it is not feasible to replace excised tissues with tissue that mimics its complex movements and changes in shape, the aim of these reconstructions is to attempt to maximize the patient's possibility for compensatory mechanisms [1]. Postoperative radiotherapy may result in unpredictable fibrosis, hampering tongue movements.

Several techniques have been developed for reconstruction of the oral cavity: secondary intention, primary closure, skin grafts, local transpositions of skin, mucosa or muscle, regional flaps and free vascularized flaps. Primary closure and secondary intention cannot strictly be categorized as reconstructive techniques, but they play a prominent role. Skin grafts are a good alternative for primary closure or granulation when there is a well-vascularized wound bed [2]. In selected cases, uni- or bilateral nasolabial flaps or infrahyoid myocutaneous flap can be used for floor of mouth defects [3, 4].

Regional flaps, e.g., the pectoralis major flap and temporalis muscle flap, still play a role in the reconstruction of medium-sized and larger defects in many institutions. The bulk of the pectoralis major flap frequently leads to modest functional results [5]. Free vascularized fasciocutaneous flaps (e.g., radial forearm flap and the anterolateral thigh flap) may be especially useful in reconstruction of medium-sized and larger oral defects [6].

Practical Tips

The main challenge in reconstruction is to avoid tethering, which may hamper normal speech and swallowing.

❶ Small defects of the lateral mobile tongue are often closed primarily with good functional results. Healing by secondary intention is a good alternative.
❷ A defect of the tip of the tongue is one of the most difficult defects to reconstruct, because often adequate contralateral functioning muscle tissue is lacking. Only if the defect is very small is primary closure or healing by secondary intention possible. In larger defects reconstruction using a fasciocutaneous free flap is often indicated to ensure optimal mobility of the remnant tongue.
❸ If the floor of mouth is involved the main challenge is avoidance of tethering of the tongue to the floor of mouth. Primary closure should therefore be avoided. Secondary healing harbors the risk of adhesion to wound surfaces. If the neck is entered reconstruction using a flap is mandatory.
❹ Split-thickness skin grafts are useful in superficial defects of the floor of mouth. These skin grafts are sutured to the mucosal margins of the defects, leaving the sutures long enough to tie a sponge on the graft for fixation to the underlying wound. This graft may prevent adhesion of the tongue to the floor of mouth. The take of the graft may be improved by using fibrin glue and quilting sutures.
❺ Generally, the fasciocutaneous skin is quadrangular shaped, but in anterior defects involving floor of mouth and tongue, a bilobed design can preserve tongue mobility more efficiently [7].
❻ Free vascularized osteocutaneous flaps, e.g., fibula flap, make it possible to use an adaptable approach for each type of bony defect, allowing dental rehabilitation [8]. An alternative method in lateral mandibular defects involves the use of mandibular reconstruction plates to bridge the defect between two segments with or without soft-tissue free flaps.
❼ A feeding tube is often advised to facilitate wound healing.

Conclusion

In this chapter, an overview of the reconstructions of small tongue and floor of mouth defects is presented and general rules and tips are given. Any given defect, however, has its own options for reconstruction, which warrants individualized treatment planning. Reconstruction with preservation of the tongue mobility is the ultimate goal, although challenging. Postoperative radiotherapy may result in unpredictable fibrosis hampering tongue movements.

References

1 de Bree R, Rinaldo A, Genden EM, Suárez C, Pablo Rodrigo J, Fagan JJ, Kowalski LP, Ferlito A, Leemans CR: Modern reconstruction techniques for oral and pharyngeal defects after tumor resection. Eur Arch Otorhinolaryngol 2008;265:1–9.
2 McGregor IA, McGrouther DA: Skin-graft reconstruction in carcinoma of the tongue. Head Neck Surg 1978;1:47–51.
3 Cohen IK, Edgerton MT: Transbuccal flap for reconstruction of the floor of mouth. Plast Reconstr Surg 1971;48:8–10.
4 Deganello A, Manciocco V, Dolivet G, Leemans CR, Spriano G: Infrahyoid fascio-myocutaneous flap as an alternative to free radial forearm flap in head and neck reconstruction. Head Neck 2007;29:285–291.
5 Ariyan S: The pectoralis major myocutaneous flap. A versatile flap for reconstruction in the head and neck. Plast Reconstr Surg 1979;63:73–81.
6 Soutar DS, Scheker LR, Tanner NS, McGregor IA: The radial forearm flap. A versatile method for intra-oral reconstruction. Br J Plast Surg 1983;36:1–8.
7 Urken ML, Biller HF: A new bilobed design for the sensate radial forearm flap to preserve tongue mobility following significant glossectomy. Arch Otolaryngol Head Neck Surg 1994;120:26–31.
8 Urken ML: Composite free flaps in oromandibular reconstruction. Arch Otolaryngol Head Neck Surg 1991;117:724–732.

Cernea CR, Dias FL, Fliss D, Lima RA, Myers EN, Wei WI (eds): Pearls and Pitfalls in Head and Neck Surgery. Basel, Karger, 2008, pp 62–63

3.2 Reconstruction of Large Tongue and Floor of Mouth Defects

Neal D. Futran

Department of Otolaryngology/Head and Neck Surgery, University of Washington School of Medicine, Seattle, Wash., USA

Pearls

- Maintaining mobility of the reconstructed tongue and floor of mouth optimizes speech and swallowing.
- Proper tissue bulk is critical in the choice of the reconstructive flap.
- Free tissue transfer provides appropriate choices for each particular defect.

Pitfalls

- Nonvascularized tissue reconstruction in defects greater than 1/3 of the tongue and floor of mouth yields poor functional results.
- Improper design of the reconstructive flap can result in impaired tongue mobility and misplaced tissue bulk.

Introduction

The soft tissues of the oral cavity are integral to speech and swallowing. Major goals to reconstruct these tissues include (1) retention of mobility in the native and reconstructed tongue, (2) restoration of lost volume, (3) maintenance of neo-tongue height, (4) separation of the tongue and floor of mouth components, (5) restoration of sensation, and (6) maximization of laryngeal protection from aspiration [1]. Specific to the floor of mouth, goals include (1) minimizing alveolar and floor of mouth soft tissue thickness and mobility, and (2) recreation of gingivolingual and gingivolabial sulci depth [2].

The normally mobile tongue may compensate for loss of some volume. As the loss increases, food bolus manipulation and articulation problems result. While the residual tongue may have unimpaired mobility, the deficient size prevents palatal and dental contact, efficient pharyngeal pressure pump activity, and effective bolus manipulation within the oral cavity. When significant portions of the mobile tongue and floor of mouth have been resected, some residual motion in the tongue base is critical to achieve an optimal functional result. Reconstructive choices should address these issues.

Practical Tips

1. When 1/3 of the tongue is resected, the reconstructive focus is on mobility and sensory restoration. Vascularized and pliable tissue is ideal. Tissue that tends to contract, such as a skin graft, limits tongue mobility.
2. With defects from 1/3 to 1/2 of the mobile tongue, restoration of tongue volume is paramount. Enough bulk must be restored to allow the patient to contact the palate with the neo-tongue.

3 Although a variety of tissues are available, the radial forearm flap has emerged as the workhorse flap [3, 4]. It has a thin, supple skin paddle, available subcutaneous tissue for added volume if needed, long pedicle, large vessels, innervation potential, and easy, two-team harvest.

4 The design of the flap should include a consideration of the geography of the defect. A bilobed design which separates the tongue and floor of mouth components is particularly useful for glossectomy defects which extend onto the floor of mouth [5]. A predictable level of sensory recovery occurs when the antebrachial cutaneous nerve is sutured to the proximal lingual nerve stump [6].

5 The thickness of this flap also varies among different individuals and across different areas of the forearm. It tends to be thinner on the distal aspect of the volar forearm in all patients.

6 The anticipated dental rehabilitation is important in reconstruction planning. A tissue-borne denture will not function if resting upon a thick, mobile soft tissue bed with inadequate gingivolabial and gingivolingual sulci stabilization. Osseointegrated implants may be required for stable dentition.

7 When greater than 1/2 of the tongue and floor of mouth volume is resected, rehabilitation focuses on the provision of a neo-tongue that allows enough anterior volume to permit contact with the palate, and enough posterior volume for the neo-tongue base to provide some protection of the laryngeal inlet and assist in the pharyngeal phase of swallowing. The latissimus dorsi and rectus abdominis flaps offer maximal bulk [7]. More recently the anterolateral thigh has supplanted these choices due to its ease of harvest and minimal donor site morbidity [8].

8 The greatest hindrance to resumption of an oral diet is protection of the larynx from aspiration during the pharyngeal phase of swallowing. Adjunctive measures including laryngeal suspension, epiglottoplasty, cricopharyngeal myotomy, or laryngoplasty may be helpful in providing a safe resumption of an oral diet.

Conclusions

Optimal reconstruction with vascularized tissue creates the best opportunity for functional restoration. The unique attributes of the radial forearm flap make it a primary choice for smaller oral cavity defects with bulkier tissue needed as defect size increases. Flap choice should be dictated by the needs of the patient and those of the site to be reconstructed.

3

References

1 Urken ML, Moscoso JF, Lawson W, Biller HF: A systematic approach to functional reconstruction of the oral cavity following partial and total glossectomy. Arch Otolaryngol Head Neck Surg 1994;120:589–601.
2 Yousif JN, Matloub HS, Sanger JR, Campbell B: Soft-tissue reconstruction of the oral cavity. Clin Plast Surg 1994;21:15–23.
3 Futran ND, Gal TJ, Farwell DG: Radial forearm free flap. Oral Maxillofac Surg Clin North Am 2003;15:577–591.
4 Soutar DS, Scheker LR, Tanner NSB, McGregor IA: The radial forearm flap: a versatile method for intraoral reconstruction. Br J Plast Surg 1983;36:1–8.
5 Uwiera T, Seikaly H, Rieger J, Chau J, Harris JR: Functional outcomes after hemiglossectomy and reconstruction with a bilobed radial forearm free flap. J Otolaryngol 2004;33:356–359.
6 Urken ML: The restoration or preservation of sensation in the oral cavity following ablative surgery. Arch Otolaryngol Head Neck Surg 1995;121:607–612.
7 Lyos AT, Evans GRD, Perez D, Schusterman MA: Tongue reconstruction: outcomes with the rectus abdominus flap. Plast Reconstr Surg 1999;103:442–449.
8 Yu P: Reinnervated anterolateral thigh flap for tongue reconstruction. Head Neck 2004;26:1038–1044.

Cernea CR, Dias FL, Fliss D, Lima RA, Myers EN, Wei WI (eds): Pearls and Pitfalls in Head and Neck Surgery. Basel, Karger, 2008, pp 64–65

3.3 How to Evaluate Surgical Margins in Mandibular Resections

Richard J. Wong

Head and Neck Service, C-1069, Department of Surgery, Memorial Sloan-Kettering Cancer Center, New York, N.Y., USA

PEARLS

- Oral cavity squamous cell carcinoma (OCSCC) may histologically invade the mandible in an erosive (EP) or infiltrative pattern (IP). The IP is associated with higher rates of positive mandibular bone margins (MBM), recurrence, and poor outcome.
- Preoperative radiographic imaging may reflect the histologic pattern of invasion.
- Intraoperative frozen section (IFS) of (1) MBM by curetting cancellous bone and (2) the proximal inferior alveolar nerve (IAN) stump may accurately reflect final margin status.

PITFALLS

- Wide MBMs should be considered for tumors with radiographic IP of invasion, which is associated with a higher positive bone margin rate.
- It may be very difficult to achieve a negative proximal IAN margin if an intraoperative biopsy returns positive on frozen section analysis.

Introduction

The potential of OCSCCs to invade the mandible may lead to significant cosmetic and functional deficits, posing a reconstructive challenge. Mandibular invasion also has a significant adverse prognostic implication, and invasion through cortical bone meets criteria for T4a status by 2003 AJCC staging criteria.

OCSCCs may gain entry into the mandible along the occlusal surface, or through open tooth sockets [1]. In cases of prior radiation therapy, routes of entry into the mandible are more variable as the periosteum loses its barrier function [1]. Once in the medullary space, SCC may progress within the mandible in one of three histologic patterns [2, 3]: EP (sharp interface between tumor and bone and a broad expansive tumor front), IP (nests of tumor cells with finger-like projections along an irregular tumor front) and a mixed pattern.

The IP is correlated with higher tumor grade, positive MBM, higher primary recurrence rates, and poorer disease-free survival [4]. Plain film radiographs of the mandible may exhibit IP or EP correlated with histologic patterns of invasion as well [5].

IFS of bone has been historically problematic due to the inability of the cryotome to section it. The assessment of MBM by conventional means involves a lengthy period of decalcification lasting from 7 to 10 days that allows the specimen to soften for sectioning. Achieving final negative margins is an important goal from an oncologic standpoint. Furthermore, in the era of mandibular reconstruction using microvascular flaps, re-resection for a positive MBM that is identified on final pathology becomes problematic. Therefore the potential application of IFS for mandibular specimens is an issue of great clinical relevance.

Practical Tips

➊ Examine preoperative plain films and CT scans of the mandible to assess for a possible IP or EP of invasion. If irregular, ragged edges are noted around the lesion suggesting an IP, plan a 1.5- to 2-cm resection margin of bone around the lesion. A 1-cm margin is probably adequate for lesions with an EP.

➋ Segmental mandibulectomy is considered appropriate for any OCSCC breaching the outer mandibular cortex and reaching the medullary space, or causing dysfunction or numbness of the IAN.

➌ After performing a segmental mandibulectomy, curette the cancellous bone on each end of the remaining mandible and send the material for IFS. The pathologist should process it in a standard cryotome. This technique is accurate and comparable to final pathology assessment of MBM [6].

➍ Identify the proximal stump of the IAN within the proximal portion of the canal, and excise a segment for IFS. However, in the event that it returns positive for carcinoma, neural invasion by the SCC may track proximally to a variable extent, and re-resection of the proximal mandible does not insure achieving a negative final nerve margin.

➎ Alternate novel methods of assessing MBM have been and will continue to be described: microwave processing with rapid decalcification [7], as well as elastic scattering spectroscopy for optical assessment of formalin-fixed margins [8]. However, their technology may not be readily available, and their application should be considered experimental.

Conclusion

An approach towards planning MBM and performing IFS of them is presented. Curettings of cancellous mandibular bone from the margins and a section of the proximal IAN stump can be readily processed and sectioned using standard IFS techniques to provide important intraoperative information regarding margin status. In the era of microvascular flap reconstruction, such information assisting in securing negative MBM is important in avoiding the need for re-resection in the setting of complex reconstruction.

References

1 McGregor AD, MacDonald DG: Routes of entry of squamous cell carcinoma to the mandible. Head Neck Surg 1988;10:294–301.

2 Carter RL, Tsao SW, Burman JF, Pittam MR, Clifford P, Shaw HJ: Patterns and mechanisms of bone invasion by squamous carcinomas of the head and neck. Am J Surg 1983;146:451–455.

3 Slootweg PJ, Muller H: Mandibular invasion by oral squamous cell carcinoma. J Craniomaxillofac Surg 1989;17:69–74.

4 Wong RJ, Keel SB, Glynn RJ, Varvares MA: Histological pattern of mandibular invasion by oral squamous cell carcinoma. Laryngoscope 2000;110:65–72.

5 Totsuka Y, Usui Y, Tei K, Fukuda H, Shindo M, Iizuka T, Amemiya A: Mandibular involvement by squamous cell carcinoma of the lower alveolus: analysis and comparative study of histologic and radiologic features. Head Neck 1991;13:40–50.

6 Forrest LA, Schuller DE, Lucas JG, Sullivan MJ: Rapid analysis of mandibular margins. Laryngoscope 1995;105:475–477.

7 Weisberger EC, Hilburn M, Johnson B, Nguyen C: Intraoperative microwave processing of bone margins during resection of head and neck cancer. Arch Otolaryngol Head Neck Surg 2001;127:790–793.

8 Jeries W, Swinson B, Johnson KS, Thomas GJ, Hopper C: Assessment of bony resection margins in oral cancer using elastic scattering spectroscopy: a study on archival material. Arch Oral Biol 2005;50:361–366.

Cernea CR, Dias FL, Fliss D, Lima RA, Myers EN, Wei WI (eds): Pearls and Pitfalls in Head and Neck Surgery. Basel, Karger, 2008, pp 66–67

3.4 How to Reconstruct Anterior Mandibular Defects in Patients with Vascular Diseases

Matthew M. Hanasono

Department of Plastic Surgery, The University of Texas M.D. Anderson Cancer Center, Houston, Tex., USA

PEARLS

- Vascularized bone flaps are indicated for anterior mandibular reconstruction whenever possible.
- Preoperative angiography or magnetic resonance angiography should be obtained in patients with an abnormal lower extremity physical exam.

PITFALLS

- Complication rates are high in reconstruction of anterior defects with titanium reconstruction plates, alone or with soft tissue flaps.
- Nonvascularized bone grafts are indicated only for short defects in nonirradiated wounds.
- In patients with very poor vascular status or a limited life expectancy, mandibular reconstruction plates with pedicled pectoralis major flap coverage can be considered.
- In cases of free flap loss, a thorough investigation for the cause of flap loss should be performed. If the cause is correctable, a second free flap is performed.

Introduction

Anterior segmental mandibular defects resulting from oncologic resection are reconstructed with vascularized bone whenever possible. Failure to reconstruct the anterior mandible results in the so-called 'Andy Gump' deformity, a condition that is disfiguring and associated with impaired mastication, pooling of saliva, and loss of oral competence.

In patients who are questionable candidates for reconstruction with microvascular free bone flaps, it is tempting to perform reconstruction with titanium reconstruction plates, alone or in combination with soft tissue flaps such as the pectoralis major flap. However, complication rates with this technique are reported to be between 21 and 87% [1]. Anterior defects are associated with a higher rate of plate extrusion than lateral defects, especially in patients treated with radiation therapy. Mandibular reconstruction that results in early fracture or plate exposure may result in a situation that is more challenging to treat than the initial defect due to difficult dissection of recipient vessels and an inability to restore accurate occlusion [2].

Autogenous bone grafts have also been used for mandibular reconstruction. Nonvascularized bone grafts are used in defects less than 5 cm long. High failure rates are generally seen in anterior defects and longer grafts. Pre- or postoperative radiation therapy is considered a contraindication due to high rates of extrusion, resorption, and infection.

Practical Tips

The fibula osseous/osteocutaneous free flap is usually our first choice for anterior mandibular reconstruction in the cancer patient [3]. Preoperative physical examination of both lower extremities, including palpation for dorsalis pedis and posterior tibial pulses, is performed to determine whether a patient is a candidate for harvest of this flap [4, 5]. When lower extremity circulation is questionable, angiography or magnetic resonance angiography should be performed [6]. In addition to pathologic conditions, it is important to rule out a peronea magna artery, an anatomic variant, present in up to 5% of patients, in which the peroneal artery is the single dominant artery supplying the distal lower extremity [7].

Alternatives to the fibula free flap include the iliac crest and scapula free flaps. However, the iliac crest flap is based on the deep circumflex iliac artery, which may be stenotic in patients with lower extremity vascular disease. In contrast, the scapula flap is based on the circumflex scapular artery, which is typically spared in atherosclerotic vascular disease. The major drawback is that the location of the scapula on the back precludes a two-teamed approach to harvesting the flap and preparation of the recipient site.

The osteocutaneous radial forearm free flap is typically not favored for anterior mandibular reconstruction due to the limited thickness of the bone that may be harvested and the risk for radial bone fracture in the forearm after harvest. However, some authors report good outcomes with this technique [8].

The pectoralis major muscle with rib or sternum can be used for anterior mandibular reconstruction [9]. The lack of reliability, limited ability to shape the soft tissue and bony flap components, and limited reach make this flap a secondary option after free bone flaps. These flaps may be considered in patients with very poor vascular status. However, distal flow to the bony component of these flaps is likely to be compromised in such patients resulting in an increased risk for flap failure.

Conclusion

For anterior mandibular reconstruction, the fibula free flap is our method of choice. If there is stenosis or hypoplasia of the vessels supplying the foot, alternative reconstructive methods must be considered. Reconstruction of the anterior mandible is challenging but important in maintaining quality of life even in patients with advanced malignancies.

References

1 Mariani PB, Kowalski LP, Magrin J: Reconstruction of large defects postmandibulectomy for oral cancer using plates and myocutaneous flaps: a long-term follow-up. Int J Oral Maxillofac Surg 2006;35:427–432.

2 Wei FC, Celik N, Yang WG, Chen IH, Chang YM, Chen H: Complications after reconstruction by plate and soft tissue free flap in composite mandibular defects and secondary salvage reconstruction with osseocutaneous flap. Plast Reconstr Surg 2003; 112:37–42.

3 Cordeiro PG, Disa JJ, Hidalgo DA, Hu Q: Reconstruction of the mandible with osseous free flaps: a 10 year experience with 150 consecutive patients. Plast Reconstr Surg 1999;104:1314–1320.

4 Disa JJ, Cordeiro PG: The current role of preoperative arteriography in free fibula flaps. Plast Reconstr Surg 1998;102:1083–1088.

5 Lutz B, Wei FC, Ng SH, Chen IH, Chen SHT: Routine donor leg angiography before vascularized free fibula transplantation is not necessary: a prospective study in 120 clinical cases. Plast Reconstr Surg 1999;103:121–127.

6 Lorenz RR, Esclamado R: Preoperative magnetic resonance angiography in fibular-free flap reconstruction of head and neck defects. Head Neck 2001;23:844–850.

7 Kim D, Orron DE, Skillman JJ: Surgical significance of popliteal artery variants: a unified angiographic classification. Ann Surg 1989;210:776–781.

8 Thoma A, Levis C, Young JEM: Oromandibular reconstruction after cancer resection. Clin Plast Surg 2005;32:361–375.

9 Robertson GA: The role of sternum in osteomyocutaneous reconstruction of major mandibular defects. Am J Surg 1986; 152:367–370.

Cernea CR, Dias FL, Fliss D, Lima RA, Myers EN, Wei WI (eds): Pearls and Pitfalls in Head and Neck Surgery. Basel, Karger, 2008, pp 68–69

3.5 Adequate Surgical Margins in Resections of Carcinomas of the Tongue

Jacob Kligerman

Instituto Nacional de Câncer, Rio de Janeiro, Brazil

PEARLS

- 5 mm is the shortest ex vivo surgical margin recommended in resections for tongue carcinomas.
- Ideally, the mucosal margins should be free of preinvasive atypical epithelial alterations.
- Intraoperative frozen section examination is conventionally the technique of choice to determine the adequacy of the margins.
- Tumors with infiltrative edge require careful measurement of the margins from the longest tumoral projection.

PITFALLS

- Stretching of the tongue while demarcating the resection lines may lead to erroneous evaluation of the margin's size.
- Inclination of the surgical blades as you cut deep into the muscle layer to get a cuneiform fragment usually diminishes the amount of tumor-free tissue between the edge of the tumor and the resection line below the mucosa.
- The deep surgical margin is the most difficult to assess at the time of resection, being usually much shorter than expected.

Introduction

The adequacy of surgical resection of a primary carcinoma of the tongue is conventionally determined intraoperatively by frozen section examination using histopathologic criteria. A 5-mm tumor-free surgical margin is the usual recommendation, although there has been some discussion in the literature on whether such a margin is or is not effective in the local control of the disease [1–6]. The well-documented fact that 10–30% of the cases with histopathologically free margins do recur is the fuel that keeps this discussion alive. In recent years, molecular biology studies have been performed to explain this occurrence [5, 7, 8]. The role of atypical preinvasive epithelial lesions in the margins has also been investigated by some authors [3, 9]. Since molecular technology is not available for intraoperative evaluation in a reasonable time frame [7, 10] and it has not yet been validated in prospective studies with a significant number of cases followed for at least 5 years, we still adhere to the 5-mm margin as a safe parameter to avoid recurrences. Nonetheless, we do believe that this molecular approach will make a great contribution to the understanding of tumor behavior and to the treatment as well, as we are sure that its use in everyday practice is quite close to becoming reality.

Practical Tips

1. Always draw the line of resection measuring between 7 and 10 mm tissue-free using visual evaluation of the mucosa and palpation of deeper tissues around the lesion.
2. If you stretch the tongue too much to draw your resection line, you may have underestimated the margins.

❸ Remember that there will be a natural retraction of the tissues due to the extensive muscular component, which may reach between 25 and 30% less than the in vivo evaluation.
❹ The recommended 5-mm margin should be measured ex vivo.
❺ The deeper you go, the more difficult it gets to calculate the amount of tumor-free tissue.
❻ Never forget to mark orientation points in the specimen before sending it to the pathologist, so that he or she can determine exactly where you should extend your incision.
❼ It is quite useful to have the pathologist in the operating room while you are removing the tumor despite the fact that demarcation of orientation points in the specimen is still necessary.
❽ Before taking the decision of extending your resection, carefully evaluate the defect you are about to impose on your patient and think of alternative therapies that could be more effective in situations such as very large tumors, tumors at the base of the tongue, or lesions of the lingual nerve.

References

1 Spiro RH, Guillamondegui O Jr, Paulino AF, Huvos AG: Pattern of invasion and margin assessment in patients with oral tongue cancer. Head Neck 1999;21:408–413.
2 Weijers M, Snow GB, van der Wal JE, van de Waal I: The status of the deep surgical margins in tongue and floor of the mouth squamous cell carcinoma and risk of local recurrence: an analysis of 68 patients. Int J Oral Maxillofac Surg 2004;33:146–149.
3 Weijers M, Snow GB, Bezemer PD, van der Wal JE, van de Waal I: The clinical relevance of epithelial dysplasia in surgical margins of tongue and floor of mouth squamous cell carcinoma: an analysis of 37 patients. J Oral Pathol Med 2002;31:11–15.
4 Brandwein-Gensler M, Teixeira MS, Lewis CM, Lee B, Rolnitzky L, Hille JJ, Genden E, Urken ML, Wang BY: Oral squamous cell carcinoma: histologic risk assessment, but not margin status, is strongly predictive of local disease-free and overall survival. Am J Surg Pathol 2005;29:167–178.
5 Upile T, Fisher C, Jerjes W, El Maayatah M, Singh S, Sudhoff H, Searle A, Archer D, Michaels L, Hopper C, Rhys-Evans P, Wright HD: Recent technological developments: in situ histopathological interrogation of surgical tissues and resection margins. Head Face Med 2007;1:3–13.
6 Bradley PJ, MacLennan K, Brakenhoff RH, Leemans CR: Status of primary tumor surgical margins in squamous head and neck cancer: prognostic implications. Curr Opin Otolaryngol Head Neck Surg 2007;15:74–81.
7 Rodrigo JP, Ferlito A, Suarez C, Shaha AR, Silver CE, Devaney KO, Bradley PJ, Bocker JM, McLaren KM, Grénman R, Rinaldo A: New molecular methods in head and neck cancer. Head Neck 2005;21:995–1003.
8 Braakhuis BJM, Tabor MP, Kummer JA, Leemans CR, Brakenhoff RH: A genetic explanation of Slaughter's concept of field cancerization. Cancer Res 2003;63:1727–1730.
9 van Es RJ, van Nieuw AN, Egyedi P: Resection margin as a predictor of recurrence at the primary site for T1 and T2 oral cancers. Evaluation of histopathologic variables. Arch Otolaryngol Head Neck Surg 1996;122:521–525.
10 Goldenberg G, Harden S, Masayesva BG, Ha P, Benoit N, Westr WH, Koch WM, Sidransky D, Califano JA: Intraoperative molecular margin analysis in head and neck cancer. Arch Otolaryngol Head Neck Surg 2004;130:39–44.

Cernea CR, Dias FL, Fliss D, Lima RA, Myers EN, Wei WI (eds): Pearls and Pitfalls in Head and Neck Surgery. Basel, Karger, 2008, pp 70–71

3.6 Practical Tips to Manage Mandibular Osteoradionecrosis

Sheng-Po Hao

Chang Gung Memorial Hospital, Chang Gung University, Taoyuan, Taiwan

PEARLS

- Prevention is the key.
- Avoid elective oral surgical procedures within an irradiated field; preoperative hyperbaric oxygen therapy (HBO) may be considered.
- Early recognition and prompt management are mandatory.
- Surgery is the mainstay treatment for osteoradionecrosis (ORN). It is not possible that the nonvital sequestrum becomes vital after HBO.

PITFALLS

- Keep in mind the difficulties to differentiate recurrent cancer from ORN.
- Occasionally, the correct diagnosis is reached only after radical surgery.

Introduction

Irradiation may cause the 3 'H' status – hypoxia, hypovascularity, hypocellularity – and impair normal collagen synthesis and cell production, which leads to tissue breakdown and a chronic nonhealing wound. ORN has been defined as exposed irradiated bone that fails to heal over a period of 3 months [1].

Practical Tips

ORN can have iatrogenic causes (81%) such as surgical trauma, tooth extraction, and poor oral hygiene, whereas only 19% are spontaneous [2].

Mandibular ORN commonly presents as an exposed necrotic mandible or a discharged fistula right under the area of disease with foul odor or severe pain [3].

Recurrent or persistent cancer may present as a chronic unhealed wound and exposed necrotic bone, which may mimic ORN. Currently, there is no useful clinical means to definitely differentiate mandibular ORN from recurrent cancer. As much as 21% of initial ORN diagnoses are corrected to recurrent cancer after several attempts of debridement or radical surgery [2].

The treatment of ORN begins with prevention. Patients with exposed bone and a lack of soft tissue coverage who undergo irradiation will invariably develop ORN. During surgery, undue soft tissue tension over the bone should be avoided. This kind of poor wound healing will directly expose the irradiated bone to contamination in the oral cavity or external environment. Mandibular ORN should be managed in a systemic and stepwise approach [2]. The first step is to diagnose and delineate the extent of the disease. We prefer magnetic resonance imaging because of its superb ability to define bone marrow and surrounding soft tissue changes of ORN.

Conservative management is indicated in mild ORN cases with repeated limited sequestrectomy and HBO. It is crucial to send the sequestrum for pathology proof. ORN should not be deemed as a disease of the bone only: the surrounding soft tissue is part of the disease process too.

The management of overlying soft tissue should be carried out carefully. Only diseased mucosa and granuloma are removed. Every effort should be made to retain its vascularity, and further tears of or injury to the normal mucosa should be avoided. Primary closure of the mucosal defect or closure with a rotational flap harvested from a neighboring area within the irradiated field is not recommended. HBO can elevate the oxygen tension within the tissue and may stimulate collagen synthesis and fibroblastic proliferation, thus facilitating the process of wound healing. HBO can minimize the extent of surgery and should be an adjunct to an aggressive management of ORN. Attempts to use HBO alone were generally unsuccessful. HBO cannot revitalize necrotic bone. The dead sequestra need to be surgically removed. Surgery is still the mainstay treatment for ORN.

We recommend radical sequestrectomy and vascularized flap reconstruction in cases of severe, extensive ORN of the mandible, such as coexistent fracture, multiple discharging fistula, and a large area of exposed bone [4]. The key to successful treatment in these extensive ORN cases is adequate and radical sequestrectomy with vascularized flap reconstruction. Removal of the full thickness of the bone and the full extent of the diseased surrounding soft tissue is usually necessary.

Conclusion

ORN of the mandible is a serious and devastating complication of radiation therapy. Prevention is the key. Once developed, early recognition and prompt management are mandatory. Always keep in mind the possibility of recurrent cancer. Mandibular ORN should be managed with a systemic and stepwise approach with conservative sequestrectomy coupled with HBO and may be followed by radical sequestrectomy and distant flap reconstruction. Radical sequestrectomy is indicated in cases of severe or extensive mandibular ORN and the tissue should be reconstructed with healthy vascularized tissue with its pedicle outside the radiation field.

References

1 Mark RE: Osteoradionecrosis: a new concept of its pathophysiology. J Oral Maxillofac Surg 1983;41:283–288.
2 Hao SP, Chen HC, Wei FC, et al: Systematic management of osteoradionecrosis in the head and neck. Laryngoscope 1999;109:1324–1327.
3 Hao SP, Tsang NM, Chang KP, Chen CK, Chao WC: Osteoradionecrosis of external auditory canal in nasopharyngeal carcinoma. Chang Gung Med J 2007;30:116–121.
4 Santamaria E, Wei FC, Chen HC: Fibula osteoseptocutaneous flap for reconstruction of osteoradionecrosis of the mandible. Plast Reconstr Surg 1998;101:921–929.

Cernea CR, Dias FL, Fliss D, Lima RA, Myers EN, Wei WI (eds): Pearls and Pitfalls in Head and Neck Surgery. Basel, Karger, 2008, pp 72–73

4.1 Practical Tips for Laser Resection of Laryngeal Cancer

F. Christopher Holsinger[a], N. Scott Howard[a], Andrew McWhorter[b]

[a] Department of Head and Neck Surgery, The University of Texas M.D. Anderson Cancer Center, Houston, Tex., and
[b] LSU Voice Center, Department of Otolaryngology – Head and Neck Surgery, Louisiana State University Health Sciences Center, Our Lady of the Lake Hospital, Baton Rouge, La., USA

PEARLS

- Laryngeal mobility is in part determined by muscle infiltration. Arytenoid fixation is predictive of deep invasion of the paraglottic space and is a contraindication for conservation surgery.
- Videostroboscopy and speech therapy assessment of rehabilitative potential are essential. Early speech therapy to prevent arytenoid ankylosis and repeat videostroboscopy to detect subtle hyperplasia, scar tissue, or vocal fold changes that may indicate recurrence should be routinely performed.
- Maintaining one functional cricoarytenoid complex and sensory innervation reduces the risk of postoperative aspiration.

PITFALLS

- Poor exposure is the most common cause of failure.
- Previously irradiated tissues will have edema and submucosal fibrosis and there will be difficulty in differentiating tumor from healthy tissue.
- At the anterior commissure, there is no conus elasticus or perichondrium, which provides a diminished natural barrier to spread. In addition, ossified cartilage has reduced resistance to tumor spread.

Introduction

Strong and Jako [1] first introduced the carbon dioxide laser to the head and neck surgeon in 1972, when they declared that the transoral laser microsurgery was 'ready for clinical trial'. Steiner and Ambrosch [2] have successfully adapted the fundamental aspects of open procedures to the endoscope with excellent results. The carbon dioxide laser is used because water absorbs this frequency of light (10,600 nm), minimizing collateral damage to nearby structures.

Conservation surgery of laryngeal cancer has excellent 5-year local control rates and good functional outcomes when compared with total laryngectomy, chemoradiation or radiation alone. Compared to open techniques, laser surgical procedures are less invasive, allow for a more rapid return to voice use, and reduce swallowing dysfunction.

Margins vary with the primary site of the tumor. For the glottic larynx, 1–3 mm may be adequate. Larger margins of 5–10 mm are more appropriate in the supraglottis. For patients undergoing TLM after radiation failure, even larger margins of resection should be taken.

Close collaboration intraoperatively with the pathologist is of paramount concern, in order to maintain proper orientation of the specimens. Reconstruction is not typically performed and healing occurs by secondary intention. Granulation tissue forms, followed by contraction and remucosalization with the contracture process helping to eliminate dead space [3].

Practical Tips

❶ Staging operative endoscopy should be performed to determine extent of disease prior to consideration of laser surgery. 0, 30 and 70° endoscopy provides the gold standard assessment of disease extent.

❷ CT or MRI of larynx should be performed to evaluate the extent of primary tumor, any evidence of spread to the preepiglottic or paraglottic space or cartilage invasion.

❸ Consider a modified barium study/FEES or esophagoscopy if obstructive symptoms exist or if there is interarytenoid or posterior involvement.

❹ Intraoperatively, the microscope allows for a better view of the surgical field and assessment of dysplastic or neoplastic changes. Intraoperative judgment afforded by this technique enables safe but close margins, while preserving as much normal tissue as possible to optimize functional outcome.

❺ Infusion of saline solution into Reinke's space may allow for improved differentiation of Tis and early invasive disease.

❻ The use of a 'pulsed', rather than a continuous, mode provides better tissue handling properties under microscopic visualization. Short pulses of laser irradiation leave a smaller thermal damage zone, which may lead to faster healing. Pulsed laser settings decrease carbonization and improve the ability of the surgeon to discern tumor from normal mucosa during microsurgery [4].

❼ Anterior commissure lesions may extend down the thyroid cartilage and extend anteriorly through the cricothyroid membrane [5]. An infrapetiolar release and exposure of the superior inner thyroid perichondrium of the thyroid cartilage may be required for proper exposure of this difficult area.

❽ Assessment of tumor extent following radiation therapy is difficult to evaluate due to fibrosis and edema causing TVC motion abnormalities, changes in imaging characteristics, and difficulty distinguishing between radionecrosis and tumor recurrence.

❾ For optimal functional and oncologic outcomes in laryngeal cancer, a multidisciplinary team approach is recommended: speech language pathology, radiation therapy, medical oncology, and dental oncology.

Recovery and Follow-Up

Oral diet may generally be resumed on the day after surgery. Wound healing is usually complete after 3–4 weeks. Video strobe assessment is scheduled at 4–6 weeks following surgery. Second-look procedures with excision of scar tissue to evaluate for residual carcinoma rests are performed at 3–6 weeks.

References

1. Strong MS, Jako GJ: Laser surgery in the larynx. Early clinical experience with continuous CO2 laser. Ann Otol Rhinol Laryngol 1972;81:791–798.
2. Steiner W, Ambrosch P: Endoscopic Laser Surgery of the Upper Aerodigestive Tract – with Special Emphasis on Cancer Surgery. New York, Thieme, 2000.
3. McWhorter AJ, Hoffman HT: Transoral laser microsurgery for laryngeal malignancies. Curr Probl Cancer 2005;29:180–189.
4. Niemz MH: Laser-Tissue Interactions: Fundamentals and Applications (Biological and Medical Physics, Biomedical Engineering). New York, Springer, 2000.
5. Kirchner J: Atlas on the Surgical Anatomy of Laryngeal Cancer. San Diego, Singular Publishing, 1998.

Cernea CR, Dias FL, Fliss D, Lima RA, Myers EN, Wei WI (eds): Pearls and Pitfalls in Head and Neck Surgery. Basel, Karger, 2008, pp 74–75

4.2 Practical Suggestions for Phonomicrosurgical Treatment of Benign Vocal Fold Lesions

Steven M. Zeitels, Gerardo Lopez Guerra

Harvard Medical School, Center for Laryngeal Surgery and Voice Rehabilitation, Massachusetts General Hospital, Boston, Mass., USA

PEARLS

- The superficial lamina propria (SLP) is the primary structural layer responsible for mucosal wave vibration, not the epithelium overlying it.
- Most microlaryngoscopic procedures are facilitated by a subepithelial infusion using saline with epinephrine, which helps to preserve the critically important SLP.
- The 532-nm KTP laser is a key state-of-the-art instrument for treating phonatory mucosa (PM) lesions associated with aberrant microcirculation.

PITFALLS

- Most unresolved hoarseness results from diminished pliability of the PM (not from aerodynamic glottal valvular incompetence), and this is the most common disabling complication from phonomicrosurgery of benign vocal fold lesions.
- Disturbing the vocal ligament (VL) is not the etiology of postoperative PM scarring and stiffness; it is caused by injudicious disturbance of the subepithelial SLP.

Introduction

Benign vocal fold lesions primarily occur within the PM [1–3], which is comprised of the SLP and the overlying epithelium. We refer to PM as the musculomembranous region rather than the membranous vocal fold since membrane is overlying all structures of the larynx. The epithelium provides negligible vibratory characteristics and assumes the viscoelastic properties of whatever aerodigestive tract tissue it encapsulates. When treating PM lesions, it is of paramount importance to minimize trauma to uninvolved epithelium and underlying SLP [1–3]. Most benign lesions are associated with phonotrauma and vocal overuse and arise within the SLP (polyps, nodules, cysts, ectasias varices). Papillomatosis [2, 4] and dysplasia [2, 4, 5] are the key noncancerous epithelial lesions.

Practical Tips

❶ It is important to place the largest laryngoscope speculum [2, 6] that can fit from the oral cavity to the glottis, preferably a triangular shape.
❷ Use a true suspension gallows [2, 5, 7, 8] rather than a fulcrum laryngoscope holder, external counterpressure with tape to enhance exposure [7].
❸ Whenever possible, the VL should not be exposed, since that would mean that the SLP has been unfavorably traumatized.
❹ Polyps, nodules, and cysts [2, 3, 9] are optimally resected by means of a subepithelial resection technique. Amputating the lesion with the overlying epithelium leaving epithelial deficits results in increased mucosal scarring.

⑤ Subsequent to the subepithelial infusion [2, 3, 5], an epithelial cordotomy should be done at the cephalad edge of the polyp, nodule, or cyst. The interface of the deep aspect of the benign lesion from the underlying normal SLP must be identified, so that it can be dissected meticulously [2, 3].

⑥ Anterior-commissure synechia will not occur unless there is bilateral loss of epithelium on the medial surface of the anterior commissure [2].

⑦ Positioning epithelial incisions laterally and away from medial lesions to avoid an incision near the medial edge is a flawed philosophy, since postoperative mucosal pliability is primarily based on not disturbing normal SLP.

⑧ When treating benign SLP lesions with the 532-nm KTP laser, it should be done with a 0.3- to 0.4-mm fiber, 450–525 mJ, a 15-ms pulse width and a 1- to 3-mm fiber-to-tissue distance [4].

⑨ The pulsed KTP laser employs very precise selective photoangiolysis, which provides the first opportunity for involution of ectasias and varices without substantially disturbing the overlying epithelium and the extravascular SLP [2, 9].

⑩ Reinke's edema [2] is comprised of excessive SLP and can be resected bilaterally as long as the incisions are confined to the superior surface. The goal of phonomicrosurgery of Reinke's edema is to diminish the mass and volume of the increased mass and volume of SLP, yet leaving the patient with mildly large vocal folds. If the VL is exposed, especially on the medial surface, severe and permanent strained hoarseness can result. This is a worse liability than the low-pitched comfortable preoperative voice.

⑪ The key objective in the treatment of epithelial diseases such as glottal papillomatosis [2, 4, 5] or dysplasia is to resect the pathological epithelium while minimally disturbing the underlying SLP or by involuting the subepithelial microcirculation with an angiolytic (i.e. 532-nm pulsed KTP) laser.

⑫ Most recalcitrant arytenoid granulomas are best treated by means of botulinum toxin injections in the lateral paraglottic musculature along with antireflux management and voice therapy. Surgical resection is minimally helpful unless there is substantial airway obstruction or the granuloma arises from a narrow pedicle.

⑬ In the not-so-distant future, SLP substitutes will be available that will restore lost mucosal pliability, which will revolutionize phonomicrosurgery for both benign and malignant lesions [1, 10].

References

1 Zeitels SM, Healy GB: Laryngology and phonosurgery. N Engl J Med 2003;349:882–892.

2 Zeitels SM: Atlas of Phonomicrosurgery and Other Endolaryngeal Procedures for Benign and Malignant Disease. San Diego, Singular, 2001.

3 Zeitels SM, Hillman RE, Desloge RB, Mauri M, Doyle PB: Phonomicrosurgery in singers and performing artists: treatment outcomes, management theories, and future directions. Ann Otol Rhinol Laryngol 2002;111(suppl 190):21–40.

4 Zeitels SM, Akst LM, Burns JA, Hillman RE, Broadhurst MS, Anderson RR: Office-based 532-nm pulsed KTP laser treatment of glottal papillomatosis and dysplasia. Ann Otol Rhinol Laryngol 2006;115:679–685.

5 Zeitels SM: Premalignant epithelium and microinvasive cancer of the vocal fold: the evolution of phonomicrosurgical management. Laryngoscope 1995;105(suppl 67):1–51.

6 Zeitels SM: A universal modular glottiscope system: the evolution of a century of design and technique for direct laryngoscopy. Ann Otol Rhinol Laryngol 1999;108(suppl 179):1–24.

7 Zeitels SM, Vaughan CW: 'External counter-pressure' and 'internal distension' for optimal laryngoscopic exposure of the anterior glottal commissure. Ann Otol Rhinol Laryngol 1994;103: 669–675.

8 Zeitels SM, Burns JA, Dailey SH: Suspension laryngoscopy revisited. Ann Otol Rhinol Laryngol 2004;113:16–22.

9 Zeitels SM, Akst LM, Burns JA, Hillman RE, Broadhurst MS, Anderson RR: Pulsed angiolytic laser treatment of ectasias and varices in singers. Ann Otol Rhinol Laryngol 2006;115:571–580.

10 Zeitels SM, Blitzer A, Hillman RE, Anderson RR: Foresight in laryngology and laryngeal surgery: a 2020 vision. Ann Otol Rhinol Laryngol 2007;116(suppl 198):1–16.

This work was generously supported by the Eugene B. Casey Foundation and the Institute of Laryngology and Voice Restoration.

Cernea CR, Dias FL, Fliss D, Lima RA, Myers EN, Wei WI (eds): Pearls and Pitfalls in Head and Neck Surgery. Basel, Karger, 2008, pp 76–77

4.3 Glottic Reconstruction after Partial Vertical Laryngectomy

Onivaldo Cervantes, Márcio Abrahão

Otorhinolaryngology and Head and Neck Department of Federal University of São Paulo – Escola Paulista de Medicina, São Paulo, Brazil

PEARLS

- Laryngeal reconstruction after partial vertical laryngectomy (PVL) is crucial for a good quality of voice.
- Reconstruction avoids chondritis and formation of granulomas.
- Initiate surgical incision with a reconstruction plan in mind.

PITFALLS

- Laryngoscopic evaluation may underestimate the extent of the tumor.
- Computed tomography may overestimate the extent of the tumor.
- The surgeon should describe the planned procedure to the patient, making clear that a total laryngectomy may be required. The final decision, however, can be made only at the time of surgery under direct visualization and with frozen-section pathologic confirmation.
- If the patient is not willing to give consent under these circumstances, limited resection should be avoided.

Introduction

The treatment of early glottic tumors is controversial: surgery or radiotherapy. The treatment plan depends on preoperative evaluation of the larynx, histology, staging (UICC, 2002), the surgical team's experience, the patient's overall clinical condition, informed consent, patient education and postoperative smoking cessation. Treatment goals are: total resection of the tumor with preservation of laryngeal physiology and function as much as possible, maintaining optimum postoperative voice quality and low rates of morbidity.

In general, partial laryngectomies enable patients to recover faster, both from the point of view of respiratory and phonatory functions. In addition, they offer rewarding outcome results. A laryngoscopic evaluation, meticulous examination, and if necessary computed tomography are needed to assess glottic tumors. Surgical considerations must always be planned in conjunction with reconstructive options. PVLs are indicated mainly for T1, T2, and perhaps some carefully selected T3 tumors. The main goal is larynx preservation and function.

Frontolateral laryngectomy is indicated for glottic tumors involving the anterior commissure, or tumors that compromise both vocal folds (with preserved mobility). Such an approach can be extended posteriorly when arytenoid cartilage involvement is confirmed.

Surgical margin assessment is fundamental to achieve complete tumor resection.

Practical Tips

❶ Some important aspects of partial laryngectomies should be highlighted: survival rates vary according to the tumor site; glottic cancer is highly curable; the staging of the disease and not the actual treatment is critical; the first treatment and clinical condition are important; the first treatment anticipates problems later; combination therapy is warranted in specific situations; patient selection is key; reconstruction considerations are paramount after resection; consistent and methodical follow-up is critical for rehabilitation and final outcome of surgery. However, the patient's life is more important than the larynx.

❷ Avoid communication between the laryngectomy incision and the tracheotomy incision. This will prevent subcutaneous emphysema and collection of secretions, potentially preventing infection. Tracheotomy performed on the third ring precludes communication between the incisions.

❸ Start thinking about the incision at the same time you review your laryngeal reconstructive options, which is critical for the best outcomes. Surgical planning is crucial, bearing in mind the different techniques available.

❹ The thyroid cartilage should be opened bearing in mind the type of resection planned. Usually, the keel must be resected. Careful opening of the cartilage is completed with parallel incisions, and opening of the glottis by hand against the side of the lesion. This allows tumor assessment and dissection of the internal perichondrium, and further resection with ample margins.

❺ An excellent option for glottal reconstruction is the sternohyoid muscle, which is dissected early on when performing a partial laryngectomy. Also, preserve most of the perichondrium of the thyroid cartilage, which must be sutured to the muscle with absorbable stitches. Other options for glottic reconstruction are: (1) lowering of the ipsilateral vestibular mucosal fold; (2) sternohyoid muscle flap with external perichondrium, and (3) lowering of the epiglottis with a myocutaneous platysma flap.

❻ Reconstruction with local mucosa will lead to an improved voice quality, offering adequate postoperative vibration.

❼ Resection of an arytenoid often leads to poorer voice quality, predisposing to dysphagia with aspiration, often leading to pulmonary infection.

Conclusions

PVL is a straightforward technically simple procedure that allows rapid recovery and voice rehabilitation. It should always include skillful reconstruction of the glottis. Protective tracheotomy with early withdrawal should be performed to preserve glottic reconstruction.

Cernea CR, Dias FL, Fliss D, Lima RA, Myers EN, Wei WI (eds): Pearls and Pitfalls in Head and Neck Surgery. Basel, Karger, 2008, pp 78–79

4.4 Suprahyoid Pharyngotomy

Eugene N. Myers, Robert L. Ferris

Department of Otolaryngology, University of Pittsburgh, School of Medicine, Pittsburgh, Pa., USA

PEARLS

- Proper patient selection and accurate tumor staging will result in adequate tumor resection together with excellent cosmesis and good quality of life.
- There is no substitute for meticulous surgical technique.
- Identification, careful dissection and retraction of the neurovascular bundle will result in good function of the tongue.

PITFALLS

- Understaging the tumor may result in inadequate tumor excision.
- Subjecting a patient with marginal motivation and significant comorbidities to a total glossectomy (TG), leaving the larynx in place, will result in recurrent pneumonia and possible death.
- Failure to isolate and protect the hypoglossal nerves and lingual arteries may result in necrosis or crippling of the tongue.

Introduction

The suprahyoid pharyngotomy (SP), introduced in the 19th century by Jeremitsch [1], provides excellent exposure for excision of small benign and malignant tumors arising in the base of the tongue (BOT), posterior pharyngeal wall and epiglottis. Little, if any, disturbance in function and excellent cosmetic results are the other important features. In 1974, Barbosa [2] of Brazil included the classic description of SP in his textbook. The use of other surgical techniques such as segmental mandibulectomy, mandibulotomy and lateral pharyngotomy may interfere with deglutition, often resulting in disabling aspiration [3].

We have used the SP in the management of T1–2 squamous cell carcinoma of the BOT for many years resulting in an excellent cure rate and good functional and cosmetic results [4]. We have also employed it in the management of benign and other malignant tumors of the BOT, lingual thyroid, posterior pharyngeal wall, and epiglottis. This approach may be used in performing a TG with preservation of the larynx [5].

Practical Tips

1. Accurate preoperative staging is essential to determine whether SP is the best approach since this technique is contraindicated for tumors of the BOT approaching the circumvallate papilla.
2. Physical examination, especially palpation of the tongue for tumor extent, remains the key to decision making.
3. MRI is the most sensitive imaging modality, providing excellent soft tissue definition for preoperative planning.
4. Direct laryngoscopy with direct visualization of the tumor, especially for early lesions of the epiglottis and posterior pharyngeal wall, is essential for preoperative planning.

5 Evaluation of the patient's performance status, especially pulmonary function, is critical since some aspiration in the early postoperative period is expected.
6 A temporary tracheostomy is important to maintain the airway in the perioperative setting and to allow adequate tracheobronchial toilet.
7 An incision in the most superior skin fold in the neck provides adequate exposure for excision of oropharyngeal lesions and good cosmesis.
8 A superiorly based apron flap is used to provide adequate exposure for the SP and to incorporate unilateral or bilateral neck dissections when appropriate.
9 The hypoglossal nerves and lingual arteries must be identified and dissected distally until they enter the tongue. This technique of mobilization and gentle retraction helps to avoid injury to these structures during the pharyngotomy. A Penrose drain may be looped around this neurovascular bundle to help with gentle retraction during excision of the BOT.
10 An incision across the mucosa of the vallecula provides entry into the pharynx. A tenaculum is then placed on the posterior aspect of the tongue drawing this structure into the wound. The lesion is then excised and the defect closed primarily.
11 Pharyngeal defects may be left to heal by second intention or by resurfacing with a split thickness skin graft or dermal graft. The disadvantage of using a skin graft is that the gauze bolus stabilizing the graft must be removed 5–7 days later, requiring another general anesthesia.
12 Intraoperative frozen section control is fundamental to assure complete tumor excision.
13 TG may be performed by undermining the mucoperiosteum of the lingual surface of the mandible and incising the mucosa of the floor of the mouth, thereby delivering the entire tongue and floor of the mouth.
14 A nasogastric tube should be inserted prior to closing the wound.

Conclusion

The SP in carefully selected patients is a valuable technique in small benign or malignant lesions of the BOT, posterior pharyngeal wall or epiglottis. Achieving good results with this procedure requires strict adherence to details in preoperative evaluation and in surgical technique. Underestimating the extent of the tumor or the patient's functional status may lead to inadequate tumor resection or difficult to manage complications.

4

References

1 Blassingame CD: The suprahyoid approach to surgical lesions at the base of tongue. Ann Otol Rhinol Laryngol 1952;61:483–489.
2 Barbosa JF: Surgical Treatment of Head and Neck Tumors. New York, Grune & Stratton, 1974.
3 Johnson JT: Mandibulotomy and oral cavity resection; in Myers EN (ed): Operative Otolaryngology: Head and Neck Surgery. Philadelphia, Saunders, 1997, pp 304–308.
4 Ferris RL, Myers EN: Suprahyoid pharyngotomy. Oper Tech Otolaryngol 2003;16:49–54.
5 Myers EN: Suprahyoid pharyngotomy; in Myers EN (ed): Operative Otolaryngology: Head and Neck Surgery, ed 1. Philadelphia, Saunders, 1997, p 242.

Cernea CR, Dias FL, Fliss D, Lima RA, Myers EN, Wei WI (eds): Pearls and Pitfalls in Head and Neck Surgery. Basel, Karger, 2008, pp 80–81

4.5 Intraoperative Maneuvers to Improve Functional Result after Supraglottic Laryngectomy

Roberto A. Lima, Fernando L. Dias

Head and Neck Service, Brazilian National Cancer Institute/INCA and Head and Neck Surgery, Catholic University of Rio de Janeiro, Rio de Janeiro, Brazil

PEARLS

- Elevate the remaining larynx by suturing the thyroid cartilage to the tongue musculature. Avoid including the lingual mucosa.
- Suture the submucosa of the lateral edge of the vocal fold to the remaining superior border of the thyroid cartilage.

PITFALLS

- The point of section of the thyroid cartilage should be carefully identified. A wrong cut of the cartilage may permanently prevent speech.
- Perform the cricopharyngeal myotomy (CM) at the posterior midline, reducing the risks of recurrent laryngeal nerve damage.

Introduction

Alonso [1] in 1947 introduced the supraglottic laryngectomy to treat selected cases of supraglottic tumors. The oncologic results are near those achieved by total laryngectomy, with preservation of the voice and deglutition. Sessions et al. [2] in a study including 438 patients who underwent supraglottic laryngectomy, total laryngectomy and radiotherapy for supraglottic cancer reported 78.2, 79.8 and 75.9% rates of normal/asymptomatic deglutition, respectively.

Supraglottic laryngectomy (horizontal partial laryngectomy) is indicated in primary lesions of the epiglottis, located either in lingual or laryngeal surface. The extent of the lesion to the base of the tongue, aryepiglottic fold or superior aspects of the false cord can be included in this surgical technique. The resection of barriers to aspiration and the supraglottic sensation may lead to improper deglutition and aspiration [3].

The major problem after supraglottic laryngectomy is the deglutition without aspiration. The resection of supraglottic structures removes the anatomical protection of the larynx tube and interrupts the sequential sensory input of the swallowing mechanism [4]. This deficiency in sensory reception can be compensated by the remaining structures, and damage to the external branch of the superior laryngeal nerve and to the recurrent laryngeal nerve should be avoided. Adequate intraoperative maneuvers can prevent important postoperative aspiration and facilitate recovery.

Practical Tips

1 Do not enter the larynx through the vallecula in cases of lingual surface lesions. If the vallecula is free of tumor, it is the most convenient site to enter the larynx because it affords better tumor visualization.

❷ The point of section of the thyroid cartilage should be carefully identified. Generally, in women, the anterior commissure is at the level of the upper third and lower two thirds of the thyroid cartilage anteriorly, as measured from the base of the thyroid notch to the inferior anterior border of the thyroid cartilage. A wrong cut of the cartilage may permanently prevent speech [5].
❸ In extended supraglottic laryngectomy with one arytenoid resection, it is important to prevent aspiration placing the remaining vocal cord in medialization by suturing it to the cricoid cartilage.
❹ Avoid including the lingual mucosa in the suture to the remaining larynx, making the suture only to the tongue muscles [6]. Position the remaining larynx as far superior and anterior under the base of the tongue. This can prevent excessive aspiration [7]. Calcaterra [8] advocated suspension of the larynx fixing the thyroid cartilage to the mentum or to the digastric muscles. We prefer to fix the thyroid cartilage to the tongue musculature.
❺ Preserving the external branch of the superior laryngeal nerve to the cricothyroid muscle is possible with careful dissection of the superior cornus of the thyroid cartilage. Avoiding injury to the superior laryngeal nerve improves the recovery of swallowing [9].
❻ Suture the submucosa of the lateral edge of the vocal fold to the remaining superior border of the thyroid cartilage. This helps to keep the tension of the vocal cord.
❼ CM may improve deglutition reducing any hypopharyngeal resistance to swallowing. Nevertheless, there is no evidence that CM improves swallowing after supraglottic laryngectomy. However, a study [10] suggested that CM helps to normalize the upper esophageal sphincter in cases of cricopharyngeal dysfunction.
❽ The CM should be done at the posterior midline to avoid lesion of the laryngeal recurrent nerve.

References

1 Alonso JM: Conservative surgery of cancer of the larynx. Trans Am Acad Ophthalmol Otolaryngol 1947;51:633–642.
2 Sessions DG, Lenox J, Spector GJ: Supraglottic laryngeal cancer: analysis of treatment results. Laryngoscope 2005;115:1402–1410.
3 Logemann JA, Gibbons P, Rademaker AW, et al: Mechanisms of recovery of swallow after supraglottic laryngectomy. J Speech Hear Res 1994;37:965–974.
4 Tucker HM: Deglutition following partial laryngectomy; in Silver CE (ed): Laryngeal Cancer. New York, Thieme, 1991, pp 197–200.
5 Thawley SE, Sessions DG, Deddins AE: Surgical therapy of supraglottic tumors; in Thawley SE, Panje WR, Batsakis JG, Lindberg RD (eds): Comprehensive Management of Head and Neck Tumors. Philadelphia, Saunders, 1999, pp 1006–1038.
6 Tucker HM: The Larynx, ed 2. New York, Thieme Medical Publishers, 1993.
7 Schweinfurth JM, Silver SM: Patterns of swallowing after supraglottic laryngectomy. Laryngoscope 2000;110:1266–1270.
8 Calcaterra TC: Laryngeal suspension after supraglottic laryngectomy. Arch Otolaryngol 1971;94:306–309.
9 Tufano RP: Open supraglottic laryngectomy; Weinstein GS (ed): Operative Techniques in Otolaryngology-Head and Neck Surgery. Philadelphia, Saunders, 2003, pp 22–26.
10 Yip HT, Leonard R, Kendall KA: Cricopharyngeal myotomy normalizes the opening size of the upper esophageal sphincter in cricopharyngeal dysfunction. Laryngoscope 2006;116:93–96.

Cernea CR, Dias FL, Fliss D, Lima RA, Myers EN, Wei WI (eds): Pearls and Pitfalls in Head and Neck Surgery. Basel, Karger, 2008, pp 82–83

4.6 Practical Tips for Performing Supracricoid Partial Laryngectomy

Gregory S. Weinstein, F. Christopher Holsinger, Ollivier Laccourreye

Department of Otorhinolaryngology Head and Neck Surgery, University of Pennsylvania, Philadelphia, Pa., USA

PEARLS

- Preserve both recurrent and superior laryngeal nerves.
- The fine points of closure, which are important to ensure good function postoperatively, include repositioning of the arytenoids and pyriform sinuses as well as proper placement of the pexy sutures.
- Use the retroarytenoid mucosa and corniculate cartilage to reconstruct a neoarytenoid when one arytenoid cartilage is resected.

PITFALLS

- Do not operate on patients with severe chronic obstructive pulmonary disease.
- Swallowing rehabilitation is significantly delayed when the patient has had prior laryngeal radiation therapy.

Introduction

There are two types of supracricoid partial laryngectomy (SCPL) which are utilized for clearly distinct indications, namely the SCPL with cricohyoidopexy (CHP) and the SCPL with cricohyoidoepiglottopexy (CHEP) [1]. While oncologically, the primary goals are local control of glottic and supraglottic cancer, the functional goals following SCPL are speech and swallowing without a permanent tracheostomy or gastrostomy tube. Although there is a commonality in terms of resection in both procedures, there are differences both in the resection and the reconstruction. For both SCPL-CHP and SCPL-CHEP, the entire thyroid cartilage, both false cords and true cords are resected, while preserving at least one arytenoid. In the SCPL with CHEP, which is utilized for selected glottic carcinomas, the petiole is also resected. In the SCPL with CHP, the entire epiglottic and preepiglottic space is removed. In both SCPLs, three sutures are placed around the cricoid. For the SCPL with CHEP, the sutures are placed through the epiglottis, tongue base and preepiglottic space. For the SCPL-CHP, there is no epiglottis and the three sutures are passed around the hyoid into the tongue base. There is a vast worldwide literature available confirming both the oncologic and functional efficacy of the SCPLs. There are now numerous and thorough reviews of the perioperative management and procedure itself. This chapter will focus on specific practical points that will optimize functional outcomes.

Practical Tips

1 Preoperative patient selection is critical, and the key issue is to avoid performing SCPL on patients with severe chronic obstructive pulmonary disease. The clinical test which is most useful is to assess the patient's ability to climb two sets of

stairs without becoming short of breath. Pulmonary function tests are not routinely ordered preoperatively.

2 The surgeon should be aware of the anatomic locations of both the superior and recurrent laryngeal nerves and avoid damaging these nerves during the procedure on both the ipsilateral and contralateral sides relative to the cancer [2].

3 During the reconstruction it is important to resuspend the arytenoid cartilages with a stitch that is essentially an air knot with a 4-0 Vicryl suture placed between the vocal process of the arytenoids and the superior-lateral aspect of the cricoid cartilage.

4 When placing the CHP or CHEP pexy sutures, it is critical to avoid going beyond 1 cm from the midline to avoid damaging the tongue neurovascular bundle.

5 Reapproximation of the constrictor muscles is done by placing a half vertical mattress suture through the cut edge of the constrictor muscles bilaterally [3].

6 The rehabilitation regimen at the University of Pennsylvania at present is as follows. With rare exception, all patients undergo preoperative percutaneous gastrostomy. The cuffed tracheostomy is changed to a cuffless No. 6 tracheostomy on postoperative day 3. The patient is discharged from the hospital on postoperative day 5 and is seen as an outpatient by a speech-language pathologist for swallowing rehabilitation on approximately postoperative day 10. The tracheostomy is downsized and corked and removed when the patient tolerates corking and/or the airway looked clinically patent via indirect laryngoscopy. In France where prolonged hospitalization is the norm a more aggressive decannulation and swallowing regimen has been safely pursued.

Conclusion

In this chapter the reader was exposed to the key points for optimizing functional outcome following SCPL. If attention is given to both patient selection as well as consistent focus on intraoperative details the chance for excellent outcomes is improved.

References

1 Weinstein GS, Laccourreye O, Brasnu D, Laccourreye H: Organ Preservation Surgery for Laryngeal Cancer. San Diego, Singular Publishing, 1999.

2 Rassekh CH, Driscoll BP, Seikaly H, Laccourreye O, Calhoun KH, Weinstein GS: Preservation of the superior laryngeal nerve in supraglottic and supracricoid partial laryngectomy. Laryngoscope 1998;108:445–447.

3 Naudo P, Laccourreye O, Weinstein G, Hans S, Laccourreye H, Brasnu D: Functional outcome and prognosis after supracricoid partial laryngectomy with cricohyoidopexy. Ann Otol Rhinol Laryngol 1997;106:291–296.

Cernea CR, Dias FL, Fliss D, Lima RA, Myers EN, Wei WI (eds): Pearls and Pitfalls in Head and Neck Surgery. Basel, Karger, 2008, pp 84–85

4.7 Intraoperative Maneuvers to Improve Functional Results after Total Laryngectomy

Javier Gavilán[a], Jesús Herranz[b]

[a] Department of Otorhinolaryngology, La Paz University Hospital, Madrid, and
[b] Juan Canalejo Hospital, La Coruña, Spain

PEARLS

- A careful tension-free suture of the hypopharynx is crucial to prevent the development of hypopharyngeal fistula.
- Create a stable, well-shaped, adequately sized and accessible stoma.
- Remember that voice rehabilitation can be achieved at the same time as total laryngectomy (TL) or at a later stage. Fit the procedure to the patient's needs and desires.

PITFALLS

- Do not attempt a primary hypopharyngeal closure if there is not enough remaining mucosa.
- Leaving tracheal cartilage uncovered at the level of the stoma results in delayed healing and infection.

Introduction

In spite of a more conservative approach for the treatment of patients with cancer of the larynx, TL is still the final option for many patients. A lung-powered voice may also be achieved through a surgically created tracheoesophageal shunt. Some technical details may result in better postoperative functional results.

Tips for a Watertight Hypopharyngeal Suture

Pharyngocutaneous fistula (PCF) is the most common complication following TL. It is associated with prolonged hospitalization and delayed oral feeding with subsequent increase in cost and discomfort for the patient. Its incidence ranges between 8 and 22% [1, 2].

1 There are two keystones to prevent PCF: meticulous closure of the hypopharynx and tension-free suture line.

2 When the resection preserves a sufficient amount of pharyngeal mucosa for direct closure, the 'tobacco pouch' technique described in 1945 by García-Hormaeche [3] is a good alternative to the classic T-shaped closure. To create the 'tobacco pouch' two parallel continuous absorbable sutures are placed around the hypopharyngeal opening. The first stitch begins below the level of the hyoid bone and is placed 2–3 mm lateral to the mucosal edge. The second suture starts above the level of the hyoid bone and runs 5 mm lateral and parallel to the first stitch. By gently pulling from both ends of the sutures the mucosal edges are approximated and turned inwards, creating a safe primary closure of the hypopharynx [4].

3 When the surgeon deals with insufficient hypopharyngeal mucosa for direct closure, the apron platysma myocutaneous flap is a fast and reliable reconstructive method with no added morbidity. Reconstruction begins by suturing the base of the

tongue to the superior base of the apron platysma flap. The lateral and inferior edges of the remaining strip of hypopharyngeal mucosa are sutured to the inner surface of the apron flap [5]. The anterior wall of the neopharynx allows a wide food passage in spite of the small amount of remaining pharyngeal mucosa.

4 Finally, leaving a Jackson-Pratt drain along the pharyngeal suture line provides early information about the development of PCF, allowing prompt intervention.

Tips for Creating a Good Stoma

A stable, adequate-sized, accessible stoma significantly improves the quality of life of the laryngectomized patient. Some technical tips may help the creation of a correct stoma.

1 Sectioning the sternal insertion of the sternocleidomastoid muscle on both sides results in a more superficial and accessible stoma, facilitating cleaning maneuvers and occlusion in patients with voice prosthesis and speaking valves.

2 Creating a half-moon section line in the superior skin flap at the level of the trachea results in a circular-shaped stoma. This also helps further manipulation of the stoma.

3 Using vertical mattress stitches in the skin of the stoma provides cutaneous coverage of the tracheal cartilage, preventing cartilage exposure and subsequent infection.

Tips for Surgical Speech Rehabilitation

Tracheoesophageal puncture (TEP) is the most common speech rehabilitation procedure after TL. It can be performed at the same time as tumor removal (primary TEP) or at a later stage (secondary TEP). The following tips refer mainly to primary TEP.

1 Try to place the puncture in the midline, 1 cm below the resection border of the trachea.

2 When the puncture is performed from outside to inside, always protect the posterior wall of the esophagus to prevent injury of the mucosa (a spoon inside the esophagus is a very useful tool).

3 Perform a posteromedial myotomy from the lower level of the oropharynx to the level of the tracheoesophageal shunt. Once sectioned, the constrictor muscles are dissected from the submucosa and retracted 1–2 cm laterally. This creates a wider and less resistant hypopharynx, facilitating air passage through the TEP [6].

References

1 Herranz J, Sarandeses A, Fernández MF, Barro CV, Vidal JM, Gavilán J: Complications after total laryngectomy in nonradiated laryngeal and hypopharyngeal carcinomas. Otolaryngol Head Neck Surg 2000;122:892–898.

2 Markou KD, Vlachtsis KC, Nikolaou AC, Petridis DG, Kouloulas AI, Daniilidis IC: Incidence and predisposing factors of pharyngocutaneous fistula formation after total laryngectomy. Is there a relationship with tumor recurrence? Eur Arch Otorhinolaryngol 2004;261:61–67.

3 García-Hormaeche D: Avance sobre un nuevo procedimiento de técnica quirúrgica para realizar las laringuectomías subtotales y totales. Rev Esp Am Laringol Otol Rinol 1945;3:99–120.

4 Gavilán C, Cerdeira MA, Gavilán J: Pharyngeal closure following total laryngectomy: the 'tobacco pouch' technique. Oper Tech Otolaryngol Head Neck Surg 1993;4:292–302.

5 Bernáldez R, Cerdeira MA, Gavilán J: Pharyngeal reconstruction with the apron platysma myocutaneous flap. Oper Tech Otolaryngol Head Neck Surg 1993;4:303–305.

6 Herranz J, Martínez-Vidal J: Primary tracheoesophageal puncture with pharyngoesophageal myotomy. Oper Tech Otolaryngol Head Neck Surg 1993;4:291–295.

Cernea CR, Dias FL, Fliss D, Lima RA, Myers EN, Wei WI (eds): Pearls and Pitfalls in Head and Neck Surgery. Basel, Karger, 2008, pp 86–87

4.8 How to Manage Tracheostomal Recurrence

Dennis H. Kraus

Memorial Sloan-Kettering Cancer Center, Head and Neck Service, New York, N.Y., USA

PEARLS

- Perform cross-sectional imaging to determine involvement of the carotid artery, pharynx, trachea, innominate artery, and mediastinum to assess resectability.
- Perform PET/CT imaging to exclude distant metastatic disease.
- Access to reconstructive surgery for pharyngeal reconstruction and extended skin replacement and thoracic surgery expertise for management of the trachea and mediastinum.

PITFALLS

- Imaging often grossly underestimates extent of disease and fails to identify the invasive nature of recurrent disease after laryngectomy.
- Wound complications, including flap necrosis and fistula formation, can manifest life-endangering events.
- Cure occurs only in 25–30% of selected patients undergoing surgical management.

Introduction

Tracheostomal recurrence after laryngectomy is an extremely challenging problem. The vast majority of these patients will have undergone chemoradiation and salvage laryngectomy. Tracheostomal disease typically represents recurrence of nodal disease in the tracheoesophageal groove. Surgical management is feasible in the minority of patients and the ability to cure is relatively remote.

Patients who are considered for surgical management should suffer limited medical comorbidities. Utilizing the Sisson staging system, stage I (suprastomal disease without pharyngeal involvement) or stage II (suprastomal disease with involvement of the pharynx) is far preferable to stage III (infrastomal disease without great vessel involvement) or stage IV (infrastomal disease with great vessel involvement) disease. Patients require complete resection of the tracheostomal disease, a portion of the trachea, pharyngeal resection, and all involved cervical skin. Reconstruction focuses on reestablishment of the pharynx, reconstruction of the cervical skin, and reconstitution of the stoma.

Postoperative complications can be life-threatening. Wound breakdown can lead to fistula formation and the risk of rupture of the carotid and/or innominate artery. Patients undergoing successful management may be considered for re-irradiation, possibly with chemotherapy. Even with aggressive treatment, approximately 25–30% patients are cured of their disease. Distant metastases remain a significant risk.

Practical Tips

A well-constructed plan is essential for the surgical management of patients with tracheostomal recurrence after prior laryngectomy. The following suggestions should be considered:

1 Cross-sectional imaging to elucidate the local extent of disease. Absolute contraindications include prevertebral fascia invasion, carotid or innominate artery encasement, or massive mediastinal involvement.
2 PET/CT imaging to exclude distant metastases.
3 Preoperative esophagoscopy excludes extensive esophageal invasion. The majority of patients will require some form of pharyngeal reconstruction. For circumferential defects, a jejunal free flap is employed. For anterior wall defects, a soft tissue free flap can be employed.
4 Resection of the trachea is associated with cervical skin resection; either pectoralis major or deltopectoral flap is employed to reconstruct the cervical skin defect and affords tracheostoma reconstruction. In this author's opinion, efforts at mediastinal tracheostomy are rarely successful and these patients almost uniformly die of postoperative complications.
5 Ipsilateral neck dissection should be performed in instances where it was not performed previously, including aggressive dissection of the tracheoesophageal groove and upper mediastinum. Preservation of both the jugular vein and the carotid arterial system allows for microvascular flap reconstruction.
6 A watertight closure of the reconstructed pharynx, as fistula formation with salivary leak is associated with life-endangering carotid or innominate artery hemorrhage.
7 Barium swallow is utilized to assess for pharyngeal leak. Prolonged enteral feeding can be utilized when necessary.
8 A significant proportion of patients develops both postoperative hypocalcemia and hypothyroidism and requires appropriate replacement.
9 Consideration of re-irradiation with or without chemotherapy is performed on a case-by-case basis.
10 Utilizing this aggressive approach, approximately 25–30% of these selected patients will be salvaged.

Conclusion

Surgical management of tracheostomal recurrence requires considerable judgment and skill. Patients must be evaluated to exclude those who have surgically unresectable disease or metastatic disease. Patients best suited for this operation have limited medical comorbidities and stage I or II disease.

Access to appropriate surgical colleagues, including plastic and reconstructive surgery, and potentially thoracic surgery, are integral to the success of this procedure. Patients must undergo complete extirpation of the tumor if there is any hope for cure. Disease is often more extensive than what is anticipated based on preoperative imaging. Patients must undergo immediate reconstruction of the pharynx, the external cervical skin and the stoma. Utilizing this approach, approximately 25–30% of patients with this advanced stage disease will have long-term disease control.

References

1 Baldwin CJ, Liddington MI: An approach to complex tracheostomal complications. J Plast Reconstr Aesthet Surg 2007, E-pub ahead of print.
2 Breneman JC, Bradshaw A, Gluckman J, Aron BS: Prevention of stomal recurrence in patients requiring emergency tracheostomy for advanced laryngeal and pharyngeal tumors. Cancer 1988;62:802–805.
3 Bignardi L, Gavioli C, Staffieri A: Tracheostomal recurrences after laryngectomy. Arch Otorhinolaryngol 1983;238:107–113.
4 Gluckman JL, Hamaker RC, Schuller DE, Weissler MC, Charles GA: Surgical salvage for stomal recurrence: a multi-institutional experience. Laryngoscope 1987;97:1025–1029.
5 McCarthy CM, Kraus DH, Cordeiro PG: Tracheostomal and cervical esophageal reconstruction with combined deltopectoral flap and microvascular free jejunal transfer after central neck exenteration. Plast Reconstr Surg 2005;115:1304–1310.
6 Sisson GA Sr: 1989 Ogura memorial lecture: mediastinal dissection. Laryngoscope 1989;99:1262–1266.
7 Yuen AP, Ho CM, Wei WI, Lam LK: Prognosis of recurrent laryngeal carcinoma after laryngectomy. Head Neck 1995;17:526–530.
8 Yuen AP, Wei WI, Ho WK, Hui Y: Risk factors of tracheostomal recurrence after laryngectomy for laryngeal carcinoma. Am J Surg 1996;172:263–266.

Cernea CR, Dias FL, Fliss D, Lima RA, Myers EN, Wei WI (eds): Pearls and Pitfalls in Head and Neck Surgery. Basel, Karger, 2008, pp 88–89

4.9 Stenosis of the Tracheostoma following Total Laryngectomy

Eugene N. Myers

Department of Otolaryngology, University of Pittsburgh, School of Medicine, Pittsburgh, Pa., USA

PEARLS

- Every effort should be made to prevent tracheostomal stenosis.
- Patients with tracheostomal stenosis should receive a trial of conservative treatment using progressively larger diameter laryngectomy tubes and stents.
- The surgical techniques used should be as simple as possible.

PITFALLS

- Peristomal recurrence of cancer should be ruled out prior to contemplating revision surgery.
- Patients who have been treated with radiation therapy should not be considered candidates for surgical revision because of the probability of poor healing and restenosis.
- Poor nutrition leads to poor wound healing so the nutritional status of the patient should be optimized prior to revision surgery.

Introduction

Stenosis of the tracheostoma is an infrequent but vexing problem which may occur despite meticulous attention to the construction of the tracheostoma. Although stenosis usually occurs within months following laryngectomy, it may also occur years later. Tracheostomal stenosis may cause respiratory insufficiency in patients with emphysema [1], difficulty in expelling mucus, the potential for complete obstruction due to excessive crusting or a mucous plug and inability to remove and insert the speaking valve.

Factors contributing to tracheostomal stenosis include radiation therapy, wound dehiscence with healing by second intention, inadequate excision of redundant peristomal skin and adipose tissue, devascularization of the trachea, postoperative infection, and excessive scar tissue formation. Stomal recurrence of cancer should be ruled out in patients with apparent peristomal stenosis. Modifications of technique may help to prevent peristomal stenosis.

Practical Tips

1. Every effort should be made to rule out peristomal recurrence of cancer prior to embarking on a treatment program.
2. Prevention of stomal stenosis should be a part of preoperative planning. Patients who have risk factors for stomal stenosis demand special attention to prevent this problem.
3. Technical modifications to prevent stenosis should include oblique section of the tracheal stump to increase the diameter of the stoma, excision of excess adipose tissue from the peristomal skin and complete coverage of the cut edge of the trachea with skin.
4. The patient is instructed to wear a No. 8 laryngectomy tube at night for 6 months while the stoma is maturing. During the day a soft silastic

stent is worn in which an opening has been placed in its posterior aspect, which makes it possible to use the speaking valve.

5 Initial management of tracheostomal stenosis should be conservative. This includes dilation of the stoma with the insertion of progressively larger laryngectomy tubes and the eventual insertion of a plastic stomal button.

6 Patients who have had radiation therapy to the larynx should be managed conservatively rather than surgically since the radiated tissues do not heal well.

7 The most common type of stenosis is a band of scar tissue which is shelf-like in appearance and concentrically narrows the stoma. The goals of revision surgery are to excise the concentric skin and to prevent it from recurring.

8 The surgical technique we first described [2] has proved to be very simple and reliable in solving the problem of tracheal stomal stenosis. This technique includes excising the shelf-like scar, defatting the surrounding skin and meticulously approximating the skin to the trachea making certain that the cartilage is completely covered. A 1-cm incision is made in the membranous posterior wall of the trachea and a small pedicle flap derived from the skin posterior to the stoma is sewn into the incision in the posterior wall of the trachea to prevent restenosis.

9 A smaller flap is necessary in patients with a tracheoesophageal speaking valve.

Conclusion

Tracheostomal stenosis is usually preventable. However, when it occurs, conservative treatment with a laryngectomy tube usually suffices. A few patients will require revision surgery which should be kept as simple as possible. Revision surgery is contraindicated in radiated patients. Peristomal recurrence of cancer should be ruled out prior to formulating a treatment program.

References

1 Wax MK, Touma J, Ramadan HH: Tracheostoma stenosis after laryngectomy: incidence and predisposing factors. Otolaryngol Head Neck Surg 1995;113:242–247.

2 Myers EN, Gallia LJ: Tracheostomal stenosis following total laryngectomy. Ann Otol Rhinol Laryngol 1982;91:450–453.

Cernea CR, Dias FL, Fliss D, Lima RA, Myers EN, Wei WI (eds): Pearls and Pitfalls in Head and Neck Surgery. Basel, Karger, 2008, pp 90–91

4.10 How to Prevent and Treat Pharyngocutaneous Fistulas after Laryngectomy

Bhuvanesh Singh

Laboratory of Epithelial Cancer Biology, Head and Neck Service, Memorial Sloan-Kettering Cancer Center, New York, N.Y., USA

PEARLS

- The rate of fistula formation (FF) nearly doubles in the setting of prior chemoradiation treatment.
- Prevention of FF is the best treatment and starts with an atraumatic surgical technique.
- A stepwise approach to pharyngeal reconstruction is advocated, beginning with tension-free horizontal closure, reinforcement of the suture line with suprahyoid and pharyngeal constrictor musculature, bolstering the closure with a pectoralis muscle-only flap and using free flaps for larger defects.

PITFALLS

- Tension or T closures are prone to FF.
- Lack of introduction of vascularized tissue can increase risk of fistulization.

Introduction

Once considered the cornerstone for the management of advanced larynx cancer, laryngectomies are now reserved for large tumors with extralaryngeal extension or, more commonly, for salvage after failure of either radiation or chemoradiation treatment. Although the initial organ preservation trials allowed selection of patients for early salvage surgery, the current state of the art is to deliver chemotherapy concomitantly with radiation, which rarely allows for early detection of failures [1–3]. The benefits from concomitant chemoradiation treatment are tempered by higher rates of short- and long-term treatment-related sequelae. This is particularly relevant in patients that fail to respond to this treatment approach, having to endure the adverse effects of treatment without any appreciable benefit. Salvage laryngeal surgery poses a complex problem for the head and neck surgeon [4]. The tissue is less vascularized and often has a reduced healing capacity, increasing the risk of FF [5–8]. Published results and our own experience suggest that the fistula rate is doubled in this setting, prompting changes in standard approaches to pharyngeal closure.

Practical Tips

1 Several intraoperative measures should be undertaken to minimize risk of FF.

a) Minimize mucosal devascularization. It is imperative to minimize the manipulation of mucosa during the course of resection. In addition, all mucosal incisions should be made with the cutting current of the Bovie (or cold steel).

b) Maximize mucosal preservation. A tension-free closure is an essential component in preventing FF. This is best accomplished by preserving as much of the mucosa as is oncologically safe. Specific attention must be paid to preservation of the pyriform sinuses and the mucosa of the lingual surface of the epiglottis.

2 Closure of the pharyngeal defect is also a key consideration.

a) As discussed above, vascularized mucosa and a tension-free closure are of paramount importance. Prior to starting the closure, examine the mucosal edges and resect any nonviable or poorly vascularized mucosa.

b) A horizontal closure is preferred over a T closure. This also has the benefit of maximizing the nasopharyngeal aperture.

c) A second layer of sutures is advocated to bolster the closure. This can be performed by approximating the pharyngeal constrictors to the suprahyoid and tongue-based musculature.

3 Introduction of vascularized tissues should be considered for any nonoptimal pharyngeal closures.

a) If adequate mucosa is present, a muscle-only pectoralis flap is an excellent way to reinforce the pharyngeal closure, while simultaneously introducing well-vascularized, nonirradiated tissues to the neck.

b) In general, when inadequate mucosa is present for a tension-free closure, a 'patch'-type closure of the defect either with a regional or free flap is not advocated. In this setting, separations between the native tissue and that brought in by the flap are a high risk.

c) A total laryngopharyngectomy is often a better option in cases where inadequate mucosa remains. Reconstruction can be performed using a variety of free flaps, including the jejunum and tubed cutaneous (lateral thigh) or mucosal (gastroomental) flaps.

4 Once a fistula develops, aggressive management is required.

a) Most fistulas will manifest within 4–10 days. Delayed fistulas can occur in chemoirradiated patients up to 4 weeks after surgery.

b) If a fistula is suspected, the wound should be controlled by widely opening and packing the wound. Healing is usually delayed in chemoirradiated patients, and a PEG tube should be considered to maintain nutrition. Wound care and packing should be continued until the fistula resolves.

c) In cases of larger or refractory fistulas, operative correction using vascularized tissue should be considered after all infection is cleared.

Conclusions

Salvage laryngectomy after concomitant chemoradiation is associated with an increased risk of FF. A graded approach, beginning with care of the local tissue during reaction, attention to the pharyngeal closure and early introduction of visualized tissues, is required to optimize surgical results.

4

References

1 Pfister DG, Laurie SA, Weinstein GS, et al: American Society of Clinical Oncology clinical practice guideline for the use of larynx-preservation strategies in the treatment of laryngeal cancer. J Clin Oncol 2006;24:3693–3704.

2 Induction chemotherapy plus radiation compared with surgery plus radiation in patients with advanced laryngeal cancer. The Department of Veterans Affairs Laryngeal Cancer Study Group. N Engl J Med 1991;324:1685–1690.

3 Forastiere AA, Goepfert H, Maor M, et al: Concurrent chemotherapy and radiotherapy for organ preservation in advanced laryngeal cancer. N Engl J Med 2003;349:2091–2098.

4 Ganly I, Patel S, Matsuo J, et al: Postoperative complications of salvage total laryngectomy. Cancer 2005;103:2073–2081.

5 Disa JJ, Pusic AL, Mehrara BJ: Reconstruction of the hypopharynx with the free jejunum transfer. J Surg Oncol 2006;94:466–470.

6 Gilbert RW, Neligan PC: Microsurgical laryngotracheal reconstruction. Clin Plast Surg 2005;32:293–301.

7 Teknos TN, Myers LL, Bradford CR, Chepeha DB: Free tissue reconstruction of the hypopharynx after organ preservation therapy: analysis of wound complications. Laryngoscope 2001;111:1192–1196.

8 Fung K, Teknos TN, Vandenberg CD, et al: Prevention of wound complications following salvage laryngectomy using free vascularized tissue. Head Neck 2007;29:425–430.

Cernea CR, Dias FL, Fliss D, Lima RA, Myers EN, Wei WI (eds): Pearls and Pitfalls in Head and Neck Surgery. Basel, Karger, 2008, pp 92–93

5.1 How to Treat Small Hypopharyngeal Primary Tumors with N3 Neck

Abrão Rapoport, Marcos Brasilino de Carvalho

Head and Neck Surgeons, Hospital Heliopolis, São Paulo, Brazil

PEARLS

- In malnourished patients, endeavor to reverse the process of weight loss before instituting any oncological therapeutic measure. Patients presenting cachexia do not benefit from standard oncological treatment; palliative measures for nutritional support and pain control offer better quality of life.

PITFALLS

- Patients with hypopharyngeal cancer are often chronic alcoholics. If surgical treatment is decided on, they may become uncooperative during the immediate postoperative period, removing the nasoenteral tube, adopting an inappropriate oral diet, neglecting bandage hygiene and also manifesting alcohol withdrawal symptoms.
- Large metastatic lymph nodes in hypopharyngeal carcinoma cases are often at level III. Extracapsular invasion may involve the carotid bulb, making the lymph nodes irresectable. The results after shaving the carotid sheath with the aim of reducing the tumor mass are ineffective in preventing recurrence, even with associated radiotherapy, and this may predispose towards vessel rupture.
- Patients with advanced metastatic disease present a great risk of recurrence, both regional and distant.

Introduction

Epidermoid carcinoma of the hypopharynx is one of the most lethal types of cancer in the head and neck region. Because of its anatomical location very close to the larynx, the therapeutic planning is almost always based on surgery and postoperative radiotherapy, usually including total laryngectomy in order to obtain adequate surgical margins [1]. This type of cancer develops in the mucosa of a region that is in permanent motion and presents a rich network of lymphatic capillaries that are quickly reached by the infiltration of the lesion. These factors, together with the fact that these tumors are generally less differentiated, explain why voluminous regional metastases related to relatively small primary lesions are frequently observed. Because the presence of lymph node metastases is the single prognostic factor that has the greatest impact, and considering that macroscopic rupture of the capsule drastically reduces disease control rates, specialists are often faced with the dilemma of recommending aggressive treatment comprising surgery, radiotherapy and/or chemotherapy, with all the associated morbidity, disproportionately set against an unsatisfactory quality of life and short survival [2]. Many studies have shown survival results equivalent to classical surgical treatment with postoperative radiotherapy, using organ preservation protocols based on a combination of chemotherapy and radiotherapy, among patients with advanced yet resectable tumors [3].

Small hypopharyngeal tumors presenting with advanced cervical metastasis should be candidates for treatment plans that offer the best possible quality of life. Therefore, partial pharyngectomy with total laryngectomy should be avoided, because the extent of the regional dissemination is an ominous prognostic factor. It is not justifiable to be preoccupied with the evolution of the primary lesion, as ultimately the condition of the lymph nodes will define the outcome. The presence of an N3 neck usually impairs regional disease control. Concomitant chemoradiotherapy regimens may offer better preservation of speech and swallowing. If, by the end of the irradiation, the lymph node metastasis has responded completely or has reduced in size and become mobile, planned selective neck dissection may be indicated, in order to remove the lymph node chains that potentially have the greatest possibility of containing residual disease. Small primary lesions generally respond well to preservation regimens, but advanced metastases present a high risk of regional and distant recurrence [4].

Practical Tips

Patients with advanced metastatic disease generally progress with inoperable regional recurrence that rapidly becomes ulcerated and necrotic, with bleeding. This leads to death with great suffering, due to cachexia or hemorrhage caused by invasion and rupture of the carotid artery. Thus, it is recommendable to anticipate these events whenever possible, so as to control or delay them, given that advanced metastatic cervical disease shortens survival and reduces the quality of the remaining life [5].

❶ The patients who come for treatment already present a significant degree of malnutrition. Insertion of a nasoenteral tube right at the first consultation may reduce the weight loss and enables the patients to receive the full irradiation dose planned [6].

❷ If, when a dose of 4,000 cGy is reached, the lymph node has reduced in size and has turned out to be mobile, the opportunity to remove it may be taken, leaving a 2-week interval in the irradiation program.

Conclusion

Initial neoplasia of the hypopharynx associated with advanced metastatic disease presents a poor prognosis, independent of the treatment method.

References

1 Moyer JS, Wolf GT, Bradford CR: Current thoughts on the role of chemotherapy and radiation in advanced head and neck cancer. Curr Opin Otolaryngol Head Neck Surg 2004;12:82–87.
2 Carvalho MB: Quantitative analysis of the extent of extracapsular invasion and its prognostic significance: prospective study of 170 cases of carcinoma of larynx and hypopharynx. Head Neck 1998;20:16–21.
3 Koch WM, Lee DJ, Eisele DW, Miller D, Poole M, Cummings CW, Forastiere A: Chemoradiotherapy for organ preservation in oral and pharyngeal carcinoma. Arch Otolayngol Head Neck Surg 1995;121:974–980.
4 Clark J, Li W, Smith G, Jackson M, Tin MM, O'Brian C: Outcome of treatment for advanced cervical metastatic squamous cell carcinoma. Head Neck 2005;27:87–94.
5 Goldstein DP, Karnell LH, Christensen AJ, Funk GF: Health related quality of life profiles based on survivorship status for head and neck cancer patients. Head Neck 2007;29:221–229.
6 Funk GF, Karnell LH, Smith RB, Christensen AJ: Clinical significance of health status assessment measures in head and neck cancer. What do quality-of-life scores mean? Arch Otolaryngol Head Neck Surg 2004;130:825–829.

Cernea CR, Dias FL, Fliss D, Lima RA, Myers EN, Wei WI (eds): Pearls and Pitfalls in Head and Neck Surgery. Basel, Karger, 2008, pp 94–95

5.2 Practical Tips to Reconstruct a Total Laryngectomy/Partial Pharyngectomy Defect

Dennis H. Kraus

Memorial Sloan-Kettering Cancer Center, Head and Neck Service, New York, N.Y., USA

PEARLS

- Endoscopic assessment preoperatively to determine extent of disease is critical.
- Access to reconstructive techniques, such as a pedicle flap (pectoralis major myocutaneous flap) or free tissue transfer (radial forearm or lateral thigh free flap) will be necessary in most patients.
- Rarely is a tension-free, primary closure feasible, given that the majority of patients represent radiation failures. The risk of fistula is extremely high, even when a flap closure is performed.

PITFALLS

- Many radiation or chemoradiation failure patients have extensive submucosal diseases, which is often underestimated.
- The majority of patients are severely malnourished, due to the impact of dysphagia from prior radiation-based treatment.
- Impaired wound healing is associated with recurrent disease in the postradiation setting, even with the use of nonirradiated flap reconstruction.

Introduction

The vast majority of patients who undergo laryngectomy with partial pharyngectomy represent chemoradiation failures. Thus, the vast majority of them will require flap reconstruction of the large soft tissue defect, which is associated with recurrent tumors in this setting. Even with the use of nonirradiated tissue transfer to close the defect, there is severe wound healing impairment, and many patients will develop a transient fistula.

Extreme care must be taken in performing closure of the combined laryngectomy/partial pharyngectomy defect. Submucosal disease is extremely common and determination of reconstructive technique should not be performed until tumor-free margins have been obtained on frozen section. The ability to perform primary closure is extremely limited. Approximately 90–95% of patients will require a patch closure of the soft tissue defect. The decision to utilize a pectoralis flap versus a free tissue transfer will be based on a number of factors: expertise and preference of the reconstructive surgeon, patient comorbidities, and availability of donor free flap vessels.

Despite all the described precautions, patients undergoing reconstruction of a laryngectomy/pharyngectomy defect remain at a high risk of fistula formation. Many of these fistulas will resolve with conservative management.

Practical Tips

Closure/reconstruction of a partial pharyngectomy/laryngectomy defect is a formidable undertaking. The following suggestions should be employed to minimize fistula formation/wound complications:

❶ Endoscopic/laryngoscopic assessment of tumor extent is critical. The propensity for submucosal disease often leads to underestimation of the extent of partial pharyngectomy.
❷ Use of frozen section margins is essential to avoid microscopic or intralymphatic residual disease.
❸ Flap choice for closure of the defect is critical. Patients who have undergone previous bilateral neck dissections or those with extensive medical comorbidities are better served with a pectoralis major myocutaneous flap reconstruction.
❹ Use of free tissue transfer is most commonly associated with patients who have limited medical comorbidities and have not undergone prior bilateral neck dissections. In performing neck dissection, every effort should be made to preserve the internal jugular vein and branches of the external carotid artery.
❺ A tension-free, water-tight seal should be performed between the native pharynx and the transferred flap. Often, localized tissues, such as the strap muscles or the sternocleidomastoid muscle, are used as a second layer closure over the anastomosis site.
❻ The majority of patients have had prior placement of a PEG feeding tube, and this allows for reinstitution of enteral feeding within 24–48 h of surgery. In addition, many patients are at high risk for hypothyroidism and consideration should be given to thyroid replacement.
❼ Due to the high risk of fistula formation, peroral feeding is delayed for 2–6 weeks. Barium swallow will successfully identify a small suture dehiscence, and oral feeding can be delayed an additional 2–3 months.
❽ In patients in whom fistulas become evident, there should be wide opening of the skin. Appropriate wound packing should be performed with acute use of antibiotics. In the majority of patients, the fistula will resolve without additional surgery. A small proportion of patients will require a secondary flap closure.
❾ Due to the high risk of fistula formation, secondary tracheoesophageal puncture is often the treatment choice for this author.

Conclusion

In this chapter, the reader was exposed to the challenging management of patients undergoing total laryngectomy with partial pharyngectomy. The vast majority of these patients will require flap closure. Despite all the previously identified precautions, a significant portion of these patients will develop fistulas and in some cases, secondary surgeries.

References

1 Kraus DH, Pfister DG, Harrison CB, Spiro RH, Strong EW, Zelefsky M, Bosl GJ, Shah JP: Salvage laryngectomy for unsuccessful larynx preservation therapy. Ann Otol Rhinol Laryngol 1995; 104:936–941.
2 Lydiatt W, Kraus DH, Cordeiro P, Hidalgo D, Shah JP: Posterior pharyngeal carcinoma resection with larynx preservation and radical forearm free flap reconstruction: a preliminary report. Head Neck Surg 1996;18:501–505.
3 Ganly I, Patel S, Matsuo J, Singh B, Kraus DH, Boyle JO, Wong R, Lee N, Pfister DG, Shaha A, Shah JP: Postoperative complications of salvage total laryngectomy. Cancer 2005;103:2073–2081.
4 Cheng E, Ho ML, Ganz C, Shaha A, Boyle JO, Singh B, Wong R, Patel SG, Shah JP, Branski RC, Kraus DH: Outcomes of primary and secondary tracheoesophageal puncture: a 16-year retrospective analysis. Ear Nose Throat J 2006;85:262, 264–267.

Cernea CR, Dias FL, Fliss D, Lima RA, Myers EN, Wei WI (eds): Pearls and Pitfalls in Head and Neck Surgery. Basel, Karger, 2008, pp 96–97

5.3 Practical Tips for Voice Rehabilitation after Pharyngolaryngectomy

Frans J.M. Hilgers[a–c], Michiel van den Brekel[a, b]

[a] Netherlands Cancer Institute – Antoni van Leeuwenhoek Hospital, [b] Academic Medical Center and
[c] Institute of Phonetic Sciences, University of Amsterdam, Amsterdam, The Netherlands

PEARLS

- Prosthetic voice rehabilitation, also after total pharyngolaryngectomy, is the method of choice for restoration of oral communication.
- When deciding about the optimal reconstruction method for the pharynx, the quality of the prosthetic voice and the possibility to restore functional speech should be taken into account, in addition to the obvious concern to restore oral intake, e.g. the use of a tubed fasciocutaneous flap instead of a jejunum transfer.

PITFALL

- Although in most instances primary tracheoesophageal puncture (TEP) with immediate insertion of an indwelling prosthesis is feasible, in case of a gastric pull-up, secondary tracheogastric puncture with immediate prosthesis insertion (e.g. after 4 weeks) is advisable to limit the risk of nonunion of the posterior wall of the trachea and the gastric tube.

Introduction

With the advent of voice prostheses, prosthetic vocal rehabilitation has gained widespread popularity, also after extensive pharyngeal resections and reconstructions [1]. The pharynx reconstruction method plays an important role in prosthetic voice quality, and a method optimal for creating a functional food passage might not be optimal for prosthetic voicing.

Practical Tips

Primary puncture with immediate insertion of an indwelling voice prosthesis is almost always an option, as long as the puncture site in the esophagus is intact, and if still present, always myotomize the cricopharyngeus muscle to prevent hypertonicity [2]. Only after a gastric pull-up, secondary puncture is to be preferred.

There are several options to reestablish a patent pharynx:

(1) After total laryngectomy, with only a strip of mucosa left that is inadequate for a circumferential closure (<2–3 cm wide), use a pectoralis major myocutaneous flap as a patch to form the anterior wall of the neopharynx. If not prohibited for oncological reasons, leaving this strip of mucosa in situ, because of its similar vibratory behavior as in a primarily closed pharynx, will result in good voice quality in many patients.

(2) After circumferential pharyngectomy without gastric pull-up, several options are available. A free revascularized jejunum interposition in combination with a voice prosthesis is not ideal. The voice is often wet and bubbly due to the continuous production of intestinal fluids and the voice is regularly blocked by the untreatable autono-

mous peristalsis. Occasionally, swallowing is problematic due to a siphon-like deformation of the graft. A better option is a free revascularized graft of the tubed greater curvature of the stomach [3]. Harvesting a portion of the greater curvature and stapling this into a tubular 3-cm diameter flap is not more difficult than obtaining a free jejunum graft. However, most head and neck surgeons do not want to increase the morbidity of the surgery by adding an abdominal procedure, and therefore prefer tubed revascularized skin flaps, e.g. the radial forearm flap or the anterolateral thigh flap [4, 5]. With both flaps, acceptable voice quality and swallowing results have been described. The risk of stenosis should not be underestimated, and some form of fish mouthing the flap into the inferior (esophageal) suture line should be attempted.

3 When circumferential pharyngolaryngectomy and esophagectomy are indicated, a gastric pull-up is required; a tubed stomach transfer is to be preferred over transposition of the complete stomach, because of the easier transfer through the mediastinum and a better diameter for prosthetic voicing. Secondary tracheogastric puncture and insertion of a mostly 12.5 mm indwelling voice prosthesis are carried out after wound healing has been completed. In case of postoperative radiotherapy (RT), the prosthesis should be inserted prior to that or, alternatively, 8–10 weeks post-RT. Even if the trachea and tubed stomach have not completely grown together during secondary TEP, the sturdy flanges of an indwelling prosthesis will keep the walls together.

Conclusion

Prosthetic voice rehabilitation after extensive pharyngolaryngectomy, just like after standard total laryngectomy, is the method of choice for reestablishing oral communication. Poor oncological prognosis, in the past often used as an argument to mainly worry about oral intake, but not about oral communication, actually is an extra valid reason to do whatever is possible to restore speech after this major surgery. The overall results are comparable to those achievable after standard total laryngectomy, but the voice quality is somewhat lower [6]. Nevertheless, prosthetic voice rehabilitation should be attempted in the vast majority of patients, in order to improve quality of life.

References

1 Hilgers FJM, Hoorweg JJ, Kroon BBR, Schaeffer B, de Boer JB, Balm AJM: Prosthetic voice rehabilitation with the Provox system after extensive pharyngeal resection and reconstruction; in Algaba J (ed): 6th International Congress on Surgical and Prosthetic Voice Restoration after Total Laryngectomy. Excerpta Medica International Congress Series, San Sebastian, 1995, pp 111–120.

2 Op de Coul BM, van den Hoogen FJ, Van As CJ, Marres HA, Joosten FB, Manni JJ, Hilgers FJ: Evaluation of the effects of primary myotomy in total laryngectomy on the neoglottis with the use of quantitative videofluoroscopy. Arch Otolaryngol Head Neck Surg 2003;129:1000–1005.

3 Genden EM, Kaufman MR, Katz B, Vine A, Urken ML: Tubed gastro-omental free flap for pharyngoesophageal reconstruction. Arch Otolaryngol Head Neck Surg 2001;127:847–853.

4 Kelly KE, Anthony JP, Singer M: Pharyngoesophageal reconstruction using the radial forearm fasciocutaneous free flap: preliminary results. Otolaryngol Head Neck Surg 1994;111:16–24.

5 Murray DJ, Gilbert RW, Vesely MJ, Novak CB, Zaitlin-Gencher S, Clark JR, Gullane PJ, Neligan PC: Functional outcomes and donor site morbidity following circumferential pharyngoesophageal reconstruction using an anterolateral thigh flap and salivary bypass tube. Head Neck 2007;29:147–154.

6 Op de Coul BM, Hilgers FJ, Balm AJ, Tan IB, van den Hoogen FJ, van TH: A decade of postlaryngectomy vocal rehabilitation in 318 patients: a single institution's experience with consistent application of provox indwelling voice prostheses. Arch Otolaryngol Head Neck Surg 2000;126:1320–1328.

Cernea CR, Dias FL, Fliss D, Lima RA, Myers EN, Wei WI (eds): Pearls and Pitfalls in Head and Neck Surgery. Basel, Karger, 2008, pp 98–99

5.4 How to Choose the Reconstructive Method after Total Pharyngolaryngectomy

William I. Wei, Jimmy Y.W. Chan

Department of Surgery, University of Hong Kong Medical Centre, Queen Mary Hospital, Hong Kong, SAR, China

PEARLS

- The reconstruction options are only determined after assessing the defect following adequate resection of the primary pathology.
- The submucosal extension of tumors in the hypopharynx after radiation is more extensive than that of those without radiotherapy. Most of these submucosal extensions are not visible macroscopically, thus a wider margin of resection is essential for salvage surgery following radiotherapy.
- Branches of the thyrocervical trunk such as the transverse cervical arteries are less frequently affected by radiation and atherosclerosis. They should be used as the recipient vessels for microvascular free flaps.

PITFALLS

- When a pedicled myocutaneous flap is turned into a tube form for reconstruction of a circumferential pharyngeal defect, the incidence of pharyngocutaneous fistula is not negligible and this is particularly so in female patients.
- The procedure of gastric pull-up is associated with some morbidity and hospital mortality and thus should only be considered when the esophagus has to be removed for tumor extirpation.
- Following reconstruction, small leakage at the anastomosis might lead to more significant dehiscence of the anastomosis through contained infection. Thus early release of the leaked saliva or construction of a controlled pharyngostome will facilitate a favorable outcome.

Introduction

The laryngopharyngeal region might be involved by malignant disease. This includes squamous cell carcinoma and very occasionally extensive carcinoma of the thyroid.

The optimal therapy for the extensive squamous cell cancers arising from this region is radical surgery followed by radiotherapy. Concurrent chemoradiation aiming to preserve the larynx can be applied in well-informed patients and in well-equipped institutions. For those patients who developed recurrences after chemoradiation, surgical salvage remains the logical option. The extent of resection depends on the extent of the primary tumor. Only after adequate resection is the optimal reconstruction modality determined.

Practical Tips

The high propensity of submucosal extension of squamous cell carcinoma arising from the laryngopharynx necessitates a wider resection margin, especially when surgery is carried out as a salvage procedure [1]. The location and size of the tumor in the hypopharynx determine the extent of resection and choice of reconstruction procedure [2]. For a small-sized tumor located in the upper part of the hypopharynx, total laryngectomy and partial pharyngectomy are adequate. Thus a strip of pharyngeal mucosa can be left behind to facilitate reconstruction. For a similar small-sized tumor in the lower part of the hypopharynx, where the lumen is smaller and the circumference of the hypopharyngeal wall short, adequate resection with a clear margin would include total laryngectomy and circumferential pharyngectomy. For tumor that is located in the lower part of the hypopharynx or in the cervical esophagus, taking a clear resection margin inferiorly would mean total esophagectomy with the laryngopharyngectomy.

The optimal reconstruction modality should have the following qualities. It should be carried out at the same setting with the resection as a one-stage procedure. Hospital mortality and morbidity should be low and there should be good return of swallowing function soon after the operation [3].

For a partial pharyngeal defect, the pedicled myocutaneous flap offers a quick and reliable method of reconstruction [4]. Sometimes, a microvascular free cutaneous flap transfer, such as the anterolateral thigh flap [5] or the rectus abdominis flap, is used. The entire operation usually takes longer and there is a small chance that the free flap might fail [6].

For a circumferential pharyngeal defect, the optimal reconstructive option is the use of a microvascular free jejunal graft [7]. To avoid going into the abdomen, a microvascular free flap such as the radial forearm flap or the anterolateral thigh flap turning into a tube for the reconstruction of the circumferential defect has also been used [8]. The stenosis at the mucocutaneous junction is not negligible and affects swallowing

Following total laryngopharyngectomy and esophagectomy, the extensive defect can be reconstructed by mobilizing the stomach into the neck. This operation however, has a definite hospital mortality and morbidity as it is a major procedure and the surgical field involves the neck, chest and abdomen [9].

For those patients who had previous operations on the stomach, a pedicled right colon with a terminal ileum could be used to bridge the gap between the oropharynx and the stomach remnant in the abdomen [10].

References

1 Ho CM, Lam KH, Wei WI, Yuen PW, Lam LK: Squamous cell carcinoma of the hypopharynx – analysis of treatment results. Head Neck 1993;15:405–412.

2 Ho CM, Ng WF, Lam KH, Wei WI, Yuen AP: Radial clearance in resection of hypopharyngeal cancer: an independent prognostic factor. Head Neck 2002;24:181–190.

3 Wei WI: The dilemma of treating hypopharyngeal carcinoma: more or less: Hayes Martin Lecture. Arch Otolaryngol Head Neck Surg 2002;128:229–232.

4 Spriano G, Pellini R, Roselli R: Pectoralis major myocutaneous flap for hypopharyngeal reconstruction. Plast Reconstr Surg 2002;110:1408–1413.

5 Yu P, Robb GL: Pharyngoesophageal reconstruction with the anterolateral thigh flap: a clinical and functional outcomes study. Plast Reconstr Surg 2005;116:1845–1855.

6 Lam LK, Wei WI, Chan VS, Ng RW, Ho WK: Microvascular free tissue reconstruction following extirpation of head and neck tumour: experience towards an optimal outcome. J Laryngol Otol 2002;116:929–936.

7 Rosenthal E, Couch M, Farwell DG, Wax MK: Current concepts in microvascular reconstruction. Otolaryngol Head Neck Surg 2007;136:519–524.

8 Yu P, Lewin JS, Reece GP, Robb GL: Comparison of clinical and functional outcomes and hospital costs following pharyngoesophageal reconstruction with the anterolateral thigh free flap versus the jejunal flap. Plast Reconstr Surg 2006;117:968–974.

9 Wei WI, Lam LK, Yuen PW, Wong J: Current status of pharyngolaryngo-esophagectomy and pharyngogastric anastomosis. Head Neck 1998;20:240–244.

10 Sartoris A, Succo G, Mioli P, Merlino G: Reconstruction of the pharynx and cervical esophagus using ileocolic free autograft. Am J Surg 1999;178:316–322.

5

Cernea CR, Dias FL, Fliss D, Lima RA, Myers EN, Wei WI (eds): Pearls and Pitfalls in Head and Neck Surgery. Basel, Karger, 2008, pp 100–101

6.1 Indications for Surgical Treatment of Nasopharyngeal Cancer

William I. Wei, Rockson Wei

Department of Surgery, University of Hong Kong Medical Centre, Queen Mary Hospital, Hong Kong, SAR, China

PEARLS

- Persistent or recurrent tumors that could be salvaged successfully are those that have not infiltrated the internal carotid artery or the skull base bone.
- Evaluation of the status of tumor in the nasopharynx should be carried out by endoscopic examination and biopsy together with imaging studies such as computed tomography (CT) and magnetic resonance imaging.
- Surgical salvage is carried out when the disease is localized at the nasopharynx and/or in the neck. Nasopharyngectomy and radical neck dissection can be carried out in one session.

PITFALLS

- Following radical resection of the disease, exposing too much bone at the skull base might lead to the development of osteoradionecrosis. A microvascular free muscle flap should be used to cover the exposed bone.
- After surgical salvage, follow-up examination of the nasopharynx at regular intervals is essential to monitor progress and to diagnose the development of a second primary tumor.

Introduction

Nasopharyngeal carcinoma (NPC) is a squamous cell carcinoma with different degrees of differentiation and has a high propensity to metastasize to cervical lymph nodes.

In most regions, NPC is uncommon while the incidence of NPC in Hong Kong, located in southern China, was 20–30/100,000 [1]. Even for those southern Chinese who have immigrated to other continents, the incidence of NPC remains high. Radiotherapy is the mainstay of treatment for locoregionally confined NPC as the tumor is radiosensitive. The tumor tends to spread to paranasopharyngeal and cervical lymph nodes, hence prophylactic nodal treatment with radiation is mandatory. The outcome of patients who were treated with radiotherapy has improved significantly in the past 4 decades [2]. In recent years, with the application of intensity-modulated radiotherapy better tumor control with reduction of late complications has been achieved [3]. For locoregionally advanced NPC, concurrent chemoradiotherapy has emerged as the treatment of choice, following the Intergroup 0099 randomized trial [4]. Despite these treatments, a small number of patients still develop persistent or recurrent disease where surgical salvage is indicated.

Practical Tips

After definitive treatment regular endoscopic examination of the nasopharynx should be performed. Evaluation of the copies of Epstein-Barr virus (EBV) DNA in the plasma should be carried out to identify the submucosal tumors. The number of copies of EBV DNA in the blood increases during radiotherapy, meaning that more viral

DNA is released after cell death [5]. Elevated levels of EBV DNA, however, were only detected in 67% of patients with locoregional recurrence when the tumor size was small and still amenable to salvage treatment [6].

The confirmation of persistent or recurrent NPC still depends on the biopsy. To plan the appropriate salvage procedure, endoscopic examination of the nasopharynx evaluates the surface extension of the tumor while the deep extension is best evaluated by imaging.

Magnetic resonance imaging with its multiplanar capability gives a three-dimensional impression of the tumor extension. It is also useful in the detection of paranasopharyngeal and deep cervical nodal metastases [7]. CT should be performed for the evaluation of tumor erosion of bone at the skull base and perineural spread through the foramen ovale. Positron emission tomography is more sensitive than CT and MR in the detection of persistent and recurrent tumors in the nasopharynx.

For small and shallow tumor localized in the nasopharynx, brachytherapy using radioactive gold grains (^{198}Au) as the radiation source can be carried out either transnasally under endoscopic guidance [8] or using the split-palate approach [9]. The procedure was not difficult and morbidity was minimal. With this form of brachytherapy employed for persistent and recurrent tumors, the 5-year local tumor control rates were 87 and 63%, respectively [10].

Brachytherapy, however, has its limitations in bulky or extensive tumor, when eustachian tube cartilage is involved, and in tumor that has extended to the paranasopharyngeal space; in these cases surgical salvage is indicated. When skull base bone or internal carotid artery was exposed following resection of the tumor in the nasopharynx, then the defect should be covered with a microvascular free muscle flap to promote healing and prevent the development of osteoradionecrosis. Nasopharyngectomy with a negative surgical margin provides a better chance of eradicating the persistent or recurrent NPC when compared to reirradiation or stereotactic radiation.

References

1 Parkin DM, Whelan SL, Ferlay J, Raymond L, Young J: Cancer Incidence in Five Continents. Lyon, International Agency for Research on Cancer (IARC Publ No 43), 1997, vol 7, pp 814–815.

2 Lee AW, Sze WM, Au JS, Leung SF, Leung TW, Chua DT, Zee BC, Law SC, Teo PM, Tung SY, Kwong DL, Lau WH: Treatment results for nasopharyngeal carcinoma in the modern era: the Hong Kong experience. Int J Radiat Oncol Biol Phys 2005;61:1107–1116.

3 Kwong DL, Pow EH, Sham JS, McMillan AS, Leung LH, Leung WK, Chua DT, Cheng AC, Wu PM, Au GK: Intensity-modulated radiotherapy for early-stage nasopharyngeal carcinoma: a prospective study on disease control and preservation of salivary function. Cancer 2004;101:1584–1593.

4 Al-Sarraf M, LeBlanc M, Giri PG, Fu KK, Cooper J, Vuong T, Forastiere AA, Adams G, Sakr WA, Schuller DE, Ensley JF: Chemoradiotherapy versus radiotherapy in patients with advanced nasopharyngeal cancer: phase III randomized intergroup study 0099. J Clin Oncol 1998;16:1310–1317.

5 Lo YM, Leung SF, Chan LY, Chan AT, Lo KW, Johnson PJ, Huang DP: Kinetics of plasma Epstein-Barr virus DNA during radiation therapy for nasopharyngeal carcinoma. Cancer Res 2000;60:2351–2355.

6 Wei WI, Yuen AP, Ng RW, Ho WK, Kwong DL, Sham JS: Quantitative analysis of plasma cell-free Epstein-Barr virus DNA in nasopharyngeal carcinoma after salvage nasopharyngectomy: a prospective study. Head Neck 2004;26:878–883.

7 Dillon WP, Mills CM, Kjos B, DeGroot J, Brant-Zawadzki M: Magnetic resonance imaging of the nasopharynx. Radiology 1984;152:731–738.

8 Harrison LB, Weissberg JB: A technique for interstitial nasopharyngeal brachytherapy. Int J Radiat Oncol Biol Phys 1987;13:451–453.

9 Wei WI, Sham JS, Choy D, Ho CM, Lam KH: Split-palate approach for gold grain implantation in nasopharyngeal carcinoma. Arch Otolaryngol Head Neck Surg 1990;116:578–582.

10 Kwong DL, Wei WI, Cheng AC, Choy DT, Lo AT, Wu PM, Sham JS: Long term results of radioactive gold grain implantation for the treatment of persistent and recurrent nasopharyngeal carcinoma. Cancer 2001;91:1105–1113.

Cernea CR, Dias FL, Fliss D, Lima RA, Myers EN, Wei WI (eds): Pearls and Pitfalls in Head and Neck Surgery. Basel, Karger, 2008, pp 102–103

6.2 Practical Tips to Perform a Maxillary Swing Approach

William I. Wei, Raymond W.M. Ng

Department of Surgery, University of Hong Kong Medical Centre, Queen Mary Hospital, Hong Kong, SAR, China

PEARLS

- The holes for the screws on miniplates are drilled before the osteotomies; this ensures precise bony reassembly on closure.
- The free mucosa graft harvests from the removed inferior turbinate on the side of the swing should be thinned to facilitate the graft take over the raw area in the nasopharynx after the maxillary swing procedure.
- The posterior portion of nasal septum is removed to enable adequate visualization and resection of the opposite nasopharynx.
- The internal carotid artery lies outside the pharyngobasilar fascia which might be quite thick after radiation. Palpation of the internal carotid artery through this might be difficult. A small additional neck incision will allow identification of the internal carotid artery in the neck; this can be traced upwards and the finger in the neck will reach superiorly to meet the finger in the nasopharynx, thus locating precisely the internal carotid artery.

PITFALLS

- The internal carotid artery might sometimes be completely exposed after nasopharyngectomy. A microvascular free muscle flap should be employed to cover the exposed internal carotid artery.
- The majority of patients develops some degree of trismus after the maxillary swing procedure, particularly if they have been irradiated. It is important to start passive stretching once wound healing has been completed to reduce this morbidity.

Introduction

Anatomically, the nasopharynx is located in the center of the head; it is difficult to get adequate exposure to remove pathologies in the region. Pathologies in the nasopharynx may arise from its wall or from the vicinity extending into the nasopharynx. These include schwannoma, sarcoma and chordoma.

The antererolateral route, the maxillary swing approach, gives good exposure of the nasopharynx and central skull base for an oncological resection. The most frequent application of this procedure is for surgical salvage of persistent or recurrent nasopharyngeal carcinoma after radiotherapy or concurrent chemoradiotherapy.

Practical Tips

As the most persistent or recurrent nasopharyngeal carcinomas are located on the lateral wall of the nasopharynx, closely associated with the orifice of the eustachian tube, a curative oncological resection should always include these structures. Step serial sectioning of nasopharyngectomy specimens has shown that persistent or recurrent nasopharyngeal carcinomas exhibit extensive submucosal spread and a wide resection of the nasopharynx is mandatory for a favorable outcome [1].

The facial incision is the Weber-Ferguson-Longmire incision as for maxillectomy and this continues between the central incisor teeth onto the hard palate. Initially, this incision on the palate continues in the midline and then turns laterally along the attachment of the soft palate to the hard palate [2]. Soft tissue over the anterior wall of the maxilla is lifted, just enough to expose a narrow strip of anterior bony wall of the maxilla for osteotomy below the orbital floor. The hard palate is divided in the midline and a curved osteotome is used to separate the maxillary tuberosity from the pterygoid plates. The maxilla attached to the cheek flap can be swung laterally as an osteocutaneous complex to expose the central skull base including the nasopharynx and paranasopharyngeal space. The pterygoid plates together with the pterygoid muscle can be removed to improve exposure of the paranasopharyngeal space. Lesions in the nasopharynx and central skull base can all be removed under direct vision [3]. The carotid artery lying external to the pharyngobasilar fascia can also be dissected from the pathology under direct vision.

After extirpation of the lesion in the nasopharynx, the maxilla attached to the anterior cheek flap can be returned and fixed to the rest of the facial skeleton using miniplates or microplates. A prefabricated dental plate is also used to facilitate the precise return of the maxilla. A nasal pack is frequently used for a few days and a nasogastric tube is inserted for 1 week for feeding.

For those patients with localized persistent or recurrent nasopharyngeal carcinoma after chemoradiation, surgical salvage offers the best outcome [4]. The 5-year actuarial control of tumors in the nasopharynx has been reported to be 65% and the 5-year disease-free survival rate was around 54% [5, 6]. Some irradiated patients developed palatal fistula; however, with modification of the palatal incision, separating soft tissue incision and the osteotomy, there was no more palatal fistula [7]. Nasopharyngectomy with this approach also does not affect the quality of life [8].

References

1. Wei WI: Carcinoma of the nasopharynx. Adv Otolaryngol Head Neck Surg 1998;12:119–132.
2. Wei WI, Lam KH, Sham JS: New approach to the nasopharynx: the maxillary swing approach. Head Neck 1991;13:200–207.
3. Wei WI, Ho CM, Yuen PW, Fung CF, Sham JS, Lam KH: Maxillary swing approach for resection of tumors in and around the nasopharynx. Arch Otolaryngol Head Neck Surg 1995;121:638–642.
4. Wei WI, Sham JS: Nasopharyngeal carcinoma. Lancet 2005;365: 2041–2054.
5. Wei WI: Nasopharyngeal cancer: current status of management. Arch Otolaryngol Head Neck Surg 2001;127:766–769.
6. Wei WI: Cancer of the nasopharynx: functional surgical salvage. World J Surg 2003;27:844–848.
7. Ng RW, Wei WI: Elimination of palatal fistula after the maxillary swing procedure. Head Neck 2005;27:608–612.
8. Ng RW, Wei WI: Quality of life of patients with recurrent nasopharyngeal carcinoma treated with nasopharyngectomy using the maxillary swing approach. Arch Otolaryngol Head Neck Surg 2006;132:309–316.

Cernea CR, Dias FL, Fliss D, Lima RA, Myers EN, Wei WI (eds): Pearls and Pitfalls in Head and Neck Surgery. Basel, Karger, 2008, pp 104–105

6.3 Management of Neck Metastases of Nasopharyngeal Carcinoma

William I. Wei, W.K. Ho

Department of Surgery, University of Hong Kong Medical Centre, Queen Mary Hospital, Hong Kong, SAR, China

PEARLS

- Over 50% of patients suffering from nasopharyngeal carcinoma present with cervical lymph node metastasis and most of them respond to concurrent chemoradiotherapy.
- When the lymph node metastases persist or recur after the primary treatment, malignant cells are found in multiple lymph nodes with extensive infiltration.
- For those extensive neck metastases which infiltrate the floor of the neck, brachytherapy in addition to radical neck dissection enhances control of neck disease.

PITFALLS

- Parallel McFee incisions are recommended for necks which were irradiated. Raising the neck skin should be done precisely, as skin necrosis might lead to significant morbidities.
- Despite positive findings on clinical examination, imaging studies and other investigations, 7% of radical neck dissection specimens showed no viable tumor cell.

Introduction

Nasopharyngeal carcinoma has a high propensity to metastasize to cervical lymph nodes. In a retrospective study reporting the clinical features of 4,768 patients, enlarged neck nodes were seen in 74.5% of the patients [1].

As nasopharyngeal carcinoma is chemoradiosensitive, the primary treatment modality of the metastatic lymph node is concurrent chemoradiation. When the neck nodes persist or recur after the primary treatment, surgical salvage is indicated. For those patients with extensive recurrent disease in the neck, brachytherapy should be employed in addition to radical neck dissection to improve the local control.

Practical Tips

The detection of cervical lymph node metastases has improved with cross-sectional imaging studies and functional imaging, such as positron emission tomography. Confirmation of the presence of malignancy in these lymph nodes can be achieved through fine needle aspiration cytology. In view of the high incidence of occult cervical lymph node metastases, prophylactic neck radiation is recommended for all patients and this has shown that locoregional control has improved [2]. In recent years, with the application of intensity-modulated radiotherapy, only 1 patient out of 83 developed failure in the regional lymph nodes at a 3-year follow-up [3]. For patients with advanced nodal disease, the incidence of failure in the neck following concurrent chemoradiation was as high as 33% [4].

For patients with nasopharyngeal carcinoma, when their cervical lymph nodes do not regress completely by 3 months after completion of concomitant chemotherapy and radiotherapy, it is likely that there was residual disease in the nodes.

Fine needle aspiration cytology of the node frequently yields inconclusive results due to the increased fibrosis and the specificity of diagnosis is around 75% [5]. Positron emission tomography has been shown to be able to detect regional recurrence in over 90% of patients [6].

The surgical procedure of salvage is radical neck dissection. The pathological behavior of these nodal metastases in nasopharyngeal carcinoma was reported through a step serial sectioning of 43 radical neck dissection specimens [7]. The findings showed that in over 70% of the specimens, there were more tumor-bearing lymph nodes than anticipated. The distribution of the nodes was in all five levels, although most of them were found in levels II and V. In over 60% of tumor-bearing lymph nodes, there was extracapsular spread and in 35%, tumor cells were seen among the nonlymphatic tissue in the neck. In over 28% of the specimens the tumor-bearing nodes were infiltrating or lying close to the spinal accessory nerve. Thus the surgical salvage procedure for the cervical lymph nodes after radiotherapy or chemoradiation should be radical neck dissection [7]. The reported 5-year tumor control rate in the neck was 66% and the 5-year actuarial survival was 38% [8].

In patients with advanced neck disease, despite adequate radical neck dissection, microscopic tumor might still be left behind. Afterloading brachytherapy could be applied to the surgical bed. The overlying skin, which was irradiated initially, might not be able to tolerate this additional brachytherapy. Thus the area of skin over the brachytherapy source had to be removed at the time of the neck dissection. This cutaneous defect should be reconstructed with nonirradiated skin such as a deltopectoral flap, lateral thoracic flap [9] or a pectoralis major myocutaneous flap. For those patients with extensive neck disease, with this form of adjuvant therapy, the local tumor control rate has been reported to be comparable to when radical neck dissection alone was performed for less extensive neck disease [10].

References

1 Lee AW, Foo W, Law SC, Poon YF, Sze WM, O SK, Tung SY, Lau WH: Nasopharyngeal carcinoma: presenting symptoms and duration before diagnosis. Hong Kong Med J 1997;3:355–361.
2 Lee AW, Lau WH, Tung SY, Chua DT, Chappell R, Xu L, Siu L, Sze WM, Leung TW, Sham JS, Ngan RK, Law SC, Yau TK, Au JS, O'Sullivan B, Pang ES, O SK, Au GK, Lau JT; Hong Kong Nasopharyngeal Cancer Study Group: Preliminary results of a randomized study on therapeutic gain by concurrent chemotherapy for regionally-advanced nasopharyngeal carcinoma: NPC-9901 Trial by the Hong Kong Nasopharyngeal Cancer Study Group. J Clin Oncol 2005;23:6966–6975.
3 Liu MT, Hsieh CY, Chang TH, Lin JP, Huang CC, Wang AY: Prognostic factors affecting the outcome of nasopharyngeal carcinoma. Jpn J Clin Oncol 2003;33:501–508.
4 Palazzi M, Guzzo M, Bossi P, Tomatis S, Cerrotta A, Cantu G, Locati LD, Licitra L: Regionally advanced nasopharyngeal carcinoma: long-term outcome after sequential chemotherapy and radiotherapy. Tumori 2004;90:60–65.
5 Toh ST, Yuen HW, Goh YH, Goh CHK: Evaluation of recurrent nodal disease after definitive radiation therapy for nasopharyngeal carcinoma: diagnostic value of fine-needle aspiration cytology and CT scan. Head Neck 2007;29:370–377.
6 Yen TC, Chang YC, Chan SC, Chang JT, Hsu CH, Lin KJ, Lin WJ, Fu YK, Ng SH: Are dual-phase 18F-FDG PET scans necessary in nasopharyngeal carcinoma to assess the primary tumour and loco-regional nodes? Eur J Nucl Med Mol Imaging 2005;32:541–548.
7 Wei WI, Ho CM, Wong MP, Ng WF, Lau SK, Lam KH: Pathological basis of surgery in the management of postradiotherapy cervical metastasis in nasopharyngeal carcinoma. Arch Otolaryngol Head Neck Surg 1992;118:923–929.
8 Wei WI, Lam KH, Ho CM, Sham JS, Lau SK: Efficacy of radical neck dissection for the control of cervical metastasis after radiotherapy for nasopharyngeal carcinoma. Am J Surg 1990;160:439–442.
9 Yuen AP, Ng WM: Surgical techniques and results of lateral cutaneous, myocutaneous, and conjoint flaps for head and neck reconstruction. Laryngoscope 2007;117:288–294.
10 Wei WI, Ho WK, Cheng AC, Wu X, Li GK, Nicholls J, Yuen PW, Sham JS: Management of extensive cervical nodal metastasis in nasopharyngeal carcinoma after radiotherapy: a clinicopathological study. Arch Otolaryngol Head Neck Surg 2001;127:1457–1462.

6

Cernea CR, Dias FL, Fliss D, Lima RA, Myers EN, Wei WI (eds): Pearls and Pitfalls in Head and Neck Surgery. Basel, Karger, 2008, pp 106–107

7.1 Practical Tips to Identify the Main Trunk of the Facial Nerve

Fernando L. Dias[a, b], Roberto A. Lima[a, b], Jorge Pinho[c]

[a] Head and Neck Surgery Department, Brazilian National Cancer Institute and
[b] Post-Graduation School of Medicine, Catholic University of Rio de Janeiro, Rio de Janeiro, and
[c] Memorial San Jose Hospital of Recife, Recife, Brazil

PEARLS

- Identification of the anatomic landmarks is paramount.
- The pointer of the tragal cartilage indicates the position of CN VII trunk.
- In reoperations or when the identification is obscured (by the tumor), try the retrograde approach.

PITFALLS

- Avoid going directly to the CN VII trunk area before identifying the anatomic landmarks.
- The styloid process is not a good landmark to retrieve the CN VII.

Introduction

The facial nerve (CN VII) exits the skull base through the stylomastoid foramen, located slightly posterolateral to the styloid process and anteromedial to the mastoid process. The main trunk of the CN VII passes through the parotid gland and, at the pes anserinus (Latin: goose's foot), divides into the temporofacial and cervicofacial divisions approximately 1.3 cm from the stylomastoid foramen [1].

Although there are several ways to develop surgical access to the CN VII (and the surgeon must be familiar with all of them), the most popular is the antegrade approach with the identification of the main trunk first [2]. Facial nerve paresis or paralysis can occur as an early complication following surgical procedures involving the parotid gland and the CN VII. Temporary paralysis occurs in 10–30% of superficial parotidectomies, while permanent CN VII paralysis occurs in less than 1% [3].

Practical Tips

It is important to keep in mind that the anatomic landmarks in the operative identification of the CN VII (posterior belly of the digastric muscle, mastoid process, timpanic bone and esternal auditory canal cartilage) should always be exposed prior to any attempt at identifying the nerve, and that the parotid parenchyma should not be incised without first locating and following the CN VII.

1 Superficial or total parotidectomy is performed under general anesthesia. Long-term paralytic agents should be avoided to allow for CN VII monitoring when indicated [2–5].

2 The nerve lies approximately 1.0–1.5 cm deep and slightly anterior and inferior to the tip of the external canal cartilage (also called 'pointer') [2–5].

3 The nerve lies approximately 1.0 cm deep to the medial attachment of the posterior belly of the digastric muscle to the digastric groove of the mastoid bone [2–5].

④ The tympanomastoid fissure, located between the mastoid and the tympanic bones, begins just distal to the suprameatal spine. The CN VII lies 6–8 mm distal to the end point of this fissure [2–5].
⑤ The CN VII usually courses superficial to the facial vein and division of this structure (as well as the division of the external jugular vein) can contribute to increasing venous bleeding during dissection of the gland [3].
⑥ The stylomandibular artery, which lies just superficial to the nerve as it enters the gland, may provoke troublesome bleeding if not ligated and divided [2].
⑦ If the proximal segment of the CN VII is obscured, retrograde dissection of one or more of the peripheral CN VII branches may be necessary to identify the main trunk [2, 3, 5].
⑧ When necessary, the CN VII can be identified in the mastoid bone by mastoidectomy and followed peripherally. This approach is usually reserved for unusual recurrences, intratympanic or large tumors [2, 3].
⑨ The use of wide-angled surgical loupes with 2.5–3.5× magnifying lenses and facial nerve monitoring may facilitate the identification of the nerve, particularly in reoperations or in situations where the anatomy is not clear [2–5].
⑩ Although recommended by some, the styloid process should not be used as a landmark for finding the trunk of the CN VII since this increases the risk of damaging the nerve [4].

Conclusion

Operative identification of the main trunk of the CN VII is a step-by-step procedure in which previous identification of the anatomic landmarks described above is highly advisable. The opening of the preauricular space allows the exposure of the tragal cartilage pointer which is the last and most important landmark for the identification of the main trunk of the CN VII.

References

1 Holsinger FC, Bui DT: Anatomy, function, and evaluation of the salivary glands; in Myers EN, Ferris RL (eds): Salivary Gland Disorders. Berlin, Springer, 2007, pp 1–16.
2 Granick MS, Hanna DC 3rd: Surgical management of salivary gland disease; in Grannick MS, Hanna DC 3rd (eds): Management of Salivary Gland Lesions. Baltimore, Williams & Wilkins, 1992, pp 145–174.
3 Wang SJ, Eisele DW: Superficial parotidectomy; in Myers EN, Ferris RL (eds): Salivary Gland Disorders. Berlin, Springer, 2007, pp 247–246.
4 Mihelke A: Surgery of the salivary glands and the extratemporal portion of the facial nerve; in Nauman HH (ed): Head and Neck Surgery: Indications, Techniques, and Pitfalls. Philadelphia, Saunders, 1980, pp 421–465.
5 Shah JP, Patel SG: Salivary glands; in Shah JP, Patel SG (eds): Head and Neck Surgery and Oncology, ed 3. Edinburgh, Mosby, 2003, pp 439–474.

Cernea CR, Dias FL, Fliss D, Lima RA, Myers EN, Wei WI (eds): Pearls and Pitfalls in Head and Neck Surgery. Basel, Karger, 2008, pp 108–109

7.2 Retrograde Approach to Facial Nerve: Indications and Technique

Flavio C. Hojaij, Caio Plopper, Claudio R. Cernea

Department of Head and Neck Surgery, University of São Paulo Medical School, São Paulo, Brazil

PEARLS

- Useful technique for peripheral tumors or for difficult identification of the facial nerve.
- Avoid wide dissections of the facial nerve in peripheral tumors.
- Use magnifying lenses and electrical neural stimulation.

PITFALLS

- It should not be used for tumors involving many branches of the facial nerve.
- Lack of constant anatomical landmarks for identification of the terminal branches, except for the mandibular marginal nerve.

Introduction

Surgical procedures on the parotid gland are challenging for head and neck surgeons for a number of reasons. About 80% of parotid gland tumors are benign, and the importance of preservation of the facial nerve in these operations cannot be overemphasized. Therefore, thorough knowledge of the anatomy of the facial nerve and its branches is absolutely necessary [1].

Usually, the facial nerve, whose primary function is facial mobility, emerges through the stylomastoid foramen, and its plane divides the gland into a superficial and a deep lobe. Most commonly, the trunk of the facial nerve divides into two main branches: temporofacial and cervicofacial divisions. However, on rare occasions it can emerge from the stylomastoid foramen already in two branches. A wide variety of branches can emerge through these main divisions. Due to these variations, the terminal divisions of the facial nerve are better named after their anatomical distribution into temporal, zygomatic, buccal, marginal mandibular and cervical nerves.

Usually, the most comfortable approach to the facial nerve in parotid gland operations is to find its main trunk. It is a larger anatomical structure, its anatomical landmarks are more constant, and dissection from the trunk to smaller branches is often safer. However, in some situations, a retrograde dissection can become necessary or preferable [2].

Practical Tips

Indications

1. Peripheral parotid lesion, localized near one or two terminal branches of the facial nerve, and with a small margin of normal salivary tissue.
2. Parotid lesion whose localization is so peripheral that long dissection from the main trunk of the facial nerve is considered too morbid [3].
3. Conditions that preclude safe identification of the facial nerve (such as fibrosis due to reoperations and infections, or tumors adjacent to the mastoid process).

Technique

The terminal branch of the facial nerve with fewer anatomical variations and determined anatomical landmarks is the marginal mandibular nerve. Peripheral identification of the other terminal branches lacks constant anatomical landmarks and depends on careful dissection in the midst of facial muscles and fascia, medial to the parotid gland (whose limits are also not well defined, making that task even more troublesome).

Some tips can be of help in those situations:

1 Use of surgical magnification lenses.

2 Use of intraoperative electrical stimulation of the branches of the facial nerve (which can be monitored visually or, more effectively, with electromyography) [4].

3 Identification of the marginal mandibular nerve with the following anatomical landmarks:

- Angle of the mandible.
- Retromandibular vein (largest branch of the external jugular vein); the nerves usually cross the vein anteriorly.

4 The nerve branches become wider as retrograde dissection progresses and other terminal branches can join the dissected one; therefore, salivary tissue division must be done more carefully to avoid nerve injury.

References

1 Fee WE, Tran LE: Evaluation of a patient with a parotid tumor. Arch Otolaryngol Head Neck Surg 2003;129:937–938.

2 Myssiorek D: Removal of the inferior half of the superficial lobe is sufficient to treat pleomorphic adenoma in the tail of the parotid gland. Arch Otolaryngol Head Neck Surg 1999;125:1164–1165.

3 López M, Quer M, León X, Orús C, Recher K, Vergés J: Usefulness of facial nerve monitoring during parotidectomy. Acta Otorrinolaringol Esp 2001;52:418–421.

4 Bhattacharyya N, Richardson ME, Gugino LD: An objective assessment of the advantages of retrograde parotidectomy. Otolaryngol Head Neck Surg 2004;131:392–396.

Cernea CR, Dias FL, Fliss D, Lima RA, Myers EN, Wei WI (eds): Pearls and Pitfalls in Head and Neck Surgery. Basel, Karger, 2008, pp 110–111

7.3 Intraoperative Decisions for Sacrificing the Facial Nerve in Parotid Surgery

Randal S. Weber, F. Christopher Holsinger

Department of Head and Neck Surgery, University of Texas M.D. Anderson Cancer Center, Houston, Tex., USA

Pearls

- In patients with a parotid neoplasms and normal facial function, facial nerve (FN) preservation should always be attempted.
- When the tumor abuts the FN, a subepineural plane of dissection is possible: the tumor may be 'peeled off' of the FN.
- For microscopic residual disease, postoperative radiotherapy is effective for achieving local control with preservation of FN function.
- When the nerve is encased or preoperative facial paralysis is present, resect all involved branches or the main trunk as necessary.

Pitfalls

- FN preservation where gross disease remains increases the risk for local recurrence.
- Parotid lymphoma may be confused with a primary parotid neoplasm and sacrifice of the FN is inappropriate for this disease.

Introduction

Malignant tumors account for 20% of neoplasms arising within the parotid gland. Signs of malignancy are pain, extension to the skin, fixation to surrounding structures, FN paresis or paralysis and lymph node metastasis. Computed tomography and magnetic resonance imaging are helpful for evaluating salivary gland tumors but do not provide consistent information for differentiating benign from malignant disease [1]. Fine needle aspiration (FNA) biopsy will correctly identify neoplasia in over 85% of patients but differentiating benign from malignant disease is more difficult and has lower accuracy. The potential for a false-positive diagnosis of malignancy by FNA and frozen section exists in 25–30% of patients and these studies should not dictate sacrifice of the FN. Ultrasound-guided core-needle biopsy and open incisional biopsy are useful adjuncts in the diagnostic armamentarium. A preoperative definitive diagnosis obtained can identify malignancy or lymphoma, thus altering either management or allowing the surgeon to better prepare the patient for FN sacrifice.

The most common primary malignancies of the parotid gland are mucoepidermoid carcinoma followed by adenoid cystic carcinoma, carcinoma ex pleomorphic adenoma, and acinic cell carcinoma. Metastasis to the parotid from a primary cutaneous tumor is also a consideration. Many tumors arising within or metastatic to the parotid gland can invade the FN by direct extension or through neurotropic spread along the nerve. Although many tumors can display perineural invasion, adenoid cystic carcinoma is the most common tumor associated with this phenomenon. In one review, half of the patients (79/160) presented with perineural invasion. Major named nerves were involved in 50% of patients; the remainder had small caliber nerve involvement [2]. Major nerve involvement is associated with both increased locoregional failure and diminished survival [2].

Practical Tips

1 Surgery with wide excision of the tumor is usually chosen as the primary treatment. Superficial parotidectomy usually provides total tumor excision unless the tumor arises within the deep lobe or there is direct extension from the superficial lobe to the deep lobe.

2 When normal FN function is present preoperatively, every effort should be made to preserve the nerve during surgery. Occasionally, salivary tumors must be sharply dissected from the FN, potentially leaving microscopic disease behind [3]. Every attempt should be made not to leave gross tumor. If microscopic residual tumor is suspected, postoperative radiation therapy to the parotid bed is indicated [4–6]. Occasionally, in advanced tumors, nerve encasement necessitates resection of the FN and adjacent structures as indicated by the extent of the tumor. The proximal and distal nerve segments should be examined by frozen section to insure complete tumor eradication. A mastoidectomy is occasionally necessary to achieve negative margins on the proximal stump of the FN.

3 Excellent local control (90%) for patients with parotid cancers treated with surgery and ipsilateral postoperative radiation, based on the M.D. Anderson Cancer Center experience [6]. A postoperative dose of 60 Gy in 30 fractions to the operative bed is recommended. When a major, named nerve is invaded, the path of the nerve is treated electively to the central nervous system or ganglion.

Conclusion

FN preservation for patients with malignant parotid tumors is an accepted contemporary management paradigm. When the nerve is encased by tumor or is not functioning preoperatively, it should be sacrificed. An acceptable surgical technique is to sharply dissect the tumor off of the nerve in the subepineural plane. If microscopic disease remains, postoperative radiation therapy is indicated. Local regional control is excellent and the patient's quality of life is improved through preservation of FN function.

References

1 Koyuncu M, Seşen T, Akan H, et al: Comparison of computed tomography and magnetic resonance imaging in the diagnosis of parotid tumors. Otolaryngol Head Neck Surg 2003;129:726–732.

2 Fordice J, Kershaw C, El-Naggar A, Goepfert H: Adenoid cystic carcinoma of the head and neck: predictors of morbidity and mortality. Arch Otolaryngol Head Neck Surg 1999;125:149–152.

3 Guillamondegui OM, Byers RM, Luna MA, et al: Aggressive surgery in treatment for parotid cancer: the role of adjunctive postoperative radiotherapy. Am J Roentgenol Radium Ther Nucl Med 1975;123:49–54.

4 Garden AS, el-Naggar AK, Morrison WH, et al: Postoperative radiotherapy for malignant tumors of the parotid gland. Int J Radiat Oncol Biol Phys 1997;37:79–85.

5 Armstrong JG, Harrison LB, Spiro RH, et al: Malignant tumors of major salivary gland origin. A matched-pair analysis of the role of combined surgery and postoperative radiotherapy. Arch Otolaryngol Head Neck Surg 1990;116:290–293.

6 Garden AS, Weber RS, Morrison WH, et al: The influence of positive margins and nerve invasion in adenoid cystic carcinoma of the head and neck treated with surgery and radiation. Int J Radiat Oncol Biol Phys 1995;32:619–626.

Cernea CR, Dias FL, Fliss D, Lima RA, Myers EN, Wei WI (eds): Pearls and Pitfalls in Head and Neck Surgery. Basel, Karger, 2008, pp 112–113

7.4 When and How to Reconstruct the Resected Facial Nerve in Parotid Surgery

Peter C. Neligan

University of Washington Medical Center, Seattle, Wash., USA

PEARLS

- Reconstruct immediately in case of intraoperative damage.
- Tension-free repair.
- Consider graft if gap exists.
- Consider static sling to hold position while awaiting nerve recovery.
- Static/dynamic reconstruction for established palsy.

PITFALLS

- Proximal injury is more likely to result in synkinesis.
- Long nerve grafts are likely to yield inferior results.
- Postoperative radiation may result in poor nerve recovery.

Introduction

Management of facial nerve problems related to parotid surgery falls under 4 headings: (1) direct repair, (2) nerve graft, (3) static slings and (4) dynamic reconstruction.

Practical Tips

1 *Direct Repair.* If the nerve is cut during parotidectomy it is best repaired directly under magnification. Recovery depends on multiple factors [1]. Synkinesis, facial spasm, and mass movement are complications particularly following proximal repairs. Direct tension-free repair is optimal.

2 *Nerve Grafting.* If a gap exists in the nerve, a graft should be considered. Donor nerve selection depends on gap length and how many cables are required. For short gaps, the greater auricular nerve or the ansa cervicalis are good donors. The sural nerve is best for larger defects. Success is multifactorial. The possibility of achieving tone makes grafting worthwhile since the donor morbidity associated with sural nerve harvest is low and significant function may be regained.

Nerve Transfer. When the proximal nerve stump is not available, alternative donor nerves may be used including the glossopharyngeal, accessory, phrenic and hypoglossal nerves. Control of facial muscles reinnervated in this way can be unnatural, uncoordinated and synkinetic. The hypoglossal nerve, the advantages and disadvantages of which have been widely reported [2], is commonly used. Tongue atrophy and associated difficulty with mastication, speech and swallowing are known complications [3]. More recently, the masseter motor nerve has been successfully used as a transfer. Donor morbidity is minimal.

Nerve transfers are also used to 'baby-sit' the facial muscles and maintain their motor end plates until a cross-facial nerve graft can be brought over from the normal side.

3 *Static Slings.* Static procedures to improve facial symmetry utilize slings of plantaris, palmar-

is longus or second or third toe extensor tendon, fascia lata or Gore-Tex that are anchored between key points in the upper lip and modiolus and the fascia overlying the zygoma or temporalis. Overcorrection is frequently required in anticipation of stretching of the sling and relaxation of the facial tissues. A static sling can improve function by correcting the commissural droop that may cause drooling particularly with liquids. It can also improve speech by holding the cheek in a better position.

④ *Dynamic Reconstruction.* Dynamic reconstruction can be achieved using a regional muscle such as the masseter or temporalis or a free muscle such as the gracilis or pectoralis minor. The excursion produced by regional muscles is disappointing. Furthermore, transfer of these muscles can produce significant morbidity, e.g. temporal hollowing following temporalis transfer. A more reliable result can be obtained using a functioning muscle transfer such as the gracilis [4] either driven by a cross-facial nerve graft from the contralateral side in a 2-stage procedure, or by the masseter motor [5] nerve from the same side in a single stage procedure.

Management of the Eye. Inability of eye closure and loss of the blink reflex render the cornea prone to injury, and may lead to blindness. The ectropic lower eyelid interferes with tear transport, resulting in epiphora. The most common procedure involves gold weight placement in the upper eyelid, anterior to and secured to the tarsal plate [6]. Complications include under or overcorrection, a visible bulge, infection and implant extrusion.

Spring devices are also available but placement and tension adjustment can be difficult and complications more common. Tarsorrhaphy may aid eye closure but the visual field is compromised and eye appearance can be unsatisfactory.

Temporalis muscle transfer can provide dynamic eyelid closure. A strip of temporalis muscle is extended with fascia or tendon, passed through the upper and lower eyelid, and fastened to the medial canthal ligament [7]. Complications include a slit-like palpebral aperture with lateral movement and skin wrinkling of the lateral lid on closure. There may be a muscle bulge over the lateral orbital margin as well as some synkinetic eyelid movement when chewing. However, forceful and full eyelid closure can result.

References

1 Eaton DA, Hirsch BE, Mansour OI: Recovery of facial nerve function after repair or grafting: our experience with 24 patients. Am J Otolaryngol 2007;28:37–41.
2 Yamamoto Y, Sekido M, Furukawa H, et al: Surgical rehabilitation of reversible facial palsy: facial-hypoglossal network system based on neural signal augmentation/neural supercharge concept. J Plast Reconstr Aesthet Surg 2007;60:223–231.
3 Malik TH, Kelly G, Ahmed A, et al: A comparison of surgical techniques used in dynamic reanimation of the paralyzed face. Otol Neurotol 2005;26:284–291.
4 Harii K: Microneurovascular free muscle transplantation for reanimation of facial paralysis. Clin Plast Surg 1979;6:361–375.
5 Manktelow RT, Tomat LR, Zuker RM, et al: Smile reconstruction in adults with free muscle transfer innervated by the masseter motor nerve: effectiveness and cerebral adaptation. Plast Reconstr Surg 2006;118:885–899.
6 Manktelow RT: Use of the gold weight for lagophthalmos. Oper Tech Plast Reconstr Surg 1999;6:157.
7 Salimbeni G: Eyelid reanimation in facial paralysis by temporalis muscle transfer. Oper Tech Plast Reconstr Surg 1999;6:159.

Cernea CR, Dias FL, Fliss D, Lima RA, Myers EN, Wei WI (eds): Pearls and Pitfalls in Head and Neck Surgery. Basel, Karger, 2008, pp 114–115

7.5 Approaches to Deep Lobe Parotid Tumors

Richard V. Smith

Department of Otorhinolaryngology – Head and Neck Surgery, Albert Einstein College of Medicine, Bronx, N.Y., USA

PEARLS

- Evaluate the position of the posterior facial vein on preoperative imaging to confirm suspicion of a deep lobe tumor.
- The fat pad deep to the superior constrictor muscle will be medial to a deep lobe parotid parapharyngeal mass.
- Most parapharyngeal parotid tumors can be removed through a transcervical approach without exposing the facial nerve or performing a mandibulotomy.
- Malignant parapharyngeal parotid tumors require mandibulotomy for resection.

PITFALLS

- Adequate counseling of a patient with a deep lobe parotid mass is essential; discuss facial nerve resection and grafting.
- Obtain preoperative needle biopsy, if possible, to facilitate discussion and decision on approach.
- Facial nerve tolerance to manipulation is capricious, so avoid unnecessary dissection of the nerve or traction on the nerve with parotid retraction.

Introduction

Accurate identification that a mass is from the deep parotid lobe is the most important aspect of its surgery. The deep lobe is defined as the parotid tissue medial to the facial nerve, and its tumors may present externally, as a parotid mass, or be a radiographic finding of a parapharyngeal space mass. The distinction between the two is the primary factor in choosing the appropriate approach, and relies upon imaging.

Either CT or MRI scans can be used to identify a deep lobe mass [1], and the choice of which to use depends upon the location of the lesion. For palpable lesions, a CT is often obtained in conjunction with a fine needle aspiration. A 'dumbbell' deep lobe tumor occupies the spaces medial and lateral to the posterior border of the mandibular ramus. Otherwise, the radiographic position of the posterior facial vein, better defined on CT imaging, is used to classify the mass, as this vein will be lateral to any deep lobe mass. MRI, on the other hand, can provide more information on the parapharyngeal deep lobe parotid tumor [2]. These tumors exist in the prestyloid parapharyngeal space, and their identification is aided by both the signal characteristics of the mass and the position of the fat pad deep to the superior constrictor muscle, an important landmark. A parapharyngeal deep lobe parotid tumor will thin and medialize that fat pad, but will rarely obliterate it or render it unobservable on MRI scans.

Practical Tips

Lateral or Dumbbell Tumors

① These are removed through a standard superficial parotidectomy approach using a preauricular incision with a cervical or rhytidectomy extension.

② Adequate exposure requires mobilization, or removal, of the superficial lobe, exposing the pertinent branches of the facial nerve.

③ Preserve as much of the superficial lobe as possible to minimize the cosmetic defect, the incidence of facial weakness, and gustatory sweating. The superficial lobe may be reflected anteriorly, away from the deep lobe mass, and can be replaced following removal of the tumor [3–5].

④ Mobilize the facial nerve sharply off the underlying mass, then dissect the tumor from the surrounding tissues through the spaces between the facial nerve branches.

⑤ Carefully retract the nerve during the dissection, taking care to avoid significant stretch, or desiccation, of the nerve.

⑥ Dumbbell tumors often require division of the stylomandibular ligament to allow excision.

Parapharyngeal Parotid Tumors

① Rarely approached directly through the parotid gland.

② Although not visualized, the facial nerve is rarely injured, but is vulnerable.

③ The transcervical approach is adequate for the majority of these, mobilizing the submandibular gland anteriorly, dividing the stylomandibular ligament, and dissecting from below.

④ Even extremely large tumors can be removed transcervically.

⑤ Any suggestion of an invasive malignancy, by needle biopsy or imaging, should prompt a paramedian mandibulotomy approach, sparing the neurovascular bundle of the mandible.

Conclusions

Deep lobe parotid tumors must be characterized as either lateral or parapharyngeal to determine the appropriate surgical approach for excision. A transparotid approach should be used for lateral or dumbbell tumors, reflecting the normal superficial lobe and replacing it to its normal anatomic position at the completion of the surgery. A transcervical approach should be employed for the majority of parapharyngeal deep lobe parotid tumors, with malignant tumors necessitating a wider approach through a paramedian mandibulotomy and mandibular 'swing'. The surgeon must be aware of the pros and cons of the various approaches to minimize unnecessary complications.

References

1 Divi V, Fatt MA, Teknos TN, Mukherji SK: Use of cross-sectional imaging in predicting surgical location of parotid neoplasms. J Comput Assist Tomogr 2005;29:315–319.

2 Som PM, Sacher M, Stollman AL, Biller HF, Lawson W: Common tumors of the parapharyngeal space: refined imaging diagnosis. Radiology 1988;169:81–85.

3 Avery CME, Fleming K, Siegmund CJ: Preservation of the superficial lobe with tumours of the deep-lobe of the parotid. Br J Oral Maxillofac Surg 2007;45:247–248.

4 Colella G, Giudice A, Rambaldi PF, Cuccurullo V: Parotid function after selective deep lobe parotidectomy. Br J Oral Maxillofac Surg 2007;45:108–111.

5 Hussain A, Murray DP: Preservation of the superficial lobe for deep-lobe parotid tumors: a better aesthetic outcome. Ear Nose Throat J 2005;84:518, 520–524.

Cernea CR, Dias FL, Fliss D, Lima RA, Myers EN, Wei WI (eds): Pearls and Pitfalls in Head and Neck Surgery. Basel, Karger, 2008, pp 116–117

7.6 Recurrent Parotid Pleomorphic Adenoma

Bruce J. Davidson

Department of Otolaryngology – Head and Neck Surgery, Georgetown University Medical Center, Washington, D.C., USA

PEARLS

- Recurrent parotid pleomorphic adenoma (RPPA) presents, on average, 15 years after the initial surgery and 3/4 of cases have a multifocal recurrence.
- Previous operative notes and pathology as well as current imaging studies should be reviewed.
- The use of intraoperative facial nerve (FN) monitoring is associated with shorter surgical times, less severe immediate paresis and shorter nerve recovery times.
- Radiotherapy (RT) is more commonly utilized after second recurrences.

PITFALLS

- The number (one to hundreds) and size (some <1 mm) of tumor foci can impair complete resection of recurrent disease (RD).
- Immediate FN paresis occurs in over 50% after surgery for RPPA.
- Second recurrences of PPA are seen in about 50% of cases at 10 years and 75% of cases at 15 years.

Introduction

When PPA were treated by enucleation, tumor recurrence rate was 10–45% [1]. With adoption of superficial parotidectomy (SP), it has dropped to 2–5% [1]. RD typically presents many years after the initial surgery [1]. In a report, the mean time from the initial surgery was 15 years with a range of 2–50 years [2]. This long period of time might influence the observation that the mean age at initial operation for patients later developing recurrent adenoma, 34 years, is about 10 years lower than of those who do not show evidence of recurrence [2]. Incomplete capsule, penetration of the tumor capsule by tumor cells, pseudopodia and satellite nodules may contribute to recurrence. Zbären and Stauffer [1] showed that one of these features was present in over 70% of pleomorphic adenoma specimens. Usually, the patient with RPPA presents with multiple masses in the parotid bed [3]. Rarely, facial weakness may be present at RPPAs, but it should raise concern for a carcinoma ex-pleomorphic adenoma. While multifocality (MF) is rare in PPAs, it is present in 73% of RPPAs [2]. The number of tumor nodules ranges from 2–20 in one series [2] and 1–266 (mean 26) in another [4]. Many of these nodules may be <1 mm, making a comprehensive resection of RD difficult. The local control rate after surgery for RPPA ranges from 65–85% [5]. Series that report using surgery with adjuvant RT in all cases report local control rates of 79–95% [5]. Certainly after a second recurrence, most would advocate the addition of adjuvant RT.

Practical Tips

1. Preoperative workup: It should include both imaging and biopsy. MRI is preferred, particularly with concern for subtle multifocal disease.

Biopsy can be performed by FNA if the nodules are large or as open incision in small nodules.

❷ Surgical planning: Previous operative notes and pathology should be reviewed to determine the following: initial tumor MF, extent of the previous surgery, eventual rupture of the tumor capsule and positive margins. Imaging evaluates present MF, amount of residual parotid tissue and its relationship with the subcutaneous tissue, the FN, the deep parotid lobe, and the parapharyngeal space.

❸ Surgical treatment: If the initial surgery was less than an SP, the surgery for recurrence will be a revision SP or total parotidectomy (TP) with FN dissection and preservation. If a standard SP was performed previously, and there is a single focus of RPPA, surgery will be limited to local resection. If the recurrence is multifocal, a TP should be performed. The previous scar is usually excised.

❹ FN management: It should be preserved unless there is documentation of malignant infiltrating disease. Preoperative facial weakness may be a clue, but occasionally infiltration may be seen in a case with normal FN function. Benign tumors may be dissected away from the nerve in the vast majority of cases, although the dissection is made considerably more difficult by scarring from prior operations. The rate of permanent FN weakness after parotidectomy for primary disease has been reported to be 6%, and involving all branches of the FN is under 1% [6]. Surgery for RPPA is associated with a rate of immediate FN paresis of 56% [4] to 100% [7]. Others have reported a 16% [7] to 21% [2] rate of permanent facial paresis. Use of intraoperative FN monitoring does not replace the need for meticulous dissection, but some added statistical benefit was reported [7]; it is therefore recommended in surgery for RPPA.

❺ Magnification: 2.5× magnification is suggested, but greater power may be helpful, particularly if nerve repair is required. The surgical microscope may also be employed, particularly to manage the FN branches within fibrosed tissue.

References

1 Zbären P, Stauffer E: Pleomorphic adenoma of the parotid gland: histopathologic analysis of the capsular characteristics of 218 tumors. Head Neck 2007;29:751–757.
2 Zbären P, Tschumi I, Nuyens M, Stauffer E: Recurrent pleomorphic adenoma of the parotid gland. Am J Surg 2005;189:203–207.
3 Leonetti JP, Marzo SJ, Petruzzelli GJ, Herr B: Recurrent pleomorphic adenoma of the parotid gland. Otolaryngol Head Neck Surg 2005;133:319–322.
4 Wittekindt C, Streubel K, Arnold G, Stennert E, Guntinas-Lichius O: Recurrent pleomorphic adenoma of the parotid gland: analysis of 108 consecutive patients. Head Neck 2007;29:822–828.
5 Chen AM, Garcia J, Bucci MK, Quivey JM, Eisele DM: Recurrent pleomorphic adenoma of the parotid gland: long-term outcome of patients treated with radiation therapy. Int J Radiat Oncol Biol Phys 2006;66:1031–1035.
6 Guntinas-Lichius O, Klussmann JP, Wittekindt C, Stennert E: Parotidectomy for benign parotid disease at a University Teaching Hospital: outcome of 963 operations. Laryngoscope 2006;116:534–540.
7 Makeieff M, Venail F, Cartier C, Garrel R, Crampette L, Guerrier B: Continuous facial nerve monitoring during pleomorphic adenoma recurrence surgery. Laryngoscope 2005;115:1310–1314.

Cernea CR, Dias FL, Fliss D, Lima RA, Myers EN, Wei WI (eds): Pearls and Pitfalls in Head and Neck Surgery. Basel, Karger, 2008, pp 118–119

7.7 How to Overcome Limitations of Fine Needle Aspiration and Frozen Section Biopsy during Operations for Salivary Gland Tumors

Alfio José Tincani, Sanford Dubner

State University of Campinas – UNICAMP, Campinas, Brazil

PEARLS

- The great majority of salivary gland tumors can be diagnosed by fine needle aspiration (FNA) and confirmed by frozen section (FS).
- The use of ultrasound to guide the FNA increases the method's accuracy.

PITFALLS

- When there is clinical suspicion of malignancy, not confirmed by FNA, FS must be performed.
- Extremely cellular tumors, inconclusive samples or tumors in which there is inadequate material submitted to FNA indicate that FS must be performed.

Introduction

Salivary gland tumors are rare neoplasms, usually benign (especially those in the parotid gland). Sometimes, they present a challenge for diagnosis and management. The role of FNA and FS in preoperative diagnosis and intraoperative management is often controversial. Many authors [1–9] describe the advantages of other methods for the differentiation of benign, malignant and inflammatory lesions. The use of FNA as well as FS can be helpful in the management of salivary tumors, as the therapeutic strategy can sometimes be changed preoperatively as well as during surgery. The FNA can be performed in an office setting, offering a rapid diagnosis. The advantages of the method are that it is minimally invasive, well-tolerated by patients, has few complications, a low possibility of seeding tumors and minimal costs [1, 9]. The false-negative or false-positive result rates may vary, depending upon the pathologist's experience as much as on the material of the collected sample. Sensitivity and specificity may vary around 73 and 91%, respectively [7]. Accuracy may be enhanced with the use of ultrasound to guide the FNA. Introperative FS often offers the first pathological diagnosis with high sensitivity, confirming or not confirming the diagnosis of the FNA, and adds information about margin status and about nerve or vessel invasion [9]. Although the FNA has a better role in the diagnosis of salivary tumors, the FS may offer better microscopic invasion parameters, the tumor's architecture and circumscription. Diagnostic dilemmas of the FNA occur mainly in extremely cellular tumors, such as pleomorphic and monomorphic adenomas, when differential diagnosis with low-grade adenoid cystic carcinoma [5, 6, 9] may be difficult; the distinction between cystic inflammatory diseases and low-grade mucoepidermoid carcinoma may also be difficult. The FS can improve the decision-making process in those situations [9].

Practical Tips

❶ The history, physical exam and imaging studies often contribute to the diagnosis [5, 6, 9].
❷ The presence of a motor deficit, especially of the facial nerve, is highly suggestive of the presence of malignancy [1, 5].
❸ When the result of the FNA is uncertain, the FS can often demonstrate the tissue's architecture and help to diagnose lymphoma and low-grade and high-grade tumors [8, 9].
❹ The use of ultrasound to guide the FNA may improve the exam's accuracy [5].

Conclusion

FNA is more sensitive whereas FS is more specific. In fact, these methods are complementary. FS can be useful to determine the extent of the surgery and to establish the diagnosis of cancer, when FNA is uncertain.

References

1 Batsakis JG, Sneige N, el-Naggar AK: Fine-needle aspiration of salivary glands: its utility and tissue effects. Ann Otol Rhinol Laryngol 1992;101:185–188.
2 Heller KS, Attie JN, Dubner S: Accuracy of frozen section in the evaluation of salivary tumors. Am J Surg 1993;166:424–427.
3 Heller KS, Dubner S, Chess Q, Attie JN: Value of fine needle aspiration biopsy of salivary gland masses in clinical decision-making. Am J Surg 1992;164:667–670.
4 Tincani AJ, Martins AS, Altemani A, Scanavini RC Jr, Barreto G, Lage HT, Valerio JB, Molina G: Parapharyngeal space tumors: considerations in 26 cases. Sao Paulo Med J 1999;117:34–37.
5 Tincani AJ, Del Negro A, Araujo PP, Akashi HK, Martins AS, Altemani AM, Barreto G: Management of salivary gland adenoid cystic carcinoma: institutional experience of a case series. Sao Paulo Med J 2006;124:26–30.
6 Tincani AJ, Altemani A, Martins AS, Barreto G, Valério JB, Del Negro A, Araújo PP: Polymorphous low-grade adenocarcinoma at the base of the tongue: an unusual location. Ear Nose Throat J 2005;84:794–795, 799.
7 Hughes JH, Volk EE, Wilbur DC; Cytopathology Resource Committee, College of American Pathologists: Pitfalls in salivary gland fine-needle aspiration cytology: lessons from the College of American Pathologists Interlaboratory Comparison Program in Nongynecologic Cytology. Arch Pathol Lab Med 2005;129:26–31.
8 Arabi Mianroodi AA, Sigston EA, Vallance NA: Frozen section for parotid surgery: should it become routine? ANZ J Surg 2006; 76:736–739.
9 Seethala RR, LiVolsi VA, Baloch ZW: Relative accuracy of fine-needle aspiration and frozen section in the diagnosis of lesions of the parotid gland. Head Neck 2005;27:217–223.

Cernea CR, Dias FL, Fliss D, Lima RA, Myers EN, Wei WI (eds): Pearls and Pitfalls in Head and Neck Surgery. Basel, Karger, 2008, pp 120–121

7.8 Practical Tips to Spare the Great Auricular Nerve in Parotidectomy

Randall P. Morton

Counties-Manukau DHB and Auckland University, Auckland, New Zealand

PEARLS

- The posterior branches of the great auricular nerve (GAN) can be preserved in more than 60% of parotidectomies.
- Surgical morbidity is reduced by preserving the posterior branches of the GAN.
- Burying the stump of a transected GAN avoids a tender amputation neuroma.

PITFALLS

- The GAN becomes more superficial as it ascends, and the posterior branches lie subcutaneously inferior to the point of attachment of the ear lobe. It is here that they are at the highest risk of inadvertent injury.
- In 5–10% of patients in whom the GAN has been sacrificed an exquisitely sensitive subcutaneous amputation neuroma may develop [1]. Less commonly neuropathic excoriation of the pinna may occur.

Introduction

The GAN is a sensory nerve arising from the 2nd and 3rd cervical rami. It emerges from the posterior margin of the sternocleidomastoid (SCM) muscle at the great auricular point (also known as McKinney's point [2] and sometimes – incorrectly – Erb's point [3]), 6.5 cm below the external auditory canal [2]. Some sketch a line from the mastoid process to the angle of the mandible, and then drop a perpendicular line at the midpoint. The great auricular point is where this line intersects with the posterior border of the SCM [3].

From the great auricular point, the GAN heads for the angle of the mandible. After crossing the anterior border of the SCM, the GAN forms anterior branches and a posterior division. The anterior branches have a variable distribution to the parotid gland and cheek and in over 50% of cases the GAN does not enter the gland at all [4]. These anterior branches are divided in parotid surgery because the ramifications to the cheek skin would inevitably be severed during skin flap elevation.

There are 2 or 3 branches of the posterior division of the GAN [5]; these supply the inferior portion of the pinna [6]. They pass directly towards the anterior attachment of the ear lobe, and lie subcutaneously just inferior to the attachment of the lobe.

The GAN posterior branches can be preserved in at least 65–70% of cases [5, 7]. Whilst postoperatively there is auricular hypoesthesia and anesthesia irrespective of whether or not the GAN is divided, there is better long-term (12-month) light touch and pain perception [6, 8, 9] and thermal sensitivity [6] if the posterior branches are preserved than if the GAN is sacrificed. One year is widely recognized as being a time limit for sensory recovery of the facial region [6].

If the posterior branches of the GAN are preserved, generally long-term sensory sequelae on the pinna may only occur in about 15% of patients compared with more than 50% where the GAN is sacrificed [5]. Preservation of the GAN posterior branches adds very little to the surgical time in my experience; others also report that it adds only 5–10 min [7, 10].

Once the GAN has been sacrificed, patients often forego wearing earrings and give up skiing because of intolerance to cold temperatures [7, 8].

Practical Tips

1. Preservation of the GAN must not compromise oncological surgical principles.
2. Make the initial skin incision through dermis but not deeper.
3. Dissect over the SCM, and identify the trunk of the GAN in the inferior part of the parotidectomy incision before raising skin flaps in the region of the pinna.
4. Follow the GAN superiorly as you would follow the trunk of the facial nerve, raising the anterior skin flap as you go.
5. Divide the anterior branches of the GAN, but free the posterior branches of their attachments, and reflect them posteriorly.
6. One of the posterior branches may pass deep and anterior to the lobule [10].
7. The parotid gland can now be separated from the pinna and the SCM in the normal manner.

Conclusion

This chapter highlights the significance of preservation of the posterior branches of the GAN in the course of parotid surgery. The sensory benefits of this technique are not immediately evident, but the advantages are well documented at 12 months. Not only is sensation in the pinna preserved, but potential complications (neuropathic excoriation [7, 10], amputation neuroma [1]) are avoided.

References

1 Moss CE, Johnston CJ, Whear NM: Amputation neuroma of the great auricular nerve after operations on the parotid gland. Br J Oral Maxillofac Surg 2000;38:537–538.
2 Brown JS, Ord RA: Preserving the great auricular nerve in parotid surgery. Br J Oral Maxillofac Surg 1989;27:459–466.
3 Leung MKS, Dieu T, Cleland H: Surgical approach to the accessory nerve in the posterior triangle of the neck. Plastic Reconstr Surg 2004;6:2067–2070.
4 Zohar Y, Siegal A, Siegal G, Halpern M, Levy B, Gal R: The great auricular nerve; does it penetrate the parotid gland? An anatomical and microscopical study. J Craniomaxillofac Surg 2002;30: 318–321.
5 Christensen NR, Jacobsen SD: Parotidectomy. Preserving the posterior branch of the great auricular nerve. J Laryngol Otol 1997;111:556–559.
6 Biglioli F, D'Orto O, Bozzetti A, Brusati R: Function of the great auricular nerve following surgery for benign parotid disorders. J Craniomaxillofac Surg 2002;30:308–317.
7 Hui Y, Wong DSY, Ho W-K, Wei WI: A prospective controlled double-blind trial of great auricular nerve preservation at parotidectomy. Am J Surg 2003;185:574–579.
8 Suen DTK, Chow T-L, Lam CYW, Wong ESW, Lam S-H: Sensation recovery improved by great auricular nerve preservation in parotidectomy: a prospective double-blind study. ANZ J Surg 2007;77:374–376.
9 Porter MJ, Wood SJ: Preservation of the great auricular nerve during parotidectomy. Clin Otolaryngol 1997;22:251–253.
10 Vieira MBM, Maia AF, Ribiero JC: Great auricular nerve preservation in parotidectomy. Arch Otolaryngol Head Neck Surg 2002;128:1191–1195.

Cernea CR, Dias FL, Fliss D, Lima RA, Myers EN, Wei WI (eds): Pearls and Pitfalls in Head and Neck Surgery. Basel, Karger, 2008, pp 122–123

7.9 Indications for Elective Neck Dissection in Parotid Cancers

Roberto A. Lima, Fernando L. Dias

Head and Neck Service, Brazilian National Cancer Institute/INCA and Head and Neck Surgery, Catholic University of Rio de Janeiro, Rio de Janeiro, Brazil

PEARLS

- In malignant parotid tumors, consider to stage the neck by dissecting level II and III. Keep in mind that most of the neck metastases that occur in these levels are easily dissected through the same classical incision [1].
- Presence of facial dysfunction along with parotid mass indicates aggressive tumors. In this case consider to electively dissect the neck [2].

PITFALLS

- Rates of complete agreement between the diagnosis based on intraoperative frozen sections and final permanent sections can be as low as 36% and depend of the pathologist's experience [3].
- If lymph node metastasis is identified on frozen sections, consider to perform a modified radical neck dissection, levels I–V.
- There are no randomized prospective studies confirming the reliability of radiotherapy in controlling neck metastasis in salivary cancer.

Introduction

The incidence of lymph node metastases in parotid carcinomas at the time of initial presentation varies from 12 to 24 [2, 4–6]. Armstrong et al. [1] reported a rate of 38% of occult neck metastasis in 90 patients who had undergone elective neck dissection. Additionally, 10 patients had periglandular positive nodal disease. Neck lymph node metastasis from salivary cancer is not common, nevertheless it has a poor prognosis. Our institution [6] reported reductions in 10-year survival rates from 77 to 34% for parotid cancer.

The characteristics that influence the risk of occult metastasis in salivary cancer are worth reviewing in any discussion of elective surgical treatment of the neck.

Spiro et al. [2] at the Memorial Sloan-Kettering Cancer Center recommended an elective neck dissection in patients with undifferentiated or squamous carcinoma due to the high rate of developing nodal metastasis, and suggested that for other high-grade tumors a staging supraomohyoid neck dissection is an appropriate adjunctive therapy.

Armstrong et al. [1] reported that high-grade tumors demonstrate increased occult lymph node metastasis in comparison with low-grade tumors, 49 versus 2%.

According to Regis et al. [7], the significant risk factors for neck metastasis in parotid carcinoma are histological type, T stage and severe desmoplasia. Additional characteristics predictive of a higher incidence of occult nodal metastasis include advanced T stage (T3, T4), tumor size 3 cm or more, and the presence of facial paralysis at presentation [5].

Practical Tips

1. Tumors classified as T3/T4 have a higher risk of neck metastasis [8].
2. Patients who present with facial nerve dysfunction on diagnosis have a higher risk of neck metastasis [8]. Consider that facial dysfunction is easy to identify when associated with parotid tumors.
3. Tumor grade is difficult to establish with frozen sections [3]. However, it has been observed that there is a relationship between histopathology and grade [9]. Primary squamous cell carcinoma, high-grade mucoepidermoid carcinoma, salivary duct carcinoma, undifferentiated carcinoma, and adenocarcinoma have a higher risk of harboring occult neck metastasis [7].
4. Selective neck dissection (levels IB, IIA, IIB, III) is appropriate surgery for patients who are at risk of neck metastasis. Upper neck areas (levels I, II, III) are easily resected through a small extension of the parotidectomy incision [10].

References

1 Armstrong JG, Harrison LB, Thaler HT, et al: The indications for elective treatment of the neck in cancer of the major salivary glands. Cancer 1992;69:615–619.
2 Spiro RH, Armstrong JG, Harrison LB, et al: Carcinoma of major salivary glands – recent trends. Arch Otolaryngol Head Neck Surg 1989;115:316–321.
3 Zbären P, Schupbach J, Nuyens M, et al: Elective neck dissection versus observation in primary parotid carcinoma. Otolaryngol Head Neck Surg 2005;132:387–391.
4 Spiro RH: Salivary neoplasms: overview of a 35-year experience with 2807 patients. Head Neck 1986;8:177–184.
5 Frankenthaler RA, Byers RM, Luna MA, et al: Predicting occult lymph node metastasis in parotid cancer. Arch Otolaryngol Head Neck Surg 1993;119:517–520.
6 Lima RA, Tavares MR, Dias FL, et al: Clinical prognostic factors in malignant parotid gland tumors. Otolaryngol Head Neck Surg 2005;133:702–708.
7 Regis De Brito Santos I, Kowalski LP, Cavalcante De Araujo V, et al: Multivariate analysis of risk factors for neck metastases in surgically treated parotid carcinomas. Arch Otolaryngol Head Neck Surg 2001;127:56–60.
8 Medina JE: Neck dissection in the treatment of cancer of the major salivary glands. Otolaryngol Clin North Am 1998;31:815–822.
9 Godballe C, Schultz JH, Krogdahl A, et al: Parotid carcinoma: impact of clinical factors on prognosis in a histologically revised series. Laryngoscope 2003;113:1411–1417.
10 McGuirt WF: Controversies regarding therapy of tumors of the parotid gland; in Thawley SE, Panje WR, Batsakis JG, Lindberg RD (eds): Comprehensive Management of Head and Neck Tumors. Philadelphia, Saunders, 1999, pp 1211–1219.

Cernea CR, Dias FL, Fliss D, Lima RA, Myers EN, Wei WI (eds): Pearls and Pitfalls in Head and Neck Surgery. Basel, Karger, 2008, pp 124–125

7.10 Indications for 'Tactical' Parotidectomy in Nonsalivary Lesions

Caio Plopper, Claudio R. Cernea

Department of Head and Neck Surgery, University of São Paulo Medical School, São Paulo, Brazil

PEARLS

- Parotid gland tissue or intraglandular lymph nodes can be compromised by malignant tumors of the anterior face and scalp.
- In these cases, superficial parotidectomy with preservation of the facial nerve is usually sufficient.

PITFALLS

- Large skin tumors usually preclude identification of the main trunk of the facial nerve, making retrograde dissection a safer and easier tactic.

Introduction

Parotid gland resections can be necessary for adequate treatment of nonsalivary tumors, usually for one of two reasons: tumors that either directly invade or are very close to the gland, or for lymph node resection.

Most often, tumors that directly invade the parotid gland are of cutaneous origin, namely basal cell and squamous cell carcinomas; however, melanomas and other rare tumors, such as desmoid tumors, dermatofibrosarcoma, or eccrine carcinomas, can also mandate some kind of parotid gland resection for their appropriate treatment [1].

The parotid gland is home to part of the lymphatic network of the head and neck, in continuity with upper level II lymph nodes. These lymph nodes are usually located in the superficial lobe of the parotid gland, and are an important basin of lymphatic drainage of the anterior face and scalp [2]. Thus, primary tumors arising from these locations with a histological high propensity for lymphatic metastases or with clinical metastatic disease to the parotid gland should also require a formal parotidectomy as part of their surgical treatment [3, 4].

Practical Tips

1 Either when indicated for direct invasion of the parotid gland or for lymph node dissection, parotid gland resection with preservation of the facial nerve and all its branches should be attempted. However, some form of nerve sacrifice can be necessary when the facial nerve is found to be compromised by primary or metastatic disease.

2 A parotidectomy should be indicated whenever a primary skin tumor invades deep to the parotid fascia. This can be necessary for facial nerve identification and preservation, as well as for tumor resection with adequate margins [5].

3 Identification of the main trunk of the facial nerve is usually easier and safer; however, when a large tumor arising from the skin of the parotid region or the auditory canal precludes the identi-

fication of the main trunk of the facial nerve, a retrograde parotidectomy can be of use.

4 Use of surgical magnification lenses and intraoperative nerve monitoring can be very important for facial nerve identification and for documenting its preservation, especially for large tumors and when retrograde facial nerve dissection is necessary.

5 Some tumors that may clinically mimic primary parotid nodes, such as lymphomas or nerve sheath tumors, can arise in the parotid gland, and a formal parotidectomy may be too extensive and morbid for these patients [6]. In these instances, preoperative fine needle aspiration biopsies are very useful and recommended for surgical planning.

6 The vast majority of parotid lymph nodes are located in the superficial lobe, lateral to the facial nerve. Thus, whenever indicated for lymph node dissection, a superficial parotidectomy is sufficient.

7 For cutaneous melanoma of the anterior scalp and face, parotid lymphatic mapping and sentinel lymph node resection are still controversial. However, the importance of facial nerve preservation in these cases cannot be overemphasized.

8 When indicated for elective or therapeutic intraglandular lymph node dissection, parotid lymph nodes should be viewed as contiguous to upper level II lymph nodes [1]. Hence, en bloc formal selective or comprehensive neck dissection should be considered.

9 When direct invasion of the parotid gland by a malignant disease or compromised parotid lymph nodes are present, adjuvant radiation therapy can be considered for improved local control [7].

References

1 Plopper C, Cernea CR, Ferraz AR, Medina dos Santos LR, Regis AB: Parotidectomy for primary nonparotid diseases. Otolaryngol Head Neck Surg 2004;131:407–412.
2 McKean ME, Lee K, McGregor IA: The distribution of lymph nodes in and around the parotid gland: an anatomical study. Br J Plast Surg 1985;38:1–5.
3 Yarington CT Jr: Metastatic malignant disease to the parotid gland. Laryngoscope 1981;91:517–519.
4 Nichols RD, Pinnock LA, Szymanowski RT: Metastases to parotid nodes. Laryngoscope 1980;90:1324–1328.
5 Lai SY, Weinstein GS, Chalian AA, Rosenthal DI, Weber RS: Parotidectomy in the treatment of aggressive cutaneous malignancies. Arch Otolaryngol Head Neck Surg 2002;128: 521–526.
6 Loggins JP, Urquhart A: Preoperative distinction of parotid lymphomas. J Am Coll Surg 2004;199:58–61.
7 Kraus DH, Carew JF, Harrison LB: Regional lymph node metastasis from cutaneous squamous cell carcinoma. Arch Otolaryngol Head Neck Surg 1998;124:582–587.

Cernea CR, Dias FL, Fliss D, Lima RA, Myers EN, Wei WI (eds): Pearls and Pitfalls in Head and Neck Surgery. Basel, Karger, 2008, pp 126–127

7.11 When Not to Operate on a Parotid Tumor

Jeffrey D. Spiro[a], Ronald H. Spiro[b, c]

[a] University of Connecticut School of Medicine, Farmington, Conn.,
[b] Head and Neck Surgery Service, Memorial Sloan-Kettering Cancer Center and
[c] Cornell University Medical College, New York, N.Y., USA

PEARLS

- Not all parotid masses are actually neoplastic.
- At least 80% of parotid neoplasms are benign.
- Fine needle aspiration biopsy (FNABx) is usually capable of distinguishing neoplastic from non-neoplastic lesions and benign from malignant neoplasms.

PITFALLS

- FNABx is not infallible, and therefore is not a substitute for clinical judgment.
- Malignant transformation of a preexisting pleomorphic adenoma (PA) is rare, but needs to be considered in the decision to perform surgery.

Introduction

The patient who presents with a mass in the parotid area usually has a primary neoplastic process arising in the parotid gland (PG). In general, clinicians will recommend a parotidectomy (PTx) in this setting. There are, however, several considerations that may impact on the decision to proceed directly with surgery.

Practical Tips

1. Not all masses arising in the PG are neoplastic in origin. Other possibilities include benign cysts or inflammatory changes and hyperplastic enlargement of lymph nodes located adjacent to, or within, the parotid capsule. Given that more than 80% of neoplasms arising in the gland will prove to be benign, the indications for resection are usually: (a) confirmation of a pathologic diagnosis, (b) concern about appearance, and (c) the possibility of malignant transformation of a preexisting benign PA.

2. FNABx can be very useful when deciding whether to proceed with parotid surgery. The accuracy of FNABx in distinguishing a neoplastic from a nonneoplastic process, and in distinguishing benign from malignant neoplasms, is generally quite high, with an overall accuracy of 84–98% [1–5]. An aspirate that is unequivocally negative for malignant cells in a patient with a clinically benign parotid mass provides additional reassurance in those cases when the patient would prefer to defer surgery. When a lymphoid aspirate suggests lymphoma, a core biopsy can provide enough tissue to establish a diagnosis without a PTx. Clearly FNABx is not infallible, and the clinical judgment of the surgeon must take priority when the results of FNABx are inconsistent with the clinical presentation.

3. PTx may be the only way to reassure the anxious patient even when a tumor is small and almost certainly benign. When a tumor is large and unsightly, surgeons and patients alike will usually favor intervention. It is worth recalling that PA, the most common neoplasm encountered in the PG, usually enlarges slowly and steadily. In

our experience, however, some patients have tumors that show no significant growth during years of observation. For this reason, watchful waiting can be a reasonable alternative in certain patients, especially those who are older or who have significant medical problems.

4 Another often cited indication for PTx is the risk of malignant transformation of a preexisting PA. The actual incidence of such a transformation is uncertain; however, it appears to be rare. Although this possibility needs to be discussed with the patient as part of the process of informed consent, we feel that it is not a compelling indication for surgery in patients with clinically benign parotid tumors.

5 There are obviously other considerations that can influence a decision to proceed with parotid surgery. Patients whose overall health precludes general anesthesia are not candidates for surgery. Some patients with neglected or high-grade cancers may have disease that is so locally extensive that it is deemed unresectable. As previously noted, the patient's level of concern will clearly be an important factor in the decision to proceed with surgery.

Conclusion

While surgical excision is usually indicated for a mass arising in the PG, there are circumstances when PTx may be deferred. A nonneoplastic process may be diagnosed by FNABx or core needle biopsy, thus avoiding surgery. In cases where a PA is either suspected clinically, or diagnosed on FNABx, the risks and benefits of PTx must be discussed with the patient, assuring that only complete extirpation can guarantee accurate pathologic analysis, and that there is a small risk of malignant transformation of benign tumors over time. If after such a discussion the patient prefers to avoid surgery, it is reasonable to follow him or her clinically. In the authors' experience, some PAs may exhibit little or no significant growth when observed over extended periods of time, thus making observation a reasonable option in carefully selected, properly informed patients.

References

1 Seethala RR, LiVolsi VA, Baloch ZW: Relative accuracy of fine-needle aspiration and frozen section in the diagnosis of lesions of the parotid gland. Head Neck 2005;27:217–223.
2 Cohen EG, Patel SG, Lin O, et al: Fine-needle aspiration biopsy of salivary gland lesions in a selected patient population. Arch Otolaryngol Head Neck Surg 2004;30:773–778.
3 Boccato P, Altavilla G, Blandamura S: Fine needle aspiration biopsy of salivary gland lesions. A reappraisal of pitfalls and problems. Acta Cytol 1998;42:888–898.
4 Al-Khafaji BM, Nestok BR, Katz RL: Fine-needle aspiration of 154 parotid masses with histologic correlation: ten year experience at the University of Texas M.D. Anderson Cancer Center. Cancer 1998;84:153–159.
5 Atula T, Greenman R, Laippala P, Klemi PJ: Fine-needle aspiration biopsy in the diagnosis of parotid gland lesions: evaluation of 438 biopsies. Diagn Cytopathol 1996;15:185–190.

Cernea CR, Dias FL, Fliss D, Lima RA, Myers EN, Wei WI (eds): Pearls and Pitfalls in Head and Neck Surgery. Basel, Karger, 2008, pp 128–129

7.12 Practical Tips on Excision of the Submandibular Gland

Kwang Hyun Kim

Department of Otolaryngology – Head and Neck Surgery, Seoul National University College of Medicine, Seoul, Korea

PEARLS

- The most important thing in submandibular gland (SMG) resection is to avoid injury of the marginal mandibular branch of the facial nerve (MMN).
- The standard technique of avoiding injury to MMN is to place the incision at least 3 cm below the lower margin of the mandible.
- Retrograde dissection of the cervical branch upwards leads to the MMN.
- Transient 'pseudoparalysis' of the MMN due to cervical branch injury can be distinguished from MMN injury.
- Intraoral excision of the SMG causes no external scar, no injury to the MMN or to the hypoglossal nerve, and no residual Wharton's duct inflammation.

PITFALLS

- Facial nerve stimulators can be used, but their safety and reliability are not absolute.
- Intraoral excision of the SMG should not be indicated for patients with malignant or huge salivary gland tumors or when there is limitation in mouth opening or floor of mouth exposure.

Introduction

Excision of the SMG has been frequently associated with neurological complications after surgery, such as damage to the MMN (7.7%), hypoglossal (2.9%), and lingual (1.4%) nerves [1]. The standard technique of avoiding injury to MMN is to place the horizontal limb of the neck dissection incision at least 3 cm below the lower margin of the mandible, ligating and dividing the common facial vein deep to the fascia, lifting the vessel along with the upper skin flap [2]. It is very easy to find the thick facial artery entering the SMG from behind. If the artery passes through the gland, it should be cut and ligated securely; otherwise, it can be saved. The lingual nerve is connected with the SMG by the submaxillary ganglion, which must be carefully cut in order to avoid nerve damage. The hypoglossal nerve is deep to the digastric muscle, thus being relatively protected during dissection. The facial vessels should be ligated and cut carefully at the upper border of the SMG. The last step is to ligate and cut the Wharton's duct. The duct should be carefully palpated before cutting to confirm stone in the resected specimen.

Alternative surgical approaches have been developed to avoid visible scarring in the upper neck and to reduce neurological risks, like intraoral removal of the SMG [3] and minimally invasive endoscopic and endo-robotic methods of SMG resection.

Practical Tips

1 A safe way of identifying the MMN is the intraoperative use of facial nerve-monitoring devices, but a slightly time-consuming preoperative setup is necessary. Both disposable intraoperative facial nerve stimulators and plexus block nerve stimulators are available, but there is some concern about their safety and reliability. The standard pulse current intensity recommended for stimulation is 1.00 mA delivered at a frequency of 1 Hz [4].

2 Just below the superficial layer of deep cervical fascia, the cervical branch of the facial nerve is identified, descending 5–10 mm anterior and parallel to the anterior border of the sternocleidomastoid muscle [5]. Retrograde dissection of this cervical branch upwards with a fine mosquito forceps leads to MMN.

3 The major advantages of the intraoral approach are no external scar, no injury to the MMN or to the hypoglossal nerve and no residual Wharton's duct inflammation [3]. The major drawback is its technical difficulty with a significant learning curve, especially when the endoscope is used for magnification. This approach has limited indications [6].

4 The platysma muscle co-functions with depressor anguli oris muscle as a lip depressor. Injury to the cervical branch in these patients results in loss of depressor function to the affected corner of the mouth. Transient lip depressor dysfunction has been a common observation in patients undergoing neck dissection with platysma excision. Transient 'pseudoparalysis' of the MMN due to cervical branch injury could be distinguished from MMN injury by the fact that those patients could still evert the lower lip because of a functioning mentalis muscle [7].

Conclusion

For a better cosmetic result after excision of SMG without neurologic deficit, especially of MMN, the reader should be aware of various available surgical options, in order to choose the most appropriate one.

References

1 Berini-Aytes L, Gay-Escoda C: Morbidity associated with removal of the submandibular gland. J Craniomaxillofac Surg 1992;20:216–219.
2 Martin H, Del Valle B, Ehrlich H, Cahan W: Neck dissection. Cancer 1951;4:441–499.
3 Hong KH, Kim YK: Intraoral removal of the submandibular gland: a new surgical approach. Otolaryngol Head Neck Surg 2000;122:798–802.
4 Sadoughi B, Hans S, de Monès E, Brasnu DF: Preservation of the marginal mandibular branch of the facial nerve using a plexus block nerve stimulator. Laryngoscope 2006;116:1713–1716.
5 Shuaib Zaidi SM: A simple nerve dissecting technique for identification of marginal mandibular nerve in radical neck dissection. J Surg Oncol 2007;96:71–72.
6 Weber SM, Wax MK, Kim JH: Transoral excision of the submandibular gland. Otolaryngol Head Neck Surg 2007;137:343–345.
7 Daane SP, Owsley JQ: Incidence of cervical branch injury with 'marginal mandibular nerve pseudo-paralysis' in patients undergoing face lift. Plast Reconstr Surg 2003;111:2414–2418.

Cernea CR, Dias FL, Fliss D, Lima RA, Myers EN, Wei WI (eds): Pearls and Pitfalls in Head and Neck Surgery. Basel, Karger, 2008, pp 130–131

8.1 Practical Tips to Perform the Subcranial Approach

Ziv Gil, Dan M. Fliss

Department of Otolaryngology – Head and Neck Surgery, Tel Aviv Sourasky Medical Center, Tel Aviv, Israel

PEARLS

- The subcranial approach is a multidisciplinary team effort.
- Use broad-spectrum antibiotic treatment perioperatively to reduce complications.
- Insert a lumbar drain after administering anesthesia to facilitate frontal lobe retraction and to reduce the risk of postoperative cerebrospinal fluid leak.
- Improve patient satisfaction by performing surgery without facial incisions, tracheostomy and shaving the hair.
- In cases of massive involvement of the palate, the pterygomaxillary fossa or the orbital apex, use combined approaches.
- Whenever possible, preserve one or both sides of the olfactory filaments.

PITFALLS

- Avoid impairment of nasal breathing by preserving the distal third of the nasal bone.
- Confirm a tight dural seal in order to prevent cerebrospinal fluid leak.
- Immediate extubation is required to allow continuous neurological monitoring.
- Never ventilate a patient with a positive pressure after extubation in order to avoid life-threatening tension pneumocephalus.
- Admit the patient to an intensive care unit for 24 h after surgery.

Introduction

The concept of a broad subcranial approach to the entire anterior skull base was first introduced as an alternative to the traditional craniofacial approach. The subcranial approach has several major advantages. (1) It affords a broad exposure of the anterior skull base from below rather than through the transfrontal route. (2) It provides an excellent access to the medial orbital walls and to the sphenoethmoidal, nasal and paranasal cavities. (3) It allows simultaneous intradural and extradural tumor removal and safe reconstruction of dural defects. (4) It does not require facial incisions. (5) It is performed with minimal frontal lobe manipulation.

Practical Tips

1 *Preoperative Evaluation and Anesthesia.* All patients scheduled for surgery should be evaluated preoperatively by a multidisciplinary surgical team. Radiological evaluation should include computed tomography (CT) and magnetic resonance imaging. Positron emission tomography-CT is also recommended [1]. Broad-spectrum antibiotics consisting of a combination of cefuroxime, vancomycin and metronidazole are instituted perioperatively. No tracheostomy is required unless free flap reconstruction is performed [2]. A lumbar spine catheter is inserted for cerebrospinal fluid drainage after administering anesthesia.

② *The Surgical Technique of the Subcranial Approach.* The skin is incised above the hairline and a coronal flap is created in a supraperiosteal plane [2]. The flap is elevated anteriorly beyond the supraorbital ridges. The pericranial flap is elevated up to the periorbits, and the supraorbital nerves and vessels are carefully separated from the supraorbital notch. The lateral and medial walls of the orbits are exposed, and the anterior ethmoidal arteries are clipped. Titanium mini-plates are applied to the frontal bones and removed before performing the osteotomies to ensure the exact repositioning of the bony segments. An osteotomy of the anterior and posterior frontal sinus walls, together with the nasal bony frame, part of the medial wall of the orbit, and a segment of the superoposterior nasal septum is performed [3]. Part of the nasal bone is preserved in order to support the nasal valve. The tumor is extirpated at this stage and the dura or brain parenchyma is resected if involved by tumor. A unilateral or bilateral medial maxillectomy is performed from above if indicated, allowing direct visualization of the maxillary sinus [4]. By means of this approach, it is possible to safely and reliably access tumors involving the medial or superior walls of the maxilla. Multilayer fascia lata flaps are routinely used for reconstruction of the dura and skull. A centripetal compression method is used to reduce the telecanthus, and stenting of the nasolacrimal duct is performed.

③ *Postsurgical Treatment.* After surgery, the patient is extubated and transferred to the critical care unit for 24 h. Stool softeners are administered to reduce the risk of Valsalva-induced increased intracranial pressure. The lumbar drain is removed 3–5 days later and the nasal packing 7 days postoperatively. Routine CT is performed at the end of the procedure and again 1 week later.

Conclusions

The subcranial approach is routinely used for extirpation of tumors involving the anterior skull base, allowing wide exposure, minimal brain retraction and no facial incisions. Detailed preoperative imaging, appropriate reconstruction, intensive postoperative care, and the cooperation of multidisciplinary teams are crucial to assure successful tumor resection and improved quality of life [5].

References

1 Gil Z, Even-Sapir E, Margalit N, Fliss DM: Integrated PET/CT system for staging and surveillance of skull base tumors. Head Neck 2007;29:537–545.

2 Gil Z, Cohen JT, Spektor S, et al: Anterior skull base surgery without prophylactic airway diversion procedures. Otolaryngol Head Neck Surg 2003;128:681–685.

3 Raveh J, Laedrach K, Speiser M, et al: The subcranial approach for fronto-orbital and anteroposterior skull base tumor. Arch Otolaryngol Head Neck Surg 1993;119:385–393.

5 Gil Z, Abergel A, Spektor S, et al: Quality of life following surgery for anterior skull base tumors. Arch Otolaryngol Head Neck Surg 2003;129:1303–1309.

6 Gil Z, Cohen JT, Spektor S, et al: The role of hair shaving in skull-base surgery. Otolaryngol Head Neck Surg 2003;128:43–47.

8

Cernea CR, Dias FL, Fliss D, Lima RA, Myers EN, Wei WI (eds): Pearls and Pitfalls in Head and Neck Surgery. Basel, Karger, 2008, pp 132–133

8.2 Facial Translocation Approach

Fernando Walder

Federal University of São Paulo – UNIFESP, São Paulo, Brazil

Pearls

- Facial anatomy presents optimal lines of separation of facial units (FU) for a surgical approach, permitting the least traumatic displacement.
- The primary blood supply to the FUs ensures their individual viability, when mobilized.
- The middle face contains multiple 'hollow' anatomic spaces that facilitate the relative ease of surgical access to the central skull base (SB).
- Offers much greater tolerance to postoperative surgical swelling, as opposed to similar displacement of the content of the neurocranium.
- Reestablishment of the normal anatomy is accomplished with repositioning of the FUs during the reconstruction phase.

Pitfalls

- Contamination of the surgical wound with oropharyngeal bacteria flora.
- The need of facial incisions with subsequent scar development.
- Emotional considerations related to surgical facial disassembly.

Introduction

Adequate exposure is the key to successful en bloc resection in any region. Due to the proximity to crucial anatomic structures, wide surgical exposure of the nasopharyngeal region of the cranial base (CB) is essential. Numerous approaches have been described for lesions of this region [1]. The approach of this region of CB utilizes facial translocations (FT) for exposure of anterior and middle CB as well as related structures [2]. This procedure utilizes the principle of vascularized facial composite units that allow rapid access, generous working space at the CB, and expedient reconstruction. Because of its modular design, it permits great versatility and accommodates the surgical needs for limited as well as complex procedures at the SB. Maximum preservation and functional/esthetic reconstruction of craniofacial anatomy are emphasized [3]. The current underlying principle of SB approaches is to minimize brain retraction while maximizing SB visualization. This concept facilitates 3D tumor resection, tumor margin verification, and functional reconstruction with appropriate esthetic concerns. Transfacial approaches create potential risks for the function and esthetics of the following structures: skin, dentition, maxillofacial skeleton, mucosal lining of the upper airway, paranasal sinus, eustachian tubes, superior pharyngeal constrictor muscle, soft and hard palate, and tongue [4].

Practical Tips

Perform a cheek flap based on the facial and a labial vascular pedicle that includes the entire cheek soft tissue, lower lid, facial nerve, and parotid gland.

1 The ipsilateral facial skin is displaced laterally and inferiorly to include upper lip split.

❷ Superior incision continues from the nose to the inferior fornix of the lower eyelid, through the lateral canthus horizontally to the preauricular area.
❸ Identify the frontal branches of the facial nerve with nerve stimulator if needed. Place them in silicone tubes; then they can be transected. During the reconstruction, they are reconnected, and their continuity is reestablished.
❹ The infraorbital nerve is electively sectioned along the floor of the orbit, tagged, and repaired at the end of the procedure.
❺ Rigid fixation is achieved with mini- and microplates.
❻ Medially extended FT can expose the ipsilateral infratemporal fossa and central and paracentral SB bilaterally. The entire clivus, optic nerves, both precavernous internal carotid arteries, and the nasopharynx become accessible.
❼ Medially and inferiorly extended FT adds significant inferior as well as upper cervical surgical access.
❽ Posteriorly extended FT incorporates the ear, temporal bone, and posterior fossa into its surgical access. This provides access to both the anterior and posterior aspect of the temporal bone with control of the key neurovascular structures.
❾ Bilateral FT exposes both infratemporal fossae, the central SB, and the entire paracentral SB. The palatal split permits a reach to the level of C2–3. If further inferior extension is needed, a mandibular split can be added so that a vertical reach to C3–4 is accomplished [4].

Conclusions

The anatomic basis for this direct approach to the SB region offers solid surgical principles. By utilizing facial soft tissue translocation and craniofacial osteotomies, the FT approach and its many extensions create a wide surgical field to the SB access. The FT approach offers previously unavailable wide and direct exposure with a potential for immediate reconstruction of this complex region. The modifications available with this approach add an element of versatility necessary to tailor the surgical approach to a specific lesion.

References

1 Maran AG: Surgical approaches to the nasopharynx. Clin Otolaryngol 1983;8:417–429.
2 Biller HF, Shugar JM, Krespi VP: A new technique for wide-field exposure of the base of skull. Arch Otolaryngol 1981;107:698–702.
3 Fish U: Infratemporal fossa approach to tumors of the temporal bone and base of the skull. J Laryngol Otol 1978;92:949–967.
4 Janecka IP, Sen C, Sekhar L, et al: Facial translocation. A new approach to the cranial base. Otolaryngol Head Neck Surg 1990;103:413–419.

Cernea CR, Dias FL, Fliss D, Lima RA, Myers EN, Wei WI (eds): Pearls and Pitfalls in Head and Neck Surgery. Basel, Karger, 2008, pp 134–135

8.3 How to Manage Large Dural Defects in Skull Base Surgery

Eduardo Vellutini, Marcos Q.T. Gomes

DFV Serviços de Neurologia e Neurocirurgia, São Paulo, Brazil

PEARLS

- Think about skull base reconstruction before skin incision.
- First step (dural reconstruction): autologous tissue (temporalis fascia, fascia lata) and watertight suture before facial approach.
- Second step (nasal and cranial cavity separation): always vascularized tissue (pericranium, temporalis muscle, microvascular free flaps) and tissue sealants.

PITFALLS

- Avoid postoperative lumbar drainage: risk of pneumoencephalus.
- Do not let the pericranium flap get dried during the surgical procedure.

Introduction

The possibility of reconstruction of extensive dural defects following tumor resection at the skull base decreased the rates of serious complications such as CSF fistula and meningitis with consequent reduction in treatment morbimortality [1–3].

Such reconstruction must be planned with a wider objective than simple reconstruction of the dural lining proper. It should also entail reduction of dead space along with an effective method of separating the paranasal sinuses-nasopharyngeal cavity and the intracranial cavity [1, 4].

The pericranium technique proposed by Van Buren et al. [5] in 1968 employs vascularized tissue and remains the most commonly used to date, probably due to ease of execution and manipulation, proving the most efficacious way of reducing the risk of CSF fistula [2].

If covering the pericranium is not possible, particularly in cases of reoperation, surgeons must look for other alternatives such as bilateral temporalis muscle graft or microvascular grafts of the rectus abdominalis or radialis, provided a microsurgical reconstruction team is available.

Practical Tips

The reconstruction should take into account tumor origin and volume, extent of intracranial invasion, primary surgery or reoperation and the possibility of microsurgical reconstruction.

Reconstitution of the meningeal lining must be performed immediately after removal of the infiltrated dura mater and/or intradural component of the tumor, prior to facial approach. Minimizing contact between the nasal cavity and subdural space reduces the risk of intraoperative contamination. Closure is carried out using free nonvascularized patient-derived grafts, such as temporalis fascia muscle or fascia lata, and continuous suture with mononylon 5.0. Synthetic dural analogs should be used only if a suitable dural edge is not available for suture.

Separation of the cranial and nasal cavities is performed after total removal of the tumor and should be based on vascularized grafts [1]. In anterior approaches, the best choice is the pericranium with its vascular pedicle through supraorbital arteries. Dissection is performed through a bicoronal incision 2 cm behind the hair line up to the level of the aponeurotic galea, followed by anterior and posterior detachment of the scalp flap. Detaching the pericranium gives enough tissue to recover the entire anterior fossa floor, from the posterior wall of the frontal sinus up to the sellar tubercle. During the procedure, the tissue must be kept moist to prevent retraction.

The fixation of the graft following tumor removal can be achieved using mononylon 5.0 stitches through small drill holes in the bone edge of the resection, either along the sphenoid plane or orbital wall, according to the extent of bone removal.

This step is complemented with fibrin glue applied between the pericranial flap and previously reconstructed dura mater.

Except in rare instances, rigid structures such as bone or titanium plates are not required to sustain the cerebral parenchyma [6].

Under circumstances precluding the use of pericranium (reoperation or tumor infiltration), alternatives available for vascularized patient-derived grafts include the two temporalis muscles, which can be shifted and stitched in order to recover the whole anterior fossa, and microvascular grafts such as abdominal rectus or radialis, requiring a reconstructive plastic microsurgical team.

In lateral approaches, the temporalis muscle can be used to fill and separate the infratemporal fossa from the maxillary and/or nasal cavity. Care should be taken to preserve the wide-based muscular flap so as not to compromise its vascularization by the deep temporal artery. The muscle can be attached to the bone edge of the resection or to the maxillary sinus mucus.

External lumbar drainage is not routinely used as prophylaxis for CSF fistula, in order to avoid frequent complications such as pneumoencephalus and meningitis.

Conclusion

Extensive dural defects should be reconstructed in two stages: closure of the dura mater prior to beginning the facial approach and, following tumor removal, separation of the paranasal and cranial cavities using vascularized tissue.

References

1 Thurnher D, Novak CB, Neligan PC, Gullane PJ: Reconstruction of lateral skull base defects after tumor ablation. Skull Base 2007;17:79–88.
2 Gil Z, Abergel A, Leider-Trejo L, Khafif A, Margalit N, Amir A, Gur E, Fliss DM: A comprehensive algorithm for anterior skull base reconstruction after oncological resections. Skull Base 2007;17:25–37.
3 Imola MJ, Sciarretta V, Schramm VL: Skull base reconstruction. Curr Opin Otolaryngol Head Neck Surg 2003;11:282–290.
4 Liu JK, Niazi Z, Couldwell WT: Reconstruction of the skull base after tumor resection: an overview of methods. Neurosurg Focus 2002;12:e9.
5 Van Buren JM, Ommaya AK, Ketcham AS: Ten years' experience with radical combined craniofacial resection of malignant tumors of the paranasal sinuses. J Neurosurg 1968;28:341–350.
6 Laedrach K, Lukes A, Raveh J: Reconstruction of skull base and fronto-orbital defects following tumor resection. Skull Base 2007;17:59–72.

Cernea CR, Dias FL, Fliss D, Lima RA, Myers EN, Wei WI (eds): Pearls and Pitfalls in Head and Neck Surgery. Basel, Karger, 2008, pp 136–137

8.4 Which Is the Best Choice to Seal the Craniofacial Diaphragm?

Ziv Gil, Dan M. Fliss

Department of Otolaryngology Head and Neck Surgery, Tel Aviv Sourasky Medical Center, Tel Aviv, Israel

PEARLS

- Resection of tumors in the anterior skull base (ASB) may create defects in the craniofacial diaphragm. To accomplish a tight seal reconstruction, tailor your reconstruction technique according to specific anatomical requirements.
- The fascia lata (FL) offers a versatile, inexpensive and reliable method of dural reconstruction using a live biological tissue graft. Its neovascularization provides long-term viability of the flap, without the need of an overlying vascularized flap.
- Use combinations of methods, including temporalis muscle (TM) or free flap (FF), to reconstruct extensive skull base (SB) defects in cases of orbital exenteration (OE) or total maxillectomy.

PITFALLS

- Be aware that failure to create adequate reconstruction harbors significant complications, among them cerebrospinal leak, meningitis and tension pneumocephalus.
- Previous surgery or perioperative radiotherapy significantly delays wound healing. In such cases, use viable biological reconstruction material as much as possible.
- Wrap the bone segment with the pericranial flap to prevent osteoradionecrosis of the frontal bone segment.
- Treat infection promptly by using broad-spectrum antibiotics.

Introduction

Resection of ASB tumors may create extensive defects that result in a free conduit between the paranasal sinuses and the intracranial compartments. Reconstruction of such defects requires precise and durable reconstruction [1]. The goals of ASB reconstruction are (1) to form a watertight dural seal, (2) to provide a barrier between the contaminated sinonasal space and the sterile subdural compartment, (3) to prevent airflow into the intracranial space, (4) to maintain a functional sinonasal system, and (5) to provide a good cosmetic outcome.

A variety of approaches have been developed to accomplish these goals, including viable, nonviable and synthetic materials [2]. However, they can induce chronic inflammation, carrying a high risk of infection, and are inferior to biological sources in terms of strength and sealing quality. On the other hand, local flaps are often inadequate, due to their limited size and their inability to produce a tight seal of the SB defect. FF is an excellent option for ASB reconstruction, but it is relatively complex and its bulk may mask local recurrence. This chapter describes a reliable and reproducible method for cranial base reconstruction based on a multilayer FL allograft [3]. The FL flap already shows signs of vascularized fibrous tissue within a few weeks after surgery, eventually providing long-term graft viability without an overlying vascularized flap [4].

Practical Tips

① The reconstruction technique is tailored to the type and size of the cranial defect, based on radiological and intraoperative assessment.

② Primary closure of the dura is performed whenever possible using tight continuous prolene sutures. A temporal fascia graft suffices if the defect is small.

③ If tumor resection results in an extensive SB defect, a large FL sheath will be needed, fitted precisely to the dimensions of the dural defect. The dural repair is then covered with a second layer of fascia that is applied against the entire undersurface of the ethmoidal roof, the sella and the sphenoidal area. Fibrin glue is used to provide additional protection against cerebrospinal fluid leak. Vaseline gauze is then applied below the dura and into the paranasal cavity for additional support against pulsation of the brain [5].

④ When adjuvant radiation therapy is planned, it is advisable to wrap the frontal bone segment with a pericranial flap, in order to prevent osteoradionecrosis [6]. The frontal sinus bone is cranialized and the bone segment is returned to its original anatomical position.

⑤ A TM flap and a split-thickness skin graft are used after extensive orbital wall resections, if OE is performed.

⑥ After a radical maxillectomy, with or without OE, a lateral thigh or a rectus abdominis FF is used to obliterate the large resultant defect.

⑦ A dacryorhinocystostomy is performed to prevent epiphora in all patients undergoing orbital wall resection or medial maxillectomy.

Conclusions

The 'dray horse' for dural reconstruction is the double layer FL, which provides a simple, inexpensive and versatile means of SB reconstruction after resection of advanced tumors. Other reconstruction methods may be used according to the SB defect. When reconstructed properly, the incidence and severity of perioperative complications, such as cerebrospinal fluid leak, intracranial infection and tension pneumocephalus, are less than 5%.

References

1 Raveh J, Turk JB, Ladrach K, et al: Extended anterior subcranial approach for skull base tumors: long-term results. J Neurosurg 1995;82:1002–1010.

2 Fliss DM, Zucker G, Cohen A, et al: Early outcome and complications of the extended subcranial approach to the anterior skull base. Laryngoscope 1999;109:153–160.

3 Amir A, Gatot A, Zucker G, et al: Harvesting of fascia lata sheaths: a rational approach. Skull Base Surg 2000;10:29–34.

4 Gil Z, Abergel A, Leider-Trejo L, et al: A comprehensive algorithm for anterior skull base reconstruction after oncological resections. Skull Base Surg 2007;17:25–38.

5 Fliss DM, Gil Z, Spektor S, et al: The double-layered fascia: a simple skull base reconstruction method for anterior subcranial resection. Neurosurg Focus 2002;12:1–7.

6 Gil Z, Fliss DM: Pericranial wrapping of the frontal bone after anterior skull base tumor resection. Plast Reconstr Surg 2005; 116:395–398.

Cernea CR, Dias FL, Fliss D, Lima RA, Myers EN, Wei WI (eds): Pearls and Pitfalls in Head and Neck Surgery. Basel, Karger, 2008, pp 138–139

8.5 Contraindications for Resection of Skull Base Tumors

Fernando L. Dias, Roberto A. Lima

Head and Neck Surgery Department, Brazilian National Cancer Institute and Post-Graduation School of Medicine, Catholic University of Rio de Janeiro, Rio de Janeiro, Brazil

PEARLS

- Be sure that the tumor is curable and that surgery will extend survival.
- Be sure that tumor histology and extent merit surgery.
- Be sure that there is an appropriate team backing you up.

PITFALLS

- Resectability does not mean that the patient will be able to tolerate and benefit from surgery.
- Do not neglect the possibility of skull base (SB) metastases from an undiscovered or previously treated malignant tumor.

Introduction

Except for situations in which debulking surgery is advocated, the main purpose of SB surgery is to achieve en bloc removal of the tumor with adequate margins of normal tissue [1–3].

Death rates associated with SB surgery range from 0 to 7.7% (average 4.4%). Major local complications were the main cause of death in 73% of cases (intracranial sepsis: 55.5%, and intracranial bleeding/hematoma: 25.9%). Major systemic complications also played an important role in mortality rates with an incidence of 27% (acute myocardial infarction: 33.3%, and cerebral infarction: 33.3%) of cases [3].

Practical Tips

Current limitations and contraindications for SB surgery are related to three areas (table 1): (1) anatomical, (2) biological and (3) patient factors.

1 a) Distant metastases from and to SB tumors are definitive contraindications. An exception may be adenoid cystic carcinoma in which palliative resection of primary SB tumor, mainly for pain, may be considered [2].

b) Unilateral cavernous sinus (CS) or internal carotid artery (ICA) invasion is not an unanimous contraindication for SB surgery but, even in 'early' cases, occult invasion of the opposite CS or ICA may exist. A staging procedure with sinus endoscopy (preferably) is advisable to establish the confinement of the disease to one sphenoid sinus [4]. Although ICA is most often encased and not invaded, en bloc resection requiring artery resection is rarely performed for cancer [2, 4].

c) Tumors involving the superior sagittal sinus (SSS) can usually be resected as long as its innermost layer is left undisturbed. It is usually safe to ligate the SSS up to the level of the coronal suture (when it rapidly increases in size). Interruption of venous flow posterior to that level usually results in quadroplegia or death [4].

d) There are multiple bridging veins from the convexity of the frontal lobes to the SSS. A few of

Table 1. Anatomic limitations/contraindications to extended procedures for paranasal sinus/SB tumors [1–3]

No longer contraindications	Relative contraindications [1]	Definitive contraindications
Pterygoid plate invasion	Dural invasion	Distant metastases
Infratemporal fossa invasion	Minimal brain invasion	Metastases to SB
Orbital invasion, unilateral	Sphenoid sinus invasion	Bilateral ICA invasion
Nasopharynx invasion	Cavernous sinus invasion	Bilateral cavernous sinus invasion
Regional metastases	Clivus invasion	SSS invasion
Unilateral ICA invasion	Vital brain bridging vein invasion	Massive brain (cortex) invasion

[1] Often contraindications with high-grade tumors.

these can be sacrificed, but ligation of more than a few can also result in the patient's death. Remember that the vein of Labbe may be the only intact drainage venous system from the ipsilateral cerebral hemisphere. Its sacrifice could result in a fatal outcome [4].

e) Any evidence of lower cranial deficits plus radiological evidence of proximity of tumor to the brain stem usually means that the patient is inoperable. Removal of vital portions of the cortex associated with a high risk of death or resulting in severe altered function (unacceptable to the patient) is also a contraindication. Although complete removal of optic chiasm can be safely achieved and is not an absolute contraindication, most patients will decline surgery if they are to be rendered blind [2, 4].

2 Attention to tumor histology. Aggressive tumors such as malignant melanoma, high-grade sarcomas and squamous carcinomas are ominous findings. Even basal cell carcinomas may acquire virulent behavior, particularly after several therapeutic attempts by means of surgery, RT and CT [1–5].

3 Good general (clinical) health is paramount. Common intercurrent diseases (between the age of 50 and 70) such as diabetes, renal, gastrointestinal, and heart diseases must be optimally controlled. Chronological age is not as important as physiological/clinical age. Patients' commitment is essential [1–5].

Conclusion

Tumors amenable to total excision with minimal (acceptable) morbidity should be excised regardless of histology. For larger tumors close to or invading important neurological or vascular structures, tumor histology will help to determine the advisability of surgery [2].

References

1 Shah JP, Patel SG: The skull base; in Shah JP, Patel SG (eds): Head and Neck Surgery and Oncology, ed 3. Edinburgh, Mosby, 2003, pp 93–148.
2 Lavertu P: An overview of indications and contraindications of extended procedures for cancer of the paranasal sinuses. Proceedings of the 4th International Conference on Head and Neck Cancer, Toronto, 1996, pp 1033–1039.
3 Dias FL, Sá GM, Kligerman J, et al: Complications of anterior craniofacial resection. Head Neck 1999;21:12–20.
4 Donald PJ: Skull base surgery for malignancy: when not to operate. Eur Arch Otolaryngol 2007;264:713–717.
5 Cernea CR, Teixeira GV, Dos Santos LRM, et al: Indications for, contraindications to, and interruption of craniofacial procedures. Ann Otol Rhinol Laryngol 1997;106:927–933.

8

Cernea CR, Dias FL, Fliss D, Lima RA, Myers EN, Wei WI (eds): Pearls and Pitfalls in Head and Neck Surgery. Basel, Karger, 2008, pp 140–141

8.6 Practical Tips about Orbital Preservation and Exenteration

Ehab Hanna

Department of Head and Neck Surgery, University of Texas M.D. Anderson Cancer Center, Houston, Tex., USA

Pearls

- Detailed neuro-ophthalmologic examination is essential.
- High-resolution CT and MRI provide critical information regarding the extent of orbital bony and soft tissue involvement, respectively.
- The decision to preserve or sacrifice the eye is sometimes made intraoperatively. Clearly discuss this with the patient and family, and obtain proper informed consent.
- Orbital preservation (OP) is feasible unless there is significant invasion of the orbital fat, muscles, nerves, or apex.
- Invasion of the bony orbit or periorbita per se is not an indication for orbital exenteration (OE).
- Meticulous reconstruction of the medial canthal ligament, lacrimal system, and orbital floor and rim will maximize functional results.

Pitfalls

- Orbital invasion by perineural spread rather than direct extension may be missed unless careful examination of the cranial nerves, especially V1 and V2, and accurate assessment of even subtle enhancement or thickening of orbital nerves on MRI are done.
- Perineural spread may extend proximally beyond the orbital apex and even to the cavernous sinus compromising local disease control.
- Bilateral orbital apex or optic chiasm involvement, especially in central skull base lesions, is usually a contraindication for surgical resection.
- Attempts at OP leaving gross residual disease usually result in poor disease control and ultimate loss of orbital function.
- If OE is contemplated, always make sure that the patient has useful vision in the contralateral eye.

Introduction

OE carries with it a significant emotional burden on patients and their families, deterring some patients from pursuing treatment, or making them chose a less effective therapy regardless of the chances for cure. Lately, the indications for OP have evolved and are more clearly defined [1]. Most studies have shown that if orbital invasion is limited to the bony orbit or the periorbita, OP is possible without compromising oncologic outcome [2–6]. OE is usually indicated when there is gross invasion of the periocular fat, extraocular muscles, or optic nerve.

Practical Tips

❶ Despite better definition of the indications for OP, the preoperative decision as to whether the orbit should be preserved or sacrificed is sometimes difficult. The presence of proptosis or diplopia may be due to displacement rather than invasion of the intraorbital contents. Decreased visual acuity or visual fields, or the presence of an afferent pupillary defect usually indicates gross invasion of the orbit.

❷ In the absence of any ocular signs or symptoms, evaluation of the extent of orbital involvement relies mainly on imaging. CT is best for evaluating bony involvement of the orbital walls and MRI to evaluate the extent of soft tissue invasion beyond the periorbita. MRI is also useful in detecting perineural spread proximally beyond the orbital apex and into the cavernous sinus [7].

The accuracy of imaging in detecting invasion of the periorbita is not completely reliable [5] and frequently, the definitive assessment of the extent of orbital invasion and decision about eye preservation has to be made intraoperatively.

3 Perform the extended lateral rhinotomy instead of the classic Weber-Fergusson incision, for total maxillectomy with OP [8]. Avoiding a subciliary incision minimizes lower eyelid complications, particularly ectropion and prolonged eyelid edema, and avoiding trifurcation of the incision reduces the risk of skin breakdown at the medial canthal area.

4 Meticulous orbital reconstruction after OP is imperative for good function [1, 9]. Careful reattachment of the medial canthal ligament will prevent telecanthus. If the lacrimal apparatus is transected, a dacryocystorhinostomy prevents postoperative epiphora. If the orbital rim or a significant portion (more than one third) of the orbital floor is removed, particularly if the periorbita is resected, bony support is essential. Bone reconstruction is best done using vascularized bone flaps. If nonvascularized bone grafts or alloplastic implants are used, they should be adequately covered with well-vascularized soft tissue to minimize infection and extrusion.

5 The function of the preserved eye will also be greatly influenced by precise dosimetry of postoperative radiation [10]. The use of 3-D conformal radiation therapy or intensity-modulated radiation therapy is particularly helpful in delivering effective radiation doses to the tumor bed while sparing ocular contents.

Conclusions

Every effort should be made to preserve the eye as long as preservation does not compromise the adequacy of oncologic resection. Careful planning of surgical incisions and meticulous orbital reconstruction will enhance the functional outcome of the preserved orbit. Precise radiation dosimetry and proper shielding of the eye will minimize ocular complications.

References

1 Hanna EY, Westfall CT: Cancer of the nasal cavity, paranasal sinuses, and orbit; in Myers EN, Suen JY, Myers JN, Hanna EY (eds): Cancer of the Head and Neck. Philadelphia, Saunders, 2003, pp 155–206.

2 Andersen PE, Kraus DH, Arbit E, Shah JP: Management of the orbit during anterior fossa craniofacial resection. Arch Otolaryngol Head Neck Surg 1996;122:1305–1307.

3 McCary WS, Levine PA, Cantrell RW: Preservation of the eye in the treatment of sinonasal malignant neoplasms with orbital involvement. A confirmation of the original treatise. Arch Otolaryngol Head Neck Surg 1996;122:657–659.

4 Carrau RL, Segas J, Nuss DW, et al: Squamous cell carcinoma of the sinonasal tract invading the orbit. Laryngoscope 1999; 109:230–235.

5 Tiwari R, van der Wal J, van der Wal I, Snow G: Studies of the anatomy and pathology of the orbit in carcinoma of the maxillary sinus and their impact on preservation of the eye in maxillectomy. Head Neck 1998;20:193–196.

6 Essig GF, Newman SA, Levine PA: Sparing the eye in craniofacial surgery for superior nasal vault malignant neoplasms: analysis of benefit. Arch Facial Plast Surg 2007;9:406–411.

7 Hanna E, Vural E, Prokopakis E, Carrau R, Snyderman C, Weissman J: The sensitivity and specificity of high-resolution imaging in evaluating perineural spread of adenoid cystic carcinoma to the skull base. Arch Otolaryngol Head Neck Surg 2007;133:541–545.

8 Vural E, Hanna E: Extended lateral rhinotomy incision for total maxillectomy. Otolaryngol Head Neck Surg 2000;123:512–513.

9 DeMonte F, Tabrizi P, Culpepper SA, Abi-Said D, Soparkar CN, Patrinely JR: Ophthalmological outcome following orbital resection in anterior and anterolateral skull base surgery. Neurosurg Focus 2001;10:E4.

10 Sheng K, Molloy JA, Larner JM, Read PW: A dosimetric comparison of non-coplanar IMRT versus helical tomotherapy for nasal cavity and paranasal sinus cancer. Radiother Oncol 2007;82:174–178.

Cernea CR, Dias FL, Fliss D, Lima RA, Myers EN, Wei WI (eds): Pearls and Pitfalls in Head and Neck Surgery. Basel, Karger, 2008, pp 142–143

8.7 Practical Tips to Approach the Cavernous Sinus

Marcos Q.T. Gomes[a, b], Eduardo Vellutini[b]

[a] Hospital das Clinicas, São Paulo University,
[b] DFV Serviços de Neurologia e Neurocirurgia, São Paulo, Brazil

PEARLS

- Extradural approach – 'peeling' of the cavernous sinus (CS).
- Try to start peeling at the superior orbital fissure (SOF).
- Fibrin glue injection into CS before opening.

PITFALLS

- Always perform an MRI to assess the carotid involvement.

Introduction

The CS is a venous structure of walls formed by dura mater containing inner neurovascular structures. The oculomotor (III), trochlear (IV), abducens (VI) nerves and the two first branches of the trigeminal nerve (V1 and V2) traverse the CS, while the third branch (V3) lies at its posterior border [1]. The internal carotid artery (ICA) passes through the CS where it continues a sinuous path to exit at the roof of the sinus.

Tumors of the paranasal sinuses and infratemporal fossa generally invade the CS due to its neurotropism, infiltrating the trigeminal branches (V2 and V3, respectively) and then expanding centripetally to the intracranial cavity reaching the CS. Intraorbital tumors may invade the skull along V1 via the SOF or the optic nerve through the optic canal.

In this type of invasion, the CS tends to be affected when intracranial invasion occurs, hampering oncologic removal, where this must be exposed to achieve an oncologically free margin.

The most frequent clinical picture of invasion of the CS is facial pain or numbness due to compromise of the trigeminal branch. If the invasion is massive, symptoms of ocular paralysis may be associated.

Practical Tips

Approach for tumors invading the CS must be elected on a case-by-case basis. In the event of ICA compromise, oncologic removal with margins cannot take place without sacrificing this vessel [2].

❶ An MRI study must always be performed to assess the extent of invasion of the CS and involvement of the ICA. If it shows signs of tumor around ICA, removal of this vessel should be considered.

❷ The CS nerves, with the exception of the VI, pass through the lateral wall of the CS [1]. If only the portion lateral or anterior to the ICA is affected, then removal without sacrificing the ICA can be attempted.

❸ The dura mater of the lateral wall of the CS has two layers: the inner one houses the nerves outlined above, whereas the external one follows the dura of the temporal convexity. This may be peeled away, leaving a thin continuous internal layer, allowing the nerves to be seen by transparency, a procedure referred to as CS 'peeling'. Described by Dolenc [1] as the extradural access pathway to CS pathologies, this approach minimizes damage to the nervous tissue, prevents the occurrence of liquor fistula and allows better identification and saving of the nerves when possible.

4 The peeling is done by cutting the dural band at the lateral edge of the SOF, together with the meningo-orbital artery. Pulling away the outer layer will detach it from the inner layer. The edge is more strongly attached and needs to be cut, particularly near V2 and V3 [1,3].

5 Although difficult, it is also possible to perform the peeling following V2, and cutting the edges superiorly and posteriorly. This is particularly useful in tumors that invade the skull through the foramen rotundum or ovale, where the nerve has to be sacrificed to achieve a free oncologic margin.

6 The peeling technique allows partial resection of the CS without lesion to the oculomotor nerves.

7 The ICA is the main limitation in removal of tumors invading the CS. Its sinuous pathway within the CS often obscures the perceived pathology extension. In malignant neoplasms, the invasion of the ICA wall, even without encasement, precludes a free oncologic margin without sacrificing the vessel. Exenteration of the CS with ICA must then be considered, involving ICA bypass and the placing of a vascularized flap to reconstruct the cranial base [2,4].

8 Bleeding of the CS is generally profuse, except in cases where it is filled by tumor. It can often be controlled using Surgicel®. Fibrin glue is extremely useful, being injected into the CS before opening, filling some of its compartments, thereby minimizing blood loss.

Conclusion

The extradural approach to the CS is the best way to reach the CS with minimum complications. If the ICA wall has not been invaded, a partial resection of the CS can be performed. If the tumor has reached the ICA, exenteration of the CS must be considered, together with an arterial bypass.

References

1 Yasuda A, Campero A, Martins C, Rhoton AL, Oliveira E, Ribas GC: Microsurgical anatomy and approaches to the cavernous sinus. Neurosurgery 2005;56(1 suppl):4–27.
2 George B, Ferrario CA, Blanquet A, Kolb F: Cavernous sinus exenteration for invasive cranial base tumors. Neurosurgery 2003;52:772–782.
3 Dolenc VV: Transcranial epidural approach to pituitary tumors extending beyond the sella. Neurosurgery 1997;41:542–552.
4 Sekhar LN, Sen CN, Jho HD: Saphenous vein graft bypass of the cavernous internal carotid artery. J Neurosurg 1990;72:35–41.

Cernea CR, Dias FL, Fliss D, Lima RA, Myers EN, Wei WI (eds): Pearls and Pitfalls in Head and Neck Surgery. Basel, Karger, 2008, pp 144–145

8.8 How to Reconstruct Large Cranial Base Defects

Patrick J. Gullane[a], Christine B. Novak[b], Kristen J. Otto[a], Peter C. Neligan[c]

[a] Department of Otolaryngology – Head and Neck Surgery, University of Toronto and
[b] Wharton Head and Neck Centre, University Health Network, Toronto, Ont., Canada;
[c] Division of Plastic Surgery, University of Washington Medical Center, Seattle, Wash., USA

PEARLS

- Consider patient comorbidities in the selection of type of reconstruction.
- A free flap (FF) provides ample well-vascularized tissue to encompass the dead space in a complex 3-D defect [1].
- Create a watertight barrier (dural seal) between intracranial and extracranial contents.
- Secure dural repair with suspension sutures to the surrounding bone.

PITFALLS

- Avoid the use of nonvascularized bone and soft tissue.
- Entry into the orbit can lead to postoperative complications such as diplopia, optic neuropathy, ectropion and enophthalmos [2].

Introduction

Management of large cranial base defects (LCBDs) presents a reconstructive challenge due to the anatomic location and the complex reconstruction that is required. The main goals are to provide soft tissue coverage and structural support that is functional and esthetically acceptable. It is necessary to obtain a watertight dural seal, to obliterate dead space, to support neural structures and to ensure coverage with well-vascularized tissue. Previously, pedicled muscle flaps (e.g., the pectoralis) were used for reconstruction of large defects. However, more recently, the advancement of microsurgery has relegated the pedicled flap to a less desirable option for LCBDs in favor of the FF in the appropriately selected patient [1, 3–5]. It provides an ample supply of vascularized soft tissue and it can be designed based upon the unique requirements of the reconstruction. An FF also provides the opportunity for two surgical teams to work simultaneously, for the tumor ablation and the harvest of the free tissue transfer.

The tumor type, location of the tumor and need for postoperative radiation will guide the selection of the optimal surgical approach [6]. Following tumor ablation, the reconstruction will depend on the size and position of the lesion and if the dura has been breached. Patient comorbidities, such as age greater than 75, diabetes, significant vascular disease or immunosuppression, may preclude the use of a free tissue transfer, but the consideration of individual patient factors is necessary.

Practical Tips

❶ *Soft Tissue Repair.* Our choice of FF includes the rectus abdominis muscle, the latissimus dorsi muscle and the anterolateral thigh flap. In the skull base, the donor vessels from the neck are commonly used and vein grafts are rarely needed. Postoperative external monitoring of pedicle patency is performed using a venous Doppler and in cases where there is no external skin paddle, an implantable venous Doppler may be used to monitor the flap.

❷ *Bony Reconstruction.* Following tumor extirpation and reconstruction, many patients with skull base tumors may require adjuvant radiotherapy, precluding the use of nonvascularized bone for reconstruction. In most patients, soft tissue will be adequate for the repair; however, when more bony support is required, vascularized bone grafts or alloplastic materials (i.e. titanium mesh) should be used. Our FF preferences are the scapular osseocutaneous (SFF) and the iliac crest (ICFF), but they have weaknesses. To harvest the SFF, the patient must be repositioned, which precludes the use of two surgical teams, increasing operative time. The ICFF is associated with increased postoperative patient morbidity and discomfort.

❸ *Dural Seal.* When the dura has been breached, a watertight seal must be established to minimize the risk of CSF fistula. Due to the unique anatomic position of the cranial base, there is a downward gravitational strain on any dural repair, posing a difficult problem to maintain the dural seal and creating more dead space. We use suspension sutures to secure the flap to the surrounding bone, placing them in the tendinous intersection of the FF to provide a more reliable attachment. Fibrin glue may be used to further secure the seal.

❹ *Orbital Reconstruction.* If the orbit is violated during the resection, controversy exists as to whether orbital reconstruction is necessary. A good rule of thumb is that reconstruction should be pursued when more than 2/3 of the orbital floor is removed. Bony repair (bone grafting or titanium mesh implants) as well as soft tissue reconstruction (repair of the periorbita) are recommended [2].

Conclusion

Reconstruction of LCBD is complex and these repairs require a watertight dural seal, obliteration of the dead space and coverage with vascularized soft tissue. Advances in diagnostic pathology, imaging and surgical technique for tumor extirpation and reconstruction have improved the treatment of these patients, minimized postoperative complications and maximized patient outcome and health-related quality of life.

References

1. Weber SM, Kim JH, Wax MK: Role of free tissue transfer in skull base reconstruction. Otolaryngol Head Neck Surg 2007;136:914–919.
2. DeMonte F, Tabrizi P, Culpepper S, Suki D, Soparker CN, Patrinely JR: Ophthalmological outcome after orbital entry during anterior and anterolateral skull base surgery. J Neurosurg 2002;97:851–856.
3. Jones NF, Schramm VL, Sekhar LN: Reconstruction of the cranial base following tumour resection. Br J Plast Surg 1987;40:155–162.
4. Neligan PC, Boyd JB: Reconstruction of the cranial base defect. Clin Plast Surg 1995;22:71–77.
5. Neligan PC, Mulholland RS, Irish J, Gullane PJ, Boyd JB, Gentili F, Brown D, Freeman J: Flap selection in cranial base reconstruction. Plast Reconstr Surg 1996;98:1159–1166.
6. Irish J, Gullane PJ, Gentili F, Freeman J, Boyd JB, Brown D, Rutka J: Tumors of the skull base: outcome and survival analysis of 77 cases. Head Neck 1994;16:3–10.

Cernea CR, Dias FL, Fliss D, Lima RA, Myers EN, Wei WI (eds): Pearls and Pitfalls in Head and Neck Surgery. Basel, Karger, 2008, pp 146–147

8.9 Surgical Management of Recurrent Skull Base Tumors

Claudio R. Cernea[a], Ehab Hanna[b]

[a] Department of Head and Neck Surgery, University of São Paulo Medical School, São Paulo, Brazil;
[b] Department of Head and Neck Surgery, University of Texas M.D. Anderson Cancer Center, Houston, Tex., USA

PEARLS

- Try to preoperatively assess operability of a recurrent skull base tumor (RSBT) with accurate imaging studies. High resolution CT and MRI are complimentary and allow accurate planning of surgical access and extent of resection.
- Discuss extensively with the patient and his/her family the potential surgical morbidity, as well as the possibility to interrupt the procedure, if necessary.
- Taylor the incision according to the features of the recurrent lesion, mainly when treating recurrent skin cancers.
- Use microvascular reconstructive techniques, especially if a wide communication between the cranium and the paranasal sinuses and/or skin was created.
- Meticulous watertight dural repair is imperative to avoid CSF fistulas.
- Consider placing metal clips to orient eventual targeted adjuvant radiotherapy.

PITFALLS

- Be very careful when indicating a reoperation in the following instances: very aggressive histologic types, extensive involvement of the cavernous sinus (CS), of the intracranial internal carotid artery (ICA), and of vital parts of the brain or of optic chiasm.
- Do not hesitate to intraoperatively abort a redo craniofacial resection, if an unexpectedly aggressive invasion is observed.

Introduction

The treatment of RSBT represents a formidable challenge. Early detection of tumor relapse may be very difficult, due to distortion of anatomical landmarks and presence of fibrosis/gliosis, as well as reconstructive flaps used at the previous operation [1, 2]. Recurrence may involve vital areas of the central nervous system, precluding radical resection with a reasonable chance of cure, while preserving life quality at a functional level [3, 4]. On the other hand, significant long-term palliation may be obtained, especially with slow-growing tumors.

Practical Tips

❶ Try to obtain data from the previous surgical procedure, as well as from the previous adjuvant treatment.

❷ Imaging studies should include high resolution CT and MRI for accurate assessment of the bony and soft tissue extent of disease, respectively. The use of PET/CT is helpful in distinguishing posttreatment effects from active tumor, and in ruling out systemic disease.

❸ Interventional radiology is indicated to perform preoperative embolization of highly vascularized tumors, mainly in the lateral skull base [5]. Carotid angiography may also be helpful in mapping out the cerebral circulation, and balloon test occlusion may guide the need for cerebral revascularization in case of injury or sacrifice of the ICA.

❹ Keep in mind that the treatment of skull base tumors requires multidisciplinary input; therefore, surgical strategy must be extensively planned by all involved teams. The feasibility of pre- or postoperative adjuvant therapy may be a critical determinant of the decision to pursue surgical resection.
❺ Frequently, the surgical approach involves atypical incisions, mandated by the extension of the recurrent lesion, especially if there is skin involvement [6].
❻ Usually, combined craniofacial resections start with the craniotomy. When dealing with recurrent tumors, do not hesitate to interrupt the procedure at this point, provided an unexpectedly extensive invasion of vital structures is noted (ICA, CS, optic chiasm, among others), especially with very aggressive histologic types [7]. Pay special attention to preserve the integrity of the cranial nerves involved with the CS, especially if the ipsilateral eye is still functional. Dural invasion is not a contraindication per se, unless the remaining defect is too basal, precluding adequate exposure for reconstruction. Similarly, brain invasion may be adequately managed, except if vital areas, like the dominant precentral gyrus, are invaded.
❼ Always perform a watertight dural closure, using grafts if necessary. In our experience, fascia lata is an excellent alternative.
❽ Do not hesitate to use microvascular flap reconstruction [8].

Conclusion

In this chapter, the reader was exposed to some considerations about the management of RSBT. It is important to emphasize that the surgical indications must be carefully debated in the scenario of a multispecialty team approach and frankly discussed with the patient and his/her family, due to the prognostic implications, the surgical risk and quality of life deterioration that may occur.

References

1 Glenn LW: Innovations in neuroimaging of skull base pathology. Otolaryngol Clin North Am 2005;38:613–629.
2 Wallace RC, Dean BL, Beals SP, Spetzler RF: Posttreatment imaging of the skull base. Semin Ultrasound CT MR 2003;24:164–181.
3 Dos Santos LR, Cernea CR, Brandao LG, Siqueira MG, et al: Results and prognostic factors in skull base surgery. Am J Surg 1994;168:481–484.
4 Cantú G, Solero CL, Mariani L, Mattavelli F, et al: A new classification for malignant tumors involving the anterior skull base. Arch Otolaryngol Head Neck Surg 1999;125:1252–1257.
5 Turowski B, Zanella FE: Interventional neuroradiology of the head and neck. Neuroimaging Clin N Am 2003;13:619–645.
6 Cernea CR, Dias FL, Lima RA, Farias T, et al: Atypical facial access: an unusually high prevalence of use among patients with skull base tumors treated at 2 centers. Arch Otolaryngol Head Neck Surg 2007;133:816–819.
7 Cernea CR, Teixeira GV, Medina dos Santos LR, Vellutini EA, et al: Indications for, contraindications to, and interruption of craniofacial procedures. Ann Otol Rhinol Laryngol 1997;106:927–933.
8 Chang DW, Langstein HN, Gupta A, De Monte F, et al: Reconstructive management of cranial base defects after tumor ablation. Plast Reconstr Surg 2001;107:1346–1355.

Cernea CR, Dias FL, Fliss D, Lima RA, Myers EN, Wei WI (eds): Pearls and Pitfalls in Head and Neck Surgery. Basel, Karger, 2008, pp 148–149

8.10 Management of Extensive Fibro-Osseous Lesions of the Skull Base

Claudio R. Cernea[a], Bert W. O'Malley, Jr.[b]

[a] Department of Head and Neck Surgery, University of São Paulo Medical School, São Paulo, Brazil;
[b] Department of Otolaryngology, University of Pennsylvania, Philadelphia, Pa., USA

PEARLS

- It is important to define the rationale for recommending surgery for any fibro-osseous lesion of the skull base.
- Indications for the surgical treatment of extensive fibro-osseous lesions of the skull base must be objectively based on factors like compression of vital structures (optic nerve), diplopia, facial disfigurement and rapid growth.
- Most surgical approaches can be performed extradurally. Aggressive lesions may require a more extensive surgical resection that must be counterbalanced with the associated risk to cranial nerves and major vessels.
- Less aggressive lesions may warrant no intervention and only observation.
- Postoperative functional rehabilitation may be surprisingly good, particularly in very young children.

PITFALLS

- Excessive drilling at the foramina or compartments which hold the cranial nerves, carotid artery, and brain and orbital soft tissues.
- Using aggressive rongeuring to remove the bony lesion at the cranial nerve foramina, near the superior and inferior orbital fissures, along the carotid canal, and at the optic canal.
- Excessive resection of bony craniofacial structures may lead to unsatisfactory cosmetic results.
- Not obtaining CT or MRI imaging and clinical follow-up on patients who receive a recommendation for observation.

Introduction

Fibro-osseous lesions of the head and neck comprise a wide clinicopathological spectrum of diseases, ranging from monostotic fibrous dysplasia to Paget's disease and even Albright's syndrome, which includes polyostotic fibrous dysplasia associated with cutaneous pigmentation and precocious sexual development [1]. Some authors consider other diseases, like ossifying fibroma, as part of this group, making diagnostic distinction sometimes rather difficult [1]. Fibro-osseous lesions of the skull base usually affect children and young adults, presenting as a slowly growing mass involving the mandible, the maxilla or the ethmoid [2]. However, local expansion may occasionally cause severe deformities as well as functional consequences, especially when there is compression of cranial nerves [3], which may lead to diplopia or visual loss, dysphagia or dysphonia, pain or paresthesias if left untreated [4]. The radiological diagnosis is of paramount importance, not only to adequately establish the extent of the disease but also to facilitate the surgical approach and requirements for reconstruction [5]. For enlarging lesions or compressive lesions, surgical treatment is the best option for intervention. However, the indications for surgery must be carefully balanced against the intraoperative risks and postoperative morbidity [6, 7].

Practical Tips

❶ Listen carefully to the clinical history, with special attention to the duration, intensity and progression of symptoms.

❷ Imaging studies should include CT and MRI to evaluate intracranial extension, orbital displacement and, especially, optic nerve or other cranial nerve compression.

❸ If the lesion has been stable for years and no major symptoms are present, observation with clinical and radiological monitoring may be preferred instead of an extensive and potentially morbid operation.

❹ Three-dimensional CT is very useful for reconstruction planning.

❺ In many cases, resection may be performed extradurally via a transfacial or subcranial approach.

❻ Another viable option would be endoscopic resection of the fibro-osseous lesion, particularly if it is within the ethmoid, maxillary, or sphenoid sinuses, the frontal recess, or the medial orbital wall or apex [8].

❼ The most critical aspect in the management of fibro-osseous lesions of the skull base is the careful approach to decompression of critical structures such as the optic nerve or carotid artery [9]. It is very important to avoid excessive drilling or aggressive rongeuring close to these structures in order to avoid inadvertent damage. Also, careful attention should be paid to the repositioning or reconstruction of the bony or soft tissues of the orbit in order to avoid diplopia, exophthalmos, or enophthalmos.

Conclusion

In this chapter, the reader was exposed to some considerations about the management of fibro-osseous lesions of the skull base. It is important to emphasize that the surgical treatment must be carefully tailored to each case and to the aggressive or slow-growing nature of each independent lesion. In some instances the intraoperative risks and postoperative morbidity may be significant and should be weighed according to the surgeon's recommendations and the patient's desire for surgery.

References

1 Barnes L, Verbin RS, Appel BN, Peel RL: Diseases of the bones and joints; in Barnes L (ed): Surgical Pathology of the Head and Neck. New York, Marcel Dekker, 2001, pp 1049–1232.

2 Lustig LR, Holliday MJ, McCarthy EF, Nager GT: Fibrous dysplasia involving the skull base and temporal bone. Arch Otolaryngol Head Neck Surg 2001;127:1239–1247.

3 Katz BJ, Nerad JA: Ophthalmic manifestations of fibrous dysplasia: a disease of children and adults. Ophthalmology 1998;105: 2207–2215.

4 Michael CB, Lee AG, Patrinely JR, Stal S, Blacklock JB: Visual loss associated with fibrous dysplasia of the anterior skull base. Case report and review of the literature. J Neurosurg 2000;92:350–354.

5 Panda NK, Parida PK, Sharma R, Jain A, Bapuraj JR: A clinicoradiologic analysis of symptomatic craniofacial fibro-osseous lesions. Otolaryngol Head Neck Surg 2007;136:928–933.

6 Becelli R, Perugini M, Cerulli G, Carboni A, Renzi G: Surgical treatment of fibrous dysplasia of the cranio-maxillo-facial area. Review of the literature and personal experience from 1984 to 1999. Minerva Stomatol 2002;51:293–300.

7 Chen YR, Noordhoff MS: Treatment of craniomaxillofacial fibrous dysplasia: how early and how extensive? Plast Reconstr Surg 1990;86:835–842.

8 Samaha M, Metson R: Image-guided resection of fibro-osseous lesions of the skull base. Am J Rhinol 2003;17:115–118.

9 Papay FA, Morales L, Flaharty P, et al: Optic nerve decompression in cranial base fibrous dysplasia. J Craniofac Surg 1995;6: 5–10.

Cernea CR, Dias FL, Fliss D, Lima RA, Myers EN, Wei WI (eds): Pearls and Pitfalls in Head and Neck Surgery. Basel, Karger, 2008, pp 150–151

9.1 Practical Tips to Manage Extensive Arteriovenous Malformations

Gresham T. Richter, James Y. Suen

Department of Otolaryngology – Head and Neck Surgery, University of Arkansas for Medical Sciences, Arkansas Children's Hospital, Little Rock, Ark., USA

Pearls

- Surgical resection complimented by preoperative embolization leads to best chance for cure.
- Supraselective embolization of the 'nidus' without incorporating the major arterial supply should be performed if embolization is the primary treatment of arteriovenous malformations (AVM).
- Free tissue transfers should occur only when anastomoses to vessels far distal to the resected AVM can be performed. Otherwise, local flaps (with prior expansion) or pedicle flaps should be used.
- Complete surgical extirpation is essential for cure.

Pitfalls

- AVM are frequently misdiagnosed as hemangiomas.
- Embolization alone or partial resection of AVM will lead to rapid progression of residual disease with recruitment of adjacent soft tissue vasculature.
- Ligation of contributing vessels without addressing the central lesion causes progressive growth and neoformation of collateral blood vessels, making further management difficult.

Introduction

AVM are rare congenital anomalies of vascular development thought to arise from persistent arteriovenous channels of early fetal life. These lesions are present at birth but may remain clinically quiescent for many years until rapid dilatation, recruitment, and collateralization of contributing arteries and veins. The result is a progressively expanding high-flow vascular lesion with devastating functional and cosmetic consequences. Intervention is necessary to prevent progression, life-threatening bleeding, and high-output cardiac failure [1, 2]. However, management decisions are met with the challenge of high recurrence rates from inadequate excision and severe deficits from radical extirpation [3, 4]. Superficial lesions are often considered just the 'tip of the iceberg'.

Rapid growth of AVM frequently occurs at the onset of puberty and during pregnancy. Continued expansion can lead to significant destruction of involved tissue and can grow to invade adjacent structures similar to malignancies. Partial excision or embolization may lead to dramatic expansion of previously unappreciated contributions to the AVM. Embolization followed by radical resection and reconstruction has shown promising results and is commonly employed by those who deal with complex AVM [4–7].

Practical Tips

1. A multidisciplinary team (interventional radiologist, otolaryngologist, and reconstructive surgeon) is essential for managing extensive head and neck AVM.
2. A thorough understanding of vascular anatomy is critical to managing large head and neck AVM as aberrant vessels often make it difficult to

map the entire area involved by the lesion. This appreciation should be met by complex radiographic imaging including MRI, MRA, and arteriograms [4, 8].

3 Preoperative embolization should be performed on AVM 1–4 days prior to undergoing surgical resection [1, 4]. Further delay can lead to rapid recruitment and collateralization of new vessels.

4 The operative surgeon should be present during embolization to help identify feeding vessels and prevent inadvertent occlusion of uninvolved tissue.

5 Total resection of small and focal AVM has a higher likelihood of cure [7, 9].

6 Incomplete resection of large AVM to avoid cosmetic and functional deficits may be indicated with the understanding that recurrence is common and repeat intervention necessary [5].

7 Urgent management of ulcerative or bleeding lesions is vital to preventing significant patient morbidity and mortality. These patients may be treated with palliative embolization or preoperative embolization prior to complete extirpation.

8 Surgeons should be prepared for complete resection at the initial procedure with expectation of long operative time, significant intraoperative bleeding, and need for reconstruction [10]. Resection should proceed with preservation of vital structures and respect for cosmetic and functional concerns.

9 Nonstick bipolar electrocautery is essential to control significant blood loss encountered when removing AVM.

10 Margins of AVM are extremely difficult to define at surgery due to increased blood flow of collateral vessels. Bleeding patterns, such as diffuse bleeding, can be helpful in defining surgical margins.

Conclusions

Extensive AVM of the head and neck are complex and debilitating lesions. Embolization is effective if followed with immediate (1–5 days) resection of all or near total disease. Respect for vital structures and functional outcome is weighed by the need for complete extirpation to achieve clinical cure. Early management of residual disease logically leads to improved long-term outcomes.

References

1 Erdmann MW, Jackson JE, Davies DM, Allison DJ: Multidisciplinary approach to the management of head and neck arteriovenous malformations. Ann R Coll Surg Engl 1995;77:53–59.
2 Sugrue M, McCollum P, O'Driscoll K, Feeley M, Shanik DG, Moore DJ: Congenital arteriovenous malformation of the scalp with high output cardiac failure: a case report. Ann Vasc Surg 1989;3:387–388.
3 Kane WJ, Morris S, Jackson IT, Woods JE: Significant hemangiomas and vascular malformations of the head and neck: clinical management and treatment outcomes. Ann Plast Surg 1995;35:133–143.
4 Seccia A, Salgarello M, Farallo E, Falappa PG: Combined radiological and surgical treatment of arteriovenous malformations of the head and neck. Ann Plast Surg 1999;43:359–366.
5 Bradley JP, Zide BM, Berenstein A, Longaker MT: Large arteriovenous malformations of the face: aesthetic results with recurrence control. Plast Reconstr Surg 1999;103:351–361.
6 Jeong HS, Baek CH, Son YI, Kim TW, Lee BB, Byun HS: Treatment for extracranial arteriovenous malformations of the head and neck. Acta Otolaryngol 2006;126:295–300.
7 Kohout MP, Hansen M, Pribaz JJ, Mulliken JB: Arteriovenous malformations of the head and neck: natural history and management. Plast Reconstr Surg 1998;102:643–654.
8 Cure JK: Imaging of vascular lesions of the head and neck. Facial Plast Surg Clin North Am 2001;9:525–549.
9 Richter GT, Suen J, North PE, James CA, Waner M, Buckmiller LM: Arteriovenous malformations of the tongue: a spectrum of disease. Laryngoscope 2007;117:328–335.
10 Buckmiller LM, Richter GT, Waner M, Suen JY: Use of recombinant factor VIIa during excision of vascular anomalies. Laryngoscope 2007;117:604–609.

Cernea CR, Dias FL, Fliss D, Lima RA, Myers EN, Wei WI (eds): Pearls and Pitfalls in Head and Neck Surgery. Basel, Karger, 2008, pp 152–153

9.2 How to Manage Extensive Lymphatic Malformations

James Y. Suen, Gresham T. Richter

Department of Otolaryngology – Head and Neck Surgery, University of Arkansas for Medical Sciences, Arkansas Children's Hospital, Little Rock, Ark., USA

PEARLS

- Rapid growth of a lymphatic malformation (LM) may occur with any local infection and should be managed initially with antibiotics and steroids for 7–10 days.
- An MRI is very helpful to determine if an LM is microcystic, macrocystic, or mixed.
- On MRI, a fluid-fluid level on T2 is usually diagnostic of LM.
- Sclerotherapy using OK-432, alcohol, doxycycline or bleomycin can be very effective for macrocystic LM.

PITFALLS

- If surgery is used to resect an LM, avoid early removal of drains because it will usually result in lymph fluid collections.
- Avoid sclerotherapy for microcystic forms of LM.
- Never remove the entire oral tongue for massive LM enlargement.

Introduction

Extensive LM are usually easy to diagnose. They typically present as painless enlargement of the face, neck and/or tongue. They often contain cystic components with lymph fluid collections. Surface vesicles are usually apparent when mucosa is involved, some of which contain blood. Extensive LM of the head and neck can grow rapidly during infancy. They can cause upper airway obstruction and often require tracheotomy for airway control [1]. Obvious enlarged cystic components can be treated with either surgery or sclerotherapy. The face, tongue and other mucosal surfaces more frequently harbor microcystic or mixed disease whereby sclerotherapy is not as useful [2]. Tongue and floor of mouth involvement may result in protrusion of the tongue out of the mouth. If treatment with antibiotics and steroids does not improve this condition, the child may require surgical reduction. If surgery is elected, primary resection should be along the medial tip and midline substance of the tongue to preserve vascular supply, innervation, and function of the tongue. A second stage reduction may be necessary in some patients.

Practical Tips

1 With extensive LM the goal is to control the disease and not necessarily cure, except when primarily macrocystic disease is present. The family and patient need to understand that this often means multiple treatments throughout life.

2 Mucosal lesions may be extensive and can be treated with the scanning device of a CO_2 laser [1, 3]. Lasering should be performed through the mucosal layer. The deep components of LM are better treated with Nd:Yag laser that can ablate deeper channels of the mucosal lesions [4]. The Nd:Yag laser setting ideal is at 20–30 W at 0.5 s in the noncontact mode.

❸ Many LM have a significant venous malformation component, so that surgical resection may encounter many large vascular channels.
❹ There is frequently a significant fibrofatty component to LM that does not respond to liposuction.
❺ It is common to have hypertrophy of the adjacent bones, such as the mandible and zygoma that may also require surgical reduction. The mandible will often elongate and can result in a significant deformity. Reshaping the mandible is commonly necessary [5].
❻ In macrocystic lesions undergoing sclerotherapy, two or more treatments may be necessary to obtain the desired result [6].
❼ Protection of the facial nerve branches and the muscles to which they innervate is critical when resecting LM that involve the face and parotid.
❽ Following surgical resection, it is important to place a suction drain and leave it for a week or more.
❾ Wound dehiscence is common.
❿ With extensive LM, the surgical goal is primarily to debulk the lesion and to do no harm.
⓫ LM involving the larynx usually infiltrates the mucosa and CO_2 laser is the treatment of choice [7].
⓬ Sclerotherapy can be employed with cysts 2 cm or greater [2, 6].
⓭ Ultrasound is best to identify and treat cysts with sclerotherapy [2].
⓮ After treatment of any kind, the patient should be placed on steroids and antibiotics for 1–2 weeks.
⓯ Dental caries is common with LM and dentists should be involved early after diagnosis [5].

Conclusion

Extensive LM are rare and a major challenge. It is better to refer these patients to a center that has experience in treating these malformations.

References

1 Edwards PD, Rahbar R, Ferraro NF, Burrows PE, Mulliken JB: Lymphatic malformation of the lingual base and oral floor. Plast Reconstr Surg 2005;115:1906–1915.
2 Peters DA, Courtemanche DJ, Heran MK, Ludemann JP, Prendiville JS: Treatment of cystic lymphatic vascular malformations with OK-432 sclerotherapy. Plast Reconstr Surg 2006;118:1441–1446.
3 April MM, Rebeiz EE, Friedman EM, Healy GB, Shapshay SM: Laser therapy for lymphatic malformations of the upper aerodigestive tract. An evolving experience. Arch Otolaryngol Head Neck Surg 1992;118:205–208.
4 Bradley PF: A review of the use of the neodymium YAG laser in oral and maxillofacial surgery. Br J Oral Maxillofac Surg 1997; 35:26–35.
5 Padwa BL, Hayward PG, Ferraro NF, Mulliken JB: Cervicofacial lymphatic malformation: clinical course, surgical intervention, and pathogenesis of skeletal hypertrophy. Plast Reconstr Surg 1995;95:951–960.
6 Alomari AI, Karian VE, Lord DJ, Padua HM, Burrows PE: Percutaneous sclerotherapy for lymphatic malformations: a retrospective analysis of patient-evaluated improvement. J Vasc Interv Radiol 2006;17:1639–1648.
7 Chan J, Younes A, Koltai PJ: Occult supraglottic lymphatic malformation presenting as obstructive sleep apnea. Int J Pediatr Otorhinolaryngol 2003;67:293–296.

Cernea CR, Dias FL, Fliss D, Lima RA, Myers EN, Wei WI (eds): Pearls and Pitfalls in Head and Neck Surgery. Basel, Karger, 2008, pp 154–155

9.3 How to Deal with Emergency Bleeding Episodes in Arteriovenous Malformations

Eduardo Noda Kihara, Mario Sergio Duarte Andrioli,
Eduardo Noda Kihara Filho

Interventional Neuroradiology Department, Hospital Albert Einstein, São Paulo, Brazil

PEARLS

- Endovascular embolization of deep seated neck and cranial arteriovenous malformations (AVM) is a feasible way to stop bleeding.
- Percutaneous embolization by drainage vein compression is the best treatment option for superficial AVM.

PITFALLS

- Previous proximal artery AVM ligature make the nidus and fistula inaccessible to embolization.
- Surgical drainage vein clamping increases intranidal pressure and risk of bleeding.

Introduction

Craniofacial and neck vascular AVM are infrequent entities. There are different types: nidus AVM, arteriovenous fistulas, venous malformations and cavernous hemangiomas. Bleeding due to AVM can occur after trauma, biopsy or during resection for curative or esthetic surgery.

Modern technology based on high resolution fluoroscopy, small microcatheters and the new embolizing materials can increase the possibility to reach the nidus of AVM or the arteriovenous fistula site, to treat the AVM or as a preoperative adjuvant therapy.

Prior angiographic evaluation of the AVM is indicated before surgical access to look for the multiple afferent arteries, presence of nidus, nidus size and draining veins.

Practical Tips

1. Deep seated AVM or fistulas can be embolized with Onyx (ethylene vinyl alcohol) or NBCA (N-butyl cyanoacrylate) placed at the nidus or at the fistula site, completely occluding the malformation.
2. High-flow fistulas can also be treated by microcatheter embolization with external compression or by balloon catheter inflation, placed at the proximal artery to reduce the flow. Ivalon (polyvinyl alcohol foam) or Gelfoam pledges are transitory occlusive particulate materials and should not be used. Coils and fibered coils are used in specific situations, when we are faced with very high-flow conditions and where we need to reduce flow velocities.
3. Superficial AVM and venous malformations can be treated by percutaneous puncture and occlusion with NBCA 50% or absolute alcohol (ethanol) during external compression using rubber bands or devices to increase the local effect and results. All these procedures are risky and must be used under high resolution fluoroscopy and extremely careful injection, avoiding pulmonary embolization or intracranial migration by dangerous anastomoses between the vertebral artery

and the external carotid artery branches and the intracranial circulation.

4 Complete digital angiographic study of an AVM followed by embolization in a high-flow lesion precludes a dangerous situation, as a bleeding condition, during a biopsy or a resection. It reduces blood loss and abbreviates both surgery and recovery time. As stated above, care must be taken with 'dangerous anastomoses' between the external carotid artery branches, vertebral artery branches and intracranial circulation.

5 Passage of the embolizing material to the jugular vein or other large draining veins can cause pulmonary embolism. Ulcerations, skin necrosis and skin color changes can occur, usually related to the material and volume used.

Conclusion

AVM are complex diseases and should be studied by a multidisciplinary team before any surgical attempt. It is feasible and safe for a well-trained interventional team to carry out endovascular and percutaneous treatment of AVM lesions. New materials, tools and devices for vascular and nidus occlusions can improve the final results excluding AVM and reducing time, bleeding and surgical risk.

References

1 Numan F, Omeroglu A, Kara B, et al: Embolization of peripheral vascular malformations with ethylene vinyl alcohol copolymer (Onyx). J Vasc Interv Radiol 2004;15:939–946.
2 Kohout MP, Hansen M, Pribaz JJ, et al: Arteriovenous malformations of the head and neck: natural history and management. Plast Reconstr Surg 1998;102:643–654.
3 Berenguer B, Burrows PE, Zurakowski D, et al: Sclerotherapy of craniofacial venous malformations: complications and results. Plast Reconstr Surg 1999;104:1–11.
4 Persky MS, Yoo HJ, Berenstein A: Management of vascular malformations of the mandible and maxilla. Laryngoscope 2003;113: 1885–1892.
5 Whiteside OJ, Monksfield P, Steventon NB, et al: Endovascular embolization of a traumatic arteriovenous fistula of the superficial temporal artery. J Laryngol Otol 2005;119:322–324.
6 Ahn HS, Kerber CW, Deeb ZL: Extra- to intracranial arterial anastomoses in therapeutic embolization: recognition and role. AJNR Am J Neuroradiol 1980;1:71–75.
7 Duncan IC, Fourie PA: Circumferential flow reduction during percutaneous embolotherapy of extracranial vascular malformations: the 'cookie-cutter' technique. AJNR Am J Neuroradiol 2003;24:1453–1455.

Cernea CR, Dias FL, Fliss D, Lima RA, Myers EN, Wei WI (eds): Pearls and Pitfalls in Head and Neck Surgery. Basel, Karger, 2008, pp 156–157

10.1 Practical Tips to Manage Branchial Cleft Cysts and Fistulas

Marcelo D. Durazzo, Gilberto de Britto e Silva Filho

Head and Neck Service, Hospital das Clínicas, Faculty of Medicine, University of São Paulo, São Paulo, Brazil

PEARLS

- Branchial cleft (BrC) cysts may initially appear in adulthood despite their presence since birth. Cysts may become evident after infection.
- Avoid surgical approach (drainage or resection) if a cyst is infected. Try to manage the infection with antibiotics.

PITFALLS

- Consider performing a facial nerve (FN) dissection when treating a first branchial cleft anomaly (BrCA).
- Dissection of the duct (or tract) must be carried out cranially when resecting a second or third BrCA.
- Recurrence is associated with incomplete resection of cysts and fistula ducts.

Introduction

BrC fistulas are diagnosed at birth in the majority of cases. BrC cysts are usually seen only after infectious processes. They may also be seen in adults despite their presence since birth [1, 2]. Both conditions are congenital and result from the nonobliteration of the cervical sinus (formed by the second, third and fourth BrCs during the embryo development). When there is a patent tract from the remnant of the cervical sinus to the skin and/or to the mucosa of the upper aerodigestive tract, a fistula appears.

BrCA are treated surgically. Surgery is ideally indicated in the absence of infection. A mass (cyst) or a cutaneous opening (fistula) may be evident at the level of the anterior border of the sternomastoid muscle. Cysts and fistulas in the preauricular region arise from the first BrC.

Infection is the main complication. It may be present in one third of the cases in the pediatric population [3].

Practical Tips

Regarding first BrCA, the tract must be dissected until it reaches the external auditory canal. The FN may be superficial to the tract, and it may be dissected if necessary [4, 5].

The following tips refer to the treatment of second BrCA. They are also useful for treating the very rare third and fourth BrCA.

1. Avoid drainage as much as possible. Avoid a surgical approach when the cyst is infected. Treat the infection with antibiotics and wait until the inflammatory signs disappear [1].
2. Under general anesthesia, proceed to a lateral incision in the neck at the level of the anterior border of the sternomastoid muscle. It may be done above or below depending on the level of the cyst or fistula. When a cutaneous orifice is present in the neck, it must be completely circumscribed by the incision [1, 2].

3 Proceed to blunt dissection of the cyst followed by a cranial isolation of the tract (or duct). Fistulas must have the external orifice included in the skin resected followed by tract dissection cephalad.

4 Follow the tract superiorly. In its upper portion, the tract passes between the internal and external carotid arteries. After that, it crosses the superior laryngeal, the XII and the IX cranial nerves, and finally reaches its opening into the pharynx at the level of the tonsil. As the tract is slightly lateral to these structures, it is not necessary to actively dissect them in order to have their control. In the deeper plane of the dissection they may be seen and preserved [1, 2].

5 After isolating the BrCA and its tract, proceed to the duct ligation at the level of the tonsil. Use of a drain is recommended [1].

6 Third BrCAs may have their tracts opening to the larynx, to the trachea or to the pharynx. The tracts reach these regions of the upper aerodigestive tract after perforating the thyrohyoid membrane. They are rare and cysts may be confused with laryngocele [1, 2].

7 Fourth BrC cysts and fistulas are extremely rare. The internal opening is located in the pyriform sinus. They are clinically evident usually at the left side of the neck [6].

Conclusion

The management of BrC cysts and fistulas involves delicate dissection of cervical structures. It must preferably be carried out by experienced surgeons. Most complications are associated with injury of the following structures: hypoglossal nerve, glossopharyngeal nerve, superior laryngeal nerve, FN and carotid arteries. Recurrence can only be avoided with complete excision of the fistula or cyst and its tract. Definitive surgical treatment is much more difficult when there is an associated infection. In these cases, surgery should be postponed until the infection has been treated.

References

1 Loré JM: An Atlas of Head and Neck Surgery. Philadelphia, Saunders, 1988, pp 686–693.
2 Peynègre R, Rugina MD, Ducroz V: Chirurgie des kystes et fistules du cou. Techniques chirurgicales – Tête et cou, 46-480. Encycl Méd Chir. Paris, Elsevier, 1995, p 12.
3 Schroeder JW Jr, Mohyuddin N, Maddalozzo J: Branchial anomalies in the pediatric population. Otolaryngol Head Neck Surg 2007;137:289–295.
4 Triglia JM, Nicollas R, Ducroz V, Koltai PJ, Garabedian EN: First branchial cleft anomalies: a study of 39 cases and a review of the literature. Arch Otolaryngol Head Neck Surg 1998;124:291–295.
5 Martinez Del Pero M, Majumdar S, Bateman N, Bull PD: Presentation of first branchial cleft anomalies: the Sheffield experience. J Laryngol Otol 2007;121:455–459.
6 Shrime M, Kacker A, Bent J, Ward RF: Fourth branchial complex anomalies: a case series. Int J Pediatr Otorhinolaryngol 2003;67:1227–1233.

Cernea CR, Dias FL, Fliss D, Lima RA, Myers EN, Wei WI (eds): Pearls and Pitfalls in Head and Neck Surgery. Basel, Karger, 2008, pp 158–159

10.2 How to Avoid Surprises in the Management of the Thyroglossal Duct Cyst

Nilton T. Herter

FAHNS, Brazilian HNSS, Argentinian HNS, Chilean HNS, Peruvian HNS, LATS Head and Neck Service, Hospital Santa Rita, Porto Alegre, Brazil

PEARLS

- Keep in mind that thyroglossal duct cyst (TGDC) may be associated with other anatomical and functional abnormalities of the thyroid gland.
- Do not operate on a patient with TGDC without previous anatomic and functional evaluation of the thyroid gland.
- Carcinoma arising in TGDC may be found in adults, so preoperative cytological evaluation is recommended in suspicious cases.

PITFALLS

- Risk of resection of the only thyroid tissue of the patient.
- Risk of hypothyroidism, either clinical or subclinical.
- Risk of finding a carcinoma in the pathologic report after surgery.

Introduction

TGDC is the main abnormality of development in the neck. Most of the patients are children or young adults and complain of a single nodule in the midline, at the level of hyoid bone. Clinical diagnosis is safe and easy [2–4]. The golden standard treatment is the Sistrunk procedure [1] which involves resection of the cyst, the central part of the hyoid bone and the embryologic remnant till the base of the tongue. Damage of the lingual artery or the hypoglossal nerves must be avoided with careful dissection. Surgical drainage of the operative field is recommended, since postoperative hematoma may be dangerous.

Associated with TGDC, we can find subclinical hypothyroidism and other abnormalities of the development of the thyroid gland, such as lingual thyroid, ectopic gland, agenesis or hemiagenesis as well as rare cases of carcinoma.

Practical Tips

Although it is usually easy to diagnose a TGDC and to perform the Sistrunk procedure, associated disorganogenetic, dishormonogenetic or carcinogenetic changes may be found and lead to some surprises for the surgeon, jeopardizing the patient's health. It is important to keep in mind some hazardous situations.

1. Consider the association between TGDC and subclinical hypothyroidism and ask for blood tests including TSH and thyroxine.
2. Consider the association between TGDC and other abnormalities of the embryologic development of the thyroid gland and ask for neck ultrasound and scintiscan of the thyroid gland.
3. Consider that in 2–3% of the TGDC we can find a carcinoma; so, ask for FNBA and cytological examination when the cyst is greater than 3 cm, when it occurs in adults [5], when there is a

solid component in the cyst, when there is rapid growth, or in the presence of local invasive signs or of a clinically evident cervical lymph node.

④ Classical Sistrunk operation is the golden standard procedure for treatment of most TGDC.

⑤ Enlarged Sistrunk procedure is recommended for TGD carcinomas as well as supraomohyoid neck dissection.

⑥ Subclinical hypothyroidism must be evaluated and treated.

Conclusion

In this chapter, the reader was exposed to a frequently overlooked complication of surgical treatment of the TGDC. TGDC may often be associated with subclinical hypothyroidism and other anatomic abnormalities of the thyroid gland, as well as with carcinoma, generally in adults. Functional, anatomical and pathologic evaluation of the cyst is recommended to prevent further complications.

References

1 Chandra RK, Madalozzo J, Kovarik P: Histological characterization of the thyroglossal tract: Implications for surgical management. Laryngoscope 2001;111:1002.

2 Herter NT, Silva GS: Carcinoma de cisto tireoglosso; relato de um caso e revisão da literatura. Rev Brás Cir Cab Pesc 1989;13:21–24.

3 Herter NT: Cistos, fístulas e neoplasias do ducto tireoglosso; in Kowalski LP (ed): Afecções Cirúrgicas do Pescoço. Col Brás Cir. São Paulo, Atheneu, 2005, vol VII, pp 105–114.

4 Livosi VA: Surgical Pathology of Thyroid. Philadelphia, Saunders, 1990, p 156.

5 Yadranko D: Thyroglossal duct cysts in the elderly population. Am J Otolaryngol 2002;23:17.

Cernea CR, Dias FL, Fliss D, Lima RA, Myers EN, Wei WI (eds): Pearls and Pitfalls in Head and Neck Surgery. Basel, Karger, 2008, pp 160–161

11.1 How to Manage Extensive Carotid Body Tumors

Nadir Ahmad, James L. Netterville

Department of Otolaryngology – Head and Neck, Vanderbilt University Medical Center, Nashville, Tenn., USA

PEARLS

- Options include surgery, observation or radiation therapy (RDT). Decisive factors are tumor size, patient age and comorbidities, among others.
- Resection of unilateral carotid body tumors (CBT) is safe, with limited morbidity in tumors <5 cm.
- Although not necessary for smaller CBT, preoperative embolization decreases blood loss, especially in larger CBT.
- Surgical resection involves a team approach, and a vascular surgeon should be alerted to the need for intraoperative carotid artery (CA) resection and bypass if required.
- Keys to low surgical morbidity: high cervical exposure, meticulous dissection and identification of regional cranial nerves (CN), with proximal and distal control of carotid system (CS).

PITFALLS

- Avoid dissection into the media layer of the CA.
- Supraadventitial dissection is often sufficient for CBT removal, but occasionally, subadventitial dissection is required and often fraught with bleeding; meticulous dissection and liberal use of bipolar cautery are recommended.
- CN injury is the most common sequela, and must be discussed with the patient before surgery in anticipation of rehabilitating possible deficits.
- First-bite syndrome (FBS) and baroreceptor failure (BF) are overlooked complications of CBT resection.

Introduction

CBT are paragangliomas arising from the carotid body (CB), a chemoreceptor located at the carotid bifurcation. The CB is attached to the bifurcation by the ligament of Mayer and is innervated by the glossopharyngeal (IX) nerve via its nerve of Hering branch. It is responsive to changes in PaO_2, $PaCO_2$, pH and blood flow by regulating ventilation.

These tumors are predominantly benign and slow-growing. The typical patient presents in the 5th decade with a painless upper neck mass; 10% of these cases have bilateral tumors and even multiple other head and neck paragangliomas. Familial cases are rare (25–50% are multifocal) [1, 2]. Apart from careful history and physical exam focusing on CN assessment, the initial workup should include either a contrast CT scan or MRI. The characteristic finding is 'lyre sign' or splaying of the external and internal CAs. This is seen classically on angiography, which can be used for preoperative embolization. Malignant CBT are rare and are usually diagnosed through the finding of a lymph node metastasis.

Surgery is the optimal treatment [2, 3]. RDT is another option and should be considered in patients that cannot tolerate surgery or the potential CN deficits. In our experience, RDT leads to regression of the tumor size, to arrest in growth, and to continued growth, respectively, in 1/3 of cases, each. Observation is a reasonable option in select cases, as these are slow-growing tumors (1–

1.5 mm/year). Complications include injury to various regional CNs, as well as FBS, which is the development of pain in the parotid region after the first bite of every meal [3, 4]. The cause of this complication is unknown but is thought to be due to interruption of regional sympathetic nerve fibers. BF can occur after unilateral or bilateral resections, and the result is lability of blood pressure and heart rate.

Practical Tips

❶ High cervical incision that passes medially over the region of hyoid bone.

❷ Perform limited selective neck dissection to sample regional nodes for metastasis and to expose the regional CNs and carotid sheath structures.

❸ Gain proximal and distal control of the CS.

❹ Dissection starts along external CA to free its branches from the tumor. It can be sacrificed if necessary.

❺ Plane of dissection can be supra or subadventitial depending on tumor invasion. Bipolar cautery is used liberally.

❻ Great care is taken to avoid dissection into the media layer, resulting in an unsafe artery. Eventually, vessel resection and bypass are performed by a vascular surgeon.

❼ Dissect along lateral surface of internal CA, rolling the tumor toward the bifurcation.

❽ Final removal often requires ligation of ascending pharyngeal artery and dissection of superior laryngeal nerve.

Conclusion

CBT are rare head and neck tumors that must be considered in the differential diagnosis of neck and parapharyngeal space masses. Surgery is the primary treatment; RDT and observation are reserved for select cases. Preoperative embolization is useful, mainly in large tumors. A vascular surgeon should be available. CN injury is uncommon. FBS and BF are less known complications of CBT surgery.

11

References

1 Cohen SM, Burkey BB, Netterville JL: Surgical management of parapharyngeal space masses. Head Neck 2005;27:669–675.
2 Pellitteri PK, Rinaldo A, Myssiorek D, et al: Paragangliomas of the head and neck. Oral Oncol 2004;40:563–575.
3 Sniezek JC, Sabri AN, Netterville JL: Paraganglioma surgery: complications and treatment. Otolaryngol Clin North Am 2001;34:993–1006.
4 Netterville JL, Reilly KM, Robertson D, et al: Carotid body tumors: a review of 30 patients with 46 tumors. Laryngoscope 1995;105:115–126.

Cernea CR, Dias FL, Fliss D, Lima RA, Myers EN, Wei WI (eds): Pearls and Pitfalls in Head and Neck Surgery. Basel, Karger, 2008, pp 162–163

11.2 How to Manage Extensive Neurogenic Tumors

Ziv Gil, Dan M. Fliss

Department of Otolaryngology – Head and Neck Surgery, Tel Aviv Sourasky Medical Center, Tel Aviv, Israel

PEARLS

- Perform a detailed imaging workup, including contrast computerized tomography and magnetic resonance imaging. Magnetic resonance angiography is occasionally added to differentiate schwannomas from paragangliomas.
- Most of the benign neurogenic tumors (NTs) are extirpated via cervical approach.
- For extensive tumors with multicompartment involvement, use combined approaches to allow adequate exposure and safe resection.

PITFALLS

- Always discuss with the patients the potential complications of surgery, which may include multiple cranial nerve palsies, bleeding, stroke and death.
- Tracheostomy should be used in patients undergoing the transmandibular approach and when the resection requires bulky reconstruction, and in all patients with expected airway impairment.
- The surgical resection of extensive NTs should always start with proximal and distal control of the great vessels of the neck and with identification, exposure and protection of all neighboring cranial nerves.
- Appropriate reconstruction should be carried out after dural, pharyngeal or extensive skin resectioning to prevent significant complications, for cosmesis and to provide good functional outcome.
- Consider immediate vocal cord medialization for patients with vagal schwannoma.

Introduction

NTs of the head and neck represent a group of uncommon lesions of benign or malignant origin. A variety of surgical approaches have been described for the management of extensive NTs [1]. Although the cervical approach permits complete tumor resection in the majority of cases, there are still situations in which the superior or inferior aspects of the tumor are not adequately accessed via conventional neck incision. For example, these tumors may infiltrate superiorly along the parapharyngeal space and invade the paranasal sinuses, orbit, pterygopalatine fossa or the infratemporal fossa. They may also grow caudally and invade the superior mediastinum. These latter cases require alternative approaches or a combination of several approaches to allow proper exposure and safe tumor resection [2].

Practical Tips

1. The selected surgical approach should be safe and should allow complete tumor resection whenever possible, while minimizing functional and cosmetic morbidity.
2. In most patients, inferior NTs are excised via the cervical approach with no need for any major reconstructive procedures [1].
3. The transmandibular approach is suitable for patients with extremely large tumors that involve the parapharyngeal space. Once the mandible is split, the two segments of the mandible are separated for exposing the tumor which is then re-

Table 1. Surgical approaches (single or combined) used for excision of extensive neurogenic skull base tumors

Tumor extension	Surgical approach
Anterior skull base, frontal/ethmoidal/sphenoidal sinuses, sphenoid clivus, planum sphenoidale	Subcranial (not requiring facial incisions)
Malignant tumors involving the inferior/anterior/lateral maxillary walls	Craniofacial or transfacial
Extension to the lateral skull base, cavernous sinus, middle fossa	Orbitozygomatic, pterional or infratemporal fossa
Extension to the orbit	Transorbital
Parapharyngeal space tumors extending to the middle fossa	Cervical-orbitozygomatic, maxillary swing

moved under direct visualization of the surrounding structures.

❹ Pterional or orbitozygomatic approaches with or without the cervical approach are used for NTs involving in the trigeminal ganglion, cavernous sinus and clivus with considerable skull base involvement [2].

❺ The middle fossa approach type A may be used in selected cases for surgical treatment of schwannomas and neurofibromas involving the jugular foramen [3].

❻ Malignant NTs (e.g., esthesioneuroblastoma, malignant peripheral nerve sheath tumor) frequently have multicompartmental invasion, requiring a multifaceted approach to the anterior skull base. Both the craniofacial or subcranial approaches can be used to access the anterior skull base, while more extensive tumors can be reached via a combined approach, based on the exact anatomical localization of the tumor (table 1) [2].

❼ Median sternotomy is required for NTs with the following indications: (1) recurrent intrathoracic tumors, (2) previous mediastinal or cardiothoracic surgery, (3) previous radiation to the neck or mediastinum,(4) malignant NTs abutting the great vessels, (5) isolated intrathoracic tumors, and (6) tumors invading below the level of the carina [4].

❽ Large defects require reconstruction with regional flaps (pectoralis major myocutaneous flap, temporalis muscle flap) or free flaps (a radial forearm fasciocutaneous flap or a scapular flap).

Conclusions

Knowledge of the differential diagnosis and a detailed presurgical workup allow careful, well thought-out planning of the surgical approach and a safe tumor resection. Surgery of NTs may be performed in most patients via the cervical approach. In a small number of patients with extremely large NTs extending to the skull base or mediastinum, and for invasive malignancies, combined approaches are used to assure safe and efficacious extirpation.

References

1 Khafif A, Segev Y, Kaplan DM, Gil Z, Fliss DM: Surgical management of parapharyngeal space tumors: a 10-year review. Otolaryngol Head Neck Surg 2005;132:401–406.

2 Fliss DM, Abergel A, Cavel O, Margalit O, Gil Z: Combined subcranial approaches for excision of complex anterior skull base tumors. Arch Otol Head Neck Surg 2007;133:888–896.

3 Shahinian H, Dornier C, Fisch U: Parapharyngeal space tumors: the infratemporal fossa approach. Skull Base Surg 1995;5:73–81.

4 Ladas G, Rhys-Evans PH, Goldstraw P: Anterior cervical-transsternal approach for resection of benign tumors at the thoracic inlet. Ann Thorac Surg 1999;67:785–789.

Cernea CR, Dias FL, Fliss D, Lima RA, Myers EN, Wei WI (eds): Pearls and Pitfalls in Head and Neck Surgery. Basel, Karger, 2008, pp 164–165

11.3 How to Choose a Surgical Approach to a Parapharyngeal Space Mass

Kerry D. Olsen

Mayo Clinic Rochester, Rochester, Minn., USA

PEARLS

- The cervical parotid approach can be used to safely remove the majority of lesions encountered in the parapharyngeal space.
- Division of the stylomandibular ligament is essential to opening the parapharyngeal space.
- Most deep lobe parotid tumors that involve the parapharyngeal space begin in the retromandibular portion of the deep lobe. Widely surrounding this portion of gland can be done without having to remove the superficial portion of the gland.

PITFALLS

- Failure to identify the facial nerve can lead to inadvertent injury when the tumor extends superior to the position of the main trunk of the facial nerve.
- Failure to obtain maximum exposure by a mandibulotomy in cases of skull base or carotid artery involvement by malignant tumors or vascular neoplasms can lead to incomplete tumor removal or significant morbidity.

Introduction

The parapharyngeal space is involved by a wide variety of benign and malignant neoplasms. The majority of cases (80%) are benign and arise from the deep lobe of the parotid gland or from nerves or paraganglia in the retrostyloid portion of the parapharynx. The goal of surgery should be to provide adequate tumor visualization that insures complete tumor removal without rupture of the tumor capsule and preservation of the surrounding nerves and vessels.

Practical Tips

The cervical parotid approach can be used to remove the majority of deep lobe parotid and extraparotid salivary gland tumors [1, 2, 3]. This approach is also used to remove most neurogenic tumors and small paragangliomas.

1. The inferior division of the facial nerve is first isolated and followed out to the level of the submandibular gland.
2. The upper jugular nodes are removed to allow for exposure of the great vessels and cranial nerves X, XI and XII.
3. The stylomandibular fascia between the parotid and in the submandibular gland is divided and the gland retracted medially.
4. The posterior belly of the digastric muscle and stylohyoid muscles are divided near the mastoid tip and reflected medially.
5. The dense stylomandibular ligament is next divided as is the external carotid artery as it enters the deep parotid tissue at the level of the styloglossus muscle.
6. If the tumor is extending around the styloid process, it is best to remove this bone to avoid inadvertent tumor capsule rupture.
7. The medial extent of the tumor can be freed from the superior constrictor muscles and the medial pterygoid muscle by blunt finger dissection.

⑧ The tumor can then be removed under direct vision with care to include a portion of the deep lobe if the tumor originates or involves a portion of the parotid gland.
⑨ Carefully look for any venous bleeding and retain a Hemovac drain for a minimum of 2 days to reduce the risk of dead space bleeding or infection.
⑩ If there is no loose areolar plane surrounding a prestyloid tumor, the lesion is either malignant or has been previously biopsied transorally with subsequent scarring along the constrictor muscle.
⑪ The cervical parotid approach can be extended posteriorly to perform a suboccipital craniotomy for tumors that extend intracranially via the retrostyloid space.
⑫ The use of a parasymphyseal mandibulotomy in combination with a cervical parotid approach is used in approximately 10% of cases.
⑬ The mandibulotomy approach is helpful for vascular tumors that involve the carotid artery or superior parapharyngeal space or for malignant tumors that invade surrounding bone or the great vessels.
⑭ A transoral approach is rarely done and reserved for isolated, small, benign extraparotid salivary tumors.

Conclusion

Surgery in the parapharyngeal space can be done safely and with good tumor exposure. The cervical parotid approach (90%) and cervical parotid approach with a parasymphyseal mandibulotomy (10%) are effective for complete tumor removal, control of bleeding, preservation of surrounding nerves, and low morbidity.

11

References

1 Olsen KD: Tumors and surgery of the parapharyngeal space. Laryngoscope 1994;104(5 Suppl 63):1–28.
2 Stell PM, Mansfield AO, Stoney PJ: Surgical approaches to tumors of the parapharyngeal space. Am J Otolaryngology 1985; 6:92–97.
3 Olsen KD: Parapharyngeal space tumors; in Gates GA (eds): Current Therapy in Otolaryngology – Head and Neck Surgery, ed 5. St Louis, Mosby, 1994, pp 243–247.

Cernea CR, Dias FL, Fliss D, Lima RA, Myers EN, Wei WI (eds): Pearls and Pitfalls in Head and Neck Surgery. Basel, Karger, 2008, pp 166–167

12.1 Practical Tips to Approach a Deep Neck Abscess

Flávio C. Hojaij, Caio Plopper

Federal Medical School of São Paulo, Department of Otorhinolaryngology and Head and Neck Surgery, São Paulo, Brazil

PEARLS

- Detect and treat the primary cause of the infection.
- When necessary, surgical treatment should not be delayed.
- Contrast-enhanced computed tomography (CECT) is the best exam to evaluate a deep neck abscess and to plan surgical intervention.

PITFALLS

- Remember that older patients with underlying diseases are more likely to have complications.
- Keep in mind that necrotizing fasciitis does not present with radiological signs of pus collection, but may be associated with gas formation within deep fascial planes.
- Deep neck infections may progress toward extensive tissue necrosis and mediastinitis with high mortality rates.

Introduction

It is very important to distinguish between superficial and deep neck infection. The former is very common and easily treated uneventfully. In contrast, the latter is more hazardous and can be life-threatening.

Deep neck abscesses (DNAs) are pus collections that develop within deep cervical spaces, separated by layers of deep cervical fascia, usually caused by dental or upper airway infection [1–5]. These abscesses can also be related to infections of salivary glands, congenital malformation or trauma. In more than 25% of patients with DNA, a clear etiology cannot be identified [1–5].

The parapharyngeal space is the most common site; unfortunately abscesses in this region are more dangerous [1–4, 6, 7]. DNAs secondary to dental infections frequently lead to sepsis or necrotizing fasciitis [8, 9].

Practical Tips

In clinical practice, it is very important to listen to patients' complaints. Cervical or oropharyngeal pain associated with fever must raise the suspicion of a possible deep neck infection. A good physical examination can easily distinguish between deep and superficial infections. Some practical tips are important in order to enable prompt and successful treatment:

1. Always keep in mind that you need to look for and to treat the primary cause of the abscess (for example dental infection, upper airway infection).
2. CECT is a useful tool to detect and to establish the treatment of neck abscesses, and should be done still in the early stage of the disease [1–7].
3. Broad-spectrum antibiotic therapy and surgical drainage are the treatment of choice for the majority of cases [1–7].

❹ For selected cases (clinically stable patients with only one cervical space abscess smaller than 3 cm), a trial of intravenous antibiotics can be made before immediate surgical drainage. In these instances, a 48-hour wait-and-watch policy, with a control CECT, will determine if surgical intervention is needed [10].
❺ Older age, diabetes mellitus, underlying systemic disease and multiple-space involvement require careful consideration about potential complications [1–3, 7].
❻ Spotted gas images and edema are common findings in patients with necrotizing fasciitis. These patients should be treated with intravenous antibiotics and early surgical debridement [8, 9].
❼ Dyspnea, dysphagia and hoarseness are poor prognostic signs, indicating the need for aggressive surgical intervention.
❽ At operation, always under general anesthesia, large incisions are generally necessary.
❾ Do not delay a new surgical intervention if there is no clinical improvement or if a new CECT still shows necrosis or pus collection.
❿ Intraoral drainage, when possible, can be safe, especially in the pediatric population.
⓫ Be aware that oral intubation can be difficult if the patient presents with trismus. Endoscopic-assisted intubation or tracheostomy under local anesthesia should be considered, in order to prevent urgent surgical airway intervention.
⓬ Special attention should be paid to mediastinum and pleura; do not hesitate to perform thoracotomy and/or chest drainage, if necessary.
⓭ It is very important to collect material for culture and antibiogram.
⓮ Seriously consider intensive care support and hyperbaric oxygen therapy.

References

1 Huang TT, Liu TC, Chen PR, Tseng FY, Yeh TH, Chen YS: Deep neck infection: analysis of 185 cases. Head Neck 2004;26:854–860.
2 Lee JK, Kim HD, Lim SC: Predisposing factors of complicated deep neck infection: an analysis of 158 cases. Yonsei Med J 2007; 48:55–62.
3 Boscolo-Rizzo P, Marchiori C, Montolli F, Vaglia A, Da Mosto MC: Deep neck infections: a constant challenge. ORL J Otorhinolaryngol Relat Spec 2006;68:259–265.
4 Parhiscar A, Har-El G: Deep neck abscess: a retrospective review of 210 cases. Ann Otol Rhinol Laryngol 2001;110:1051–1054.
5 Sethi DS, Stanley RE: Deep neck abscesses – changing trends. J Laryngol Otol 1994;108:138–143.
6 Oh JH, Kim Y, Kim CH: Parapharyngeal abscess: comprehensive management protocol. ORL J Otorhinolaryngol Relat Spec 2007; 69:37–42.
7 Mazita A, Hazim MY, Megat Shiraz MA, Primuharsa Putra SH: Neck abscess: five year retrospective review of Hospital University Kebangsaan Malaysia experience. Med J Malaysia 2006; 61: 151–156.
8 Edwards JD, Sadeghi N, Najam F, Margolis M: Craniocervical necrotizing fasciitis of odontogenic origin with mediastinal extension. Ear Nose Throat J 2004;83:579–582.
9 Balbierz JM, Ellis K: Streptococcal infection and necrotizing fasciitis – implications for rehabilitation: a report of 5 cases and review of the literature. Arch Phys Med Rehabil 2004;85:1205–1209.
10 Boscolo-Rizzo P, Marchiori C, Zanetti F, Vaglia A, Da Mosto MC: Conservative management of deep neck abscesses in adults: the importance of CECT findings. Otolaryngol Head Neck Surg 2006;135:894–899.

Cernea CR, Dias FL, Fliss D, Lima RA, Myers EN, Wei WI (eds): Pearls and Pitfalls in Head and Neck Surgery. Basel, Karger, 2008, pp 168–169

12.2 Management of Necrotizing Fasciitis

Dorival De Carlucci, Jr.

Cerqueira César, São Paulo, Brazil

PEARLS

- Keep in mind that necrotizing fasciitis (NF) is a rare but aggressive soft tissue infection.
- It is commonly associated with other debilitating conditions.
- The clinical manifestations and physical findings are not specific but are often typical.

PITFALLS

The management of cervical NF needs a multiple approach:

- Local aggressive radical debridement.
- Systemic-level broad-spectrum antibiotics.
- Intensive supportive care, such as hyperbaric oxygen.

Introduction

One of the most dangerous complications of deep abscesses of the head and neck is NF, which is a relatively uncommon but aggressive soft tissue infection characterized by progressive destruction of fascia and adipose tissue that may not involve the skin [1].

NF was first observed during the American Civil War in 1871 by Joseph Jones [2], a Confederate Army surgeon, who described hospital cases of gangrene characterized by skin discoloration with loss of superficial and deep tissue. The term NF was first used by Wilson [3] in 1952 to describe cases with staphylococcal infection.

NF can develop in patients of all ages with no predilection for sex or race [4]. A history of operation, minor trauma or dental procedures represents common causes of infection. Other associated antecedent events included skin biopsy, tracheostomy wound, and even fish bone ingestion. However, in many cases, not even a tiny trauma inlet could be identified.

The predisposing factors include diabetes mellitus, arteriosclerosis, alcoholism, chronic renal failure, malignancy and intravenous drug abuse. Most patients showed at least one debilitating condition [5].

The exact mechanism of this rapidly spreading gangrenous infection has not been established. The releases of enzymes, such as hyaluronidase, and proteolytic portions of cell membranes have been shown to be contributing factors in the necrosis. The relative lack of vascularity of the relevant fascial planes has also been hypothesized as a contributing factor [6].

Polymicrobial infections are reported in most recent series. Causative organisms include mixed aerobes and anaerobes, most commonly Streptococcus spp., Staphylococcus spp., Bacteroides spp., Fusobacterium spp. and Peptostreptococcus spp. [5].

Practical Tips

❶ Early recognition and management are essential to a better prognosis [6].

❷ A number of signs and symptoms should alert clinicians, such as shortness of breath, dysphagia, and odynophagia. At the time of presentation, most patients are toxic with high fever. In case shock, organ dysfunction, or gas in tissue (radiography or palpation) are present, immediate surgery is indicated [7].

❸ Complications include pneumonia, lung abscess, internal jugular vein thrombosis, meningitis, mediastinitis, arterial erosion and mandible necrosis. Recent reports suggested that the mortality rate ranged from 16.5 to 20% [8, 9].

❹ Computed tomography (CT) is the imaging modality of choice, providing information on the localization and extension of the disease. It confirms the presence or absence of gas and provides detailed anatomic information. Magnetic resonance imaging can also be helpful in delineating the extent of intramuscular or subcutaneous abscesses [5].

❺ The key to successful treatment is early diagnosis, which, when combined with aggressive treatment, can substantially improve the outcome. An extensive excision, debridement and drainage of the involved necrotic skin, fascia and muscle are the most important aspects of therapy.

❻ Parenteral antibiotics should be instituted without delay. As the infection always exhibits a fulminant course, it is not advisable to wait for culture results. Empirical initial coverage should include broad-spectrum antibiotics. The treatment generally includes penicillinase-resistant penicillins plus additional coverage for anaerobic organisms.

❼ Hyperbaric oxygen is considered an adjunctive therapy. It inhibits anaerobes and helps break the vicious synergistic cycle between anaerobes and aerobes and limits the debridement by demarcating the border between devitalized and healthy tissue [10].

Conclusions

❶ NF of the head and neck is a rare but aggressive soft tissue infection, commonly associated with other debilitating conditions.

❷ The clinical manifestations and physical findings are not specific but are often typical. A high index of suspicion for NF should be maintained.

❸ CT is helpful for an early diagnosis and for planning therapy.

❹ The key to successful treatment is early diagnosis combined with aggressive surgical treatment and administration of parenteral antibiotics.

❺ Hyperbaric oxygen is an adjunctive therapy to surgery and antibiotics.

❻ There is still a high mortality rate (25%) despite aggressive management.

12

References

1 Sellers BJ, Woods ML, Morris SE, Saffle JR: Necrotizing group A streptococcal infections associated with streptococcal toxic shock syndrome. Am J Surg 1996;172:523–528.

2 Jones J: Investigation upon the nature, causes and treatment of hospital gangrene as it prevailed in the Confederate Armies 1861–1865; in Hamilton FH (ed): Surgical Memoirs of the War of Rebellion. New York, Riverside, 1871, pp 146–170.

3 Wilson B: Necrotizing fasciitis. Am Surg 1952;18:416–431.

4 Reed JM, Vinod KA: Odontogenic cervical necrotizing fasciitis with intrathoracic extension. Otolaryngol Head Neck Surg 1992;107:596–600.

5 Skitarelic N, Mladina R, Morovic M, Skitarelic N: Cervical necrotizing fasciitis: sources and outcomes. Infection 2003;31:39–44.

6 Greinwald JH, Wilson JF, Haggerty PG: Peritonsillar abscess: an unlikely cause of necrotizing fasciitis. Ann Otol Rhinol Laryngol 1995;104:133–137.

7 Lin C, Yeh FL, Lin JT, Ma H, Hwang CH, Shen BH, Fang RH: Necrotizing fasciitis of the head and neck: an analysis of 47 cases. Plast Reconstr Surg 2001;107:1684–1693.

8 Haywood CT, McGeer A, Low DE: Clinical experience with 20 cases of group A Streptococcus necrotizing fasciitis and myonecrosis: 1995 to 1997. Plast Reconstr Surg 1999;103:1567–1573.

9 Marty-Ané CH, Berthet JP, Alric P, Pegis JD, Rouvière P, Mary H: Management of descending necrotizing mediastinitis: an aggressive treatment for an aggressive disease. Ann Thorac Surg 1999;68:212–217.

10 Kirby SD, Deschler DG: Hyperbaric oxygen therapy: application in diseases of the head and neck. Gen Otolaryngol 1999;7:137.

Cernea CR, Dias FL, Fliss D, Lima RA, Myers EN, Wei WI (eds): Pearls and Pitfalls in Head and Neck Surgery. Basel, Karger, 2008, pp 170–171

13.1 Minimizing Complications in Tracheotomy

Eugene N. Myers

Department of Otolaryngology, University of Pittsburgh, School of Medicine, Pittsburgh, Pa., USA

PEARLS

- Most complications of tracheotomy are preventable.
- Securing the airway is fundamental to the success of the procedure and preventing complications.
- Meticulous surgical technique is the key feature in preventing complications.

PITFALLS

- Failure to insert the tracheotomy cannula under direct vision can lead to a false passage between the anterior wall of the trachea and the sternum which will result in death if not recognized.
- Bleeding or injury to vital structures may occur if dissection is not limited to the midline.
- An unrepaired laceration of the posterior wall of the trachea may result in a tracheoesophageal fistula.

Introduction

Tracheotomy may be one of the easiest or one of the most difficult, dangerous, and frustrating of surgical procedures. The highest priority before performing a tracheotomy is securing the airway [1] since the risk factors for complications increase when the procedure is performed under less than ideal circumstances. Prevention of complications is much easier than their management.

Practical Tips

❶ Once the incision is made, dissecting in the midline will prevent bleeding from structures such as the anterior jugular veins, carotid arteries, aberrant innominate arteries or thyroid isthmus.

❷ Keeping dissection in the midline will also minimize the possibility of pneumomediastinum or pneumothorax or injury to the recurrent laryngeal nerves [2].

❸ A false passage between the trachea and the sternum can be avoided by inserting the tracheotomy tube into the trachea under direct vision using retractors and good illumination [3].

❹ Subcutaneous emphysema can be prevented by securing the airway prior to the tracheotomy with an endotracheal tube, avoiding excess dissection of the paratracheal tissues and not closing the skin incision tightly or packing the wound.

❺ A displaced tracheotomy tube is a potentially lethal problem [4]. Prevention includes the use of traction sutures in the trachea and sewing the neck plate of the tracheotomy tube to the peristomal skin. Tube size and configuration is also important since an ill-fitting tube may be associated with increased morbidity and death [5].

❻ Tracheal stenosis is usually related to the cuff of an endotracheal tube. The use of high volume, low pressure cuffs has greatly decreased the problem. Avoiding injury to the cricoid cartilage by keeping the tracheotomy at the level of the 2nd to 3rd tracheal ring helps to prevent stenosis.

Conclusions

Most complications of tracheotomy are preventable. Securing the airway prior to tracheotomy is the highest priority. Meticulous attention to the details of the surgery is of paramount importance. Complications such as a displaced tracheotomy tube are potentially fatal and require immediate attention.

References

1 Walkevekar R, Myers EN: Techniques and Complications in Tracheostomy in Adults. San Diego, Plural Publishing, 2007.
2 Rabuzzi DD, Reed GF: Intrathoracic complications following tracheotomy in children. Laryngoscope 1971;81:939–946.
3 Durbin CG Jr: Early complications of tracheostomy. Respir Care 2005;50:511–515.
4 Parnes SM, Myers EN: Traction sutures in a tracheostomy using a ligature passer. Trans Am Acad Ophthalmol Otolaryngol 1976; 82:479–485.
5 Grillo HC: Management of non-neoplastic diseases of the trachea; in Shields TW, LoCicero J 3rd, Ponn RB (eds): General Thoracic Surgery, ed 5. Philadelphia, Lippincott Williams & Wilkins, 2000, vol 1, pp 885–897.

13

Cernea CR, Dias FL, Fliss D, Lima RA, Myers EN, Wei WI (eds): Pearls and Pitfalls in Head and Neck Surgery. Basel, Karger, 2008, pp 172–173

13.2 Emergency Upper Airway Obstruction: Cricothyroidotomy or Tracheotomy?

Carlos N. Lehn

Head and Neck Surgery Service, Hospital Heliópolis, São Paulo, Brazil

PEARLS

- Orotracheal intubation should be attempted first in patients with upper airway obstruction; only a few patients will require tracheotomy or cricothyroidotomy.
- Try to establish the cause of obstruction: edema, trauma, foreign body, infection or tumor.
- In cancer patients and in trauma with suspected laryngotracheal disjunction a tracheotomy is preferred.

PITFALLS

- Performing a cricothyroidotomy in a larynx cancer patient may be disastrous: you will disrupt the tumor and may start a bleeding.
- Cricothyroidotomy in acute laryngeal disease does not provide adequate ventilation.

Introduction

The management of emergency upper airway obstruction depends on its cause. Edema, trauma, foreign body, infection and tumor can lead to this condition [1]. In head and neck surgery specifically the presence of a growing tumor may lead to this condition but it can be expected and prevented with elective tracheotomy.

In most trauma patients airway problems can be managed with orotracheal intubation and only a few require open techniques. Today tracheotomy is not and should not be an emergency procedure owing to the huge complication and mortality rate of emergency tracheotomy and the existence of alternative routes to obtain immediate airway control in the acutely obstructed upper airway [2, 3].

The complication rates for emergency cricothyroidotomy and tracheotomy are similar (20 and 21%). Inpatients requiring an emergency surgical airway had a higher complication rate (32 vs. 0%) but better overall survival (91 vs. 46%) than patients treated in the emergency department. Some authors describe a complication rate of 32% in emergency cricothyroidotomy [4, 5].

Practical Tips

1. Most patients with emergency upper airway obstruction can be managed with orotracheal intubation or rapid sequence intubation techniques and only a few will require tracheotomy or cricothyroidotomy [3, 6].
2. Try to establish the cause of airway obstruction: the approach may be different depending on whether the patient has a larynx tumor or a foreign body [1].
3. Remember that the hyoid bone is higher in children than in adults.
4. In larynx cancer patients tracheotomy is the method of choice.
5. In trauma patients, if laryngotracheal disjunction is suspected avoid cricothyroidotomy [7].

⑥ The conversion of a cricothyroidotomy into a tracheotomy can be performed if the patient is not in a life-threatening condition. Some authors do not agree that all cricothyroidotomies should be converted [4].
⑦ Subglottic stenosis does not occur in all cases of cricothyroidotomy.

Conclusion

In this chapter we discussed the indications for tracheotomy and cricothyroidotomy in emergency airway obstruction. It is important to state that in these cases we can expect a high rate of complications but an even higher rate of survival of a life-threatening condition. The ability to differentiate individual cases (tumor, trauma, infection, foreign body and edema) and the skill to perform one or other technique of airway assessment are crucial. The main goal of these tips is to guide the reader how to evaluate the best option for each patient, depending on the primary cause of the airway impairment.

References

1. Linscott MS, Horton WC: Management of upper airway obstruction. Otolaryngol Clin North Am 1979;12:351–373.
2. Goldenberg D, Golz A, Netzer A, Joachims HZ: Tracheotomy: changing indications and a review of 1,130 cases. J Otolaryngol 2002;31:211–215.
3. Bair AE, Panacek EA, Wisner DH, Bales R, Sakles JC: Cricothyrotomy: a 5-year experience at one institution. J Emerg Med 2003;24:151–156.
4. Gillespie MB, Eisele DW: Outcomes of emergency surgical airway procedures in a hospital-wide setting. Laryngoscope 1999; 109:1766–1769.
5. McGill J, Clinton JE, Ruiz E: Cricothyrotomy in the emergency department. Ann Emerg Med 1982;11:361–364.
6. Bair AE, Filbin MR, Kulkarni RG, Walls RM: The failed intubation attempt in the emergency department: analysis of prevalence, rescue techniques, and personnel. J Emerg Med 2002;23: 131–140.
7. Weissler MC, Couch ME: Tracheotomy and intubation; in Bailey BJ, Johnson JT, Newlands SD (eds): Head and Neck Surgery and Otolaryngology. Philadelphia, Lippincott Williams & Wilkins, 2006.

Cernea CR, Dias FL, Fliss D, Lima RA, Myers EN, Wei WI (eds): Pearls and Pitfalls in Head and Neck Surgery. Basel, Karger, 2008, pp 174–175

13.3 Avoidance of Complications in Conventional Tracheotomy and Percutaneous Dilatational Tracheotomy

David W. Eisele

Department of Otolaryngology – Head and Neck Surgery, University of California, San Francisco, Calif., USA

PEARLS

- Avoid a high tracheotomy through or near the cricoid cartilage.
- Carefully select patients and use endoscopic guidance for percutaneous dilatational tracheotomy (PDT).
- Carefully secure the tracheotomy tube (TT) and exercise precautions to avoid accidental decannulation.

PITFALLS

- Inadequate safety precautions can result in a surgical fire.
- A small, sutured, or packed tracheotomy incision can result in subcutaneous emphysema or pneumothorax (PT).
- Hemorrhage from a tracheoinnominate artery fistula can be fatal.

Introduction

Conventional tracheotomy (CT) is indicated for emergency airway control and is the standard method for elective tracheotomy.

Recently, PDT has become a widely accepted and efficient method of tracheotomy for select patients who require prolonged intubation and mechanical ventilation. Contraindications include emergency airway access, children, obscuration of anatomic landmarks, tracheal deformity, high ventilation pressures, and uncorrectable coagulopathy [1].

CT became standardized by Chevalier Jackson [2] and others. Complications occur in 5–40% of patients and relate to the specific patient population, indication, surgical technique and emergency setting [3–5]. The most common complications include hemorrhage, tube obstruction, and accidental decannulation. PT, airway stenosis, and tracheoesophageal fistula are uncommon complications. Some complications are life-threatening, thus requiring prompt recognition and proper management.

Practical Tips for Open Tracheotomy

1. The surgeon must communicate with the anesthesiologist and other members of the operating team prior to the procedure.
2. The patient should be properly identified and positioned.
3. Prevent a surgical fire. Wait to drape until all flammable prep solutions have dried [6]. Stop supplemental oxygen for 1 min prior to use of electrocautery if possible. Be cognizant of possible oxygen enrichment under the drapes.
4. Either a vertical or horizontal neck incision, adequately sized, works well.
5. Carefully divide the thyroid isthmus with electrocautery [7]. Ligatures are used as needed.
6. Avoid a high tracheotomy near or through the cricoid cartilage.
7. Never use electrocautery to enter the trachea [8].
8. Creation of a circular or square tracheal window or a Bjork flap facilitates TT reinsertion should accidental decannulation occur.

9 Have the endotracheal tube (ET) withdrawn to just above the tracheal opening for TT placement. If there is difficulty in placing the TT, the ET can be advanced into the distal trachea for ventilation.
10 Select the proper TT based on the patient's characteristics. For obese patients, perform subcutaneous fat excision.
11 Do not suture or pack the tracheotomy wound to avoid subcutaneous emphysema or PT.
12 Carefully secure the TT by suturing the tube flange to the skin, with snugly secured ties, and with cuff inflation to avoid accidental decannulation.
13 A routine postoperative (PO) chest radiograph is not indicated [9].
14 Postoperatively administer humidified air.
15 Monitor TT cuff pressures and keep the cuff pressure less that 25 mm Hg to prevent tracheal mucosa injury.
16 Keep a spare TT and instruments necessary for tube replacement at the bedside postoperatively.
17 All instances of PO hemorrhage must be carefully evaluated and managed. A tracheoinnominate artery fistula must be excluded to avoid fatal hemorrhage.

Practical Tips for PDT

If PDT is performed, an endoscopist uses the flexible bronchoscope (FB) for endoscopic guidance and general anesthesia is administered.
1 Have all instruments and kit components.
2 Have a standard tracheotomy tray available.
3 Make the neck incision the same length as used for open tracheotomy.
4 Dissect bluntly to the trachea.
5 Visualize the trachea with the FB after the tip of the ET is withdrawn to the proximal trachea.
6 Be wary of oxygen desaturation with use of the bronchoscope.
7 Use transillumination and palpation of anatomic landmarks to place the needle through the anterior tracheal wall. Avoid the thyroid isthmus. Avoid puncture of the membranous trachea. Confirm proper needle placement endoscopically.
8 Pass the guide wire, dilators, and TT under endoscopic inspection.
9 Never force the dilators or TT.
10 Confirm proper tube placement with FB.
11 Confirm that the tracheotomy cuff has not been damaged.
12 The TT should not be removed until maturation of the tract has occurred [1]. For accidental decannulation within 1 week of the procedure, orotracheal intubation may be preferred because of potential difficulty with TT reinsertion [3].

Conclusion

Complications of CT and PDT should be carefully avoided. Proper patient selection, bronchoscopic guidance and proper technique, and adherence to postprocedure principles increase the safety of PDT.

References

1 Bhatti N, Tatlipinar A, Mirski M, et al: Percutaneous dilational tracheotomy in intensive care unit patients. Otolaryngol Head Neck Surg 2007;136:938–941.
2 Jackson C: High tracheotomy and other errors: the chief causes of chronic laryngeal stenosis. Surg Gynecol Obstet 1923;32:392–398.
3 Kost KM: Endoscopic percutaneous dilatational tracheotomy: a prospective evaluation of 500 consecutive cases. Laryngoscope 2005;115:1–30.
4 Goldenberg D, Gov-Ari E, Golz A, et al: Tracheotomy complications: a retrospective study of 1130 cases. Otolaryngol Head Neck Surg 2000;123:495–500.
5 Gillespie MB, Eisele DW: Outcomes of emergency surgical procedures in a hospital-wide setting. Laryngoscope 1999;109:1766–1769.
6 Weber SM, Hargunani CA, Wax MK: Duraprep and the risk of fire during tracheostomy. Head Neck 2006;28:649–652.
7 Calhoun KH, Weiss RL, Scott B, et al: Management of the thyroid isthmus in tracheostomy: a prospective and retrospective study. Otolaryngol Head Neck Surg 1994;111:450–452.
8 Tykocinski M, Thomson P, Hooper R: Airway fire during tracheotomy. ANZ J Surg 2006;76:195–197.
9 Hamburger MD, Wolf JS, Berry JA, Molter D: Appropriateness of routine chest radiography after tracheotomy. Arch Otolaryngol Head Neck Surg 2000;126:649–651.
10 Swanson GJ, Meleca RJ, Bander J, Stackler RJ: The utility of chest radiography following percutaneous dilational tracheotomy. Arch Otolaryngol Head Neck Surg 2002;128:1253–1254.

Cernea CR, Dias FL, Fliss D, Lima RA, Myers EN, Wei WI (eds): Pearls and Pitfalls in Head and Neck Surgery. Basel, Karger, 2008, pp 176–177

14.1 Practical Tips to Perform a Microvascular Anterolateral Thigh Flap

Luiz Carlos Ishida, Luis Henrique Ishida

Plastic Surgery Division, Faculty of Medicine, University of São Paulo, São Paulo, Brazil

PEARLS

- Very versatile thin flap with a large amount of skin available.
- Low donor site morbidity, both esthetically and functionally.
- Long vascular pedicle that allows microvascular anastomosis far from the defect site.

PITFALLS

- There is a small chance (1%) of an absence of perforator vessels originating from the descending branch of the lateral circumflex artery.
- Overweight and female patients may have thicker subcutaneous tissue in the anterolateral thigh area.

Introduction

Since its first description [1], the anterolateral thigh (ALT) flap has become a very important resource in head and neck reconstructions and a workhorse for soft tissue reconstructions [2]. This flap has very interesting characteristics for the reconstructive surgery, such as one of the greatest extensions of skin, one of the longest pedicles, and one of the lowest morbidities at the donor site when compared to the traditionally used microsurgical flaps [3].

The ALT flap is based on the perforator vessels of the descending branch of the lateral circumflex femoral artery (DBLCFA). There are up to 4 perforators per thigh, all in a 6-cm radius from the midpoint between the anterosuperior iliac spine (ASIS) and the lateral border of the patella (LBP). The average pedicle length is about 12 cm. The artery and vein diameter at the origin of the DBLCFA is about 2.5 mm, which is very suitable for microanastomosis. The perforator pedicles are musculocutaneous in 75% of the thighs and septocutaneous in 25%. Among the musculocutaneous pedicles, 87% have direct and 13% indirect intramuscular trajectory [3–5]. The unique characteristics of the ALT flap increase the reliability of this flap and reduce surgical time.

Practical Tips

Usually the dissection of perforator flaps is more difficult than of traditional flaps. The ALT flap is not different, and the tiny perforators and the intramuscular dissection may increase surgical time. About 35% of the thighs have septocutaneous or direct musculocutaneous perforators and 65% have indirect musculocutaneous ones [3]. Only the former impose some additional difficulties during flap dissection, whereas with the first two types dissection is no different from any other fasciocutaneous flap. On the other hand, the advantages of this flap, such as the donor site [6], easily surpass possible intraoperatory difficulties.

❶ The perforator vessels to the ALT flap are found in an area of 6 cm of diameter around the middle point between the ASIS and the LBP [3, 5].

❷ The exact perforator locations can be plotted with a 5.3-MHz Doppler ultrasound; even though it is not necessary for ALT flap raising, it may reduce the dissection time.

❸ The dissection should start by finding the DBLCFA between the rectus femoralis and the vastus lateralis muscles. In this way, the perforator vessel locations are easily found distally.

❹ The fascia lata can be raised along with the cutaneous flap, providing a vascularized fascial tissue and facilitating the perforator dissection.

❺ When necessary, muscular flaps can be raised along on the same pedicle of the ALT flap, specially the vastus lateralis (chimeric flaps) [7].

❻ More than one cutaneous flap can be raised separately depending on the number and location of the perforator vessels [7].

❼ Overweight and female patients tend to have thicker subcutaneous tissue in the ALT area. The ALT flap can be thinned on its deeper subcutaneous portion as the main vascularization is through the subdermal plexus [8].

❽ In case of an absence of perforator vessels from the DBLCFA, which may occur in 1% of the patients, the surgeon can use on the same donor site perforator flaps based on the transverse branch of the lateral circumflex artery or direct branches from the femoral artery [9, 10].

❾ The perforator branches are extremely delicate and sensitive to torsions; the surgeon must avoid cauterizing nearby vessels, always preferring mechanical hemostasis.

Conclusion

Perforator flaps offer a whole new perspective in reconstructive surgery. They allow the reconstructive surgeon to transfer almost any tissue in the human body. Any segment of the skin can be transferred nowadays as a perforator flap, and among all the skin flaps, the ALT flap is one of the most reliable ones with a well-known and predictable anatomy. It can provide a thin cutaneous flap on a very long pedicle with a relatively low morbidity at the donor site.

References

1 Song YG, Chen GZ, Song YL: The free thigh flap: a new flap concept based on the septocutaneous artery. Br J Plast Surg 1984; 37:149–159.
2 Wei FC, Vivek J, Celik N, Chen HC, Chuang DCC, Lin CH: Have we found an ideal soft-tissue flap? An experience with 672 anterolateral thigh flaps. Plast Reconstr Surg 2002;109:2219–2226.
3 Ishida LC, Ishida LH, Munhoz AM, Martins DS, Besteiro JM, Cernea CR, Ferreira MC: Utilização do retalho perfurante anterolateral da coxa na reconstrução de cabeça e pescoço: estudo anatômico e aplicações clínicas. Rev Bras Cir Cab Pesc 2002;27: 7–16.
4 Ishida LH, Ishida LC, Munhoz AM, Morais J: Retalhos perfurantes em cirurgia de cabeça e pescoço; in Mélega JM (ed): Cirurgia plástica fundamentos e arte: cirurgia reparadora de cabeça e pescoço. Medsi, Rio de Janeiro, 2002, pp 1046–1050.
5 Xu DC, Zhong SZ, Kong JM, Wang GY, Liu MZ, Luo LS, Gao JH: Applied anatomy of the anterolateral femoral flap. Plast Reconstr Surg 1988;82:305–310.
6 Kimata Y, Uchiyama K, Ebihara S, Sakuraba M, Iida H, Nakatsuka T, Harii K: Anterolateral thigh flap donor-site complications and morbidity. Plast Reconstr Surg 2000;106:584–589.
7 Koshima I, Yamamoto H, Hosoda M, et al: Free combined composite flaps using the lateral circumflex femoral system for repair of massive defects of the head and neck regions: an introduction to the chimeric flap principle. Plast Reconstr Surg 1993; 92:411.
8 Nojima K, Brown SA, Acikel G, Arbique G, Ozturk S, Chao J, Kurihara K, Rohrich RJ: Defining vascular supply and territory of thinned perforator flaps. I. Anterolateral thigh perforator flap. Plast Reconstr Surg 2005;116:182–193.
9 Kimata Y, Uchiyama K, Ebihara S, Nakatsuka T, Harii K: Anatomic variations and technical problems of the anterolateral thigh flap: a report of 74 cases. Plast Reconstr Surg 1998;102: 1517–1523.
10 Kawai K, Imanishi N, Nakajima H, Aiso S, Kakibuchi N, Hosokawa K: Vascular anatomy of the anterolateral thigh flap. Plast Reconstr Surg 2004;114:1108–1117.

Cernea CR, Dias FL, Fliss D, Lima RA, Myers EN, Wei WI (eds): Pearls and Pitfalls in Head and Neck Surgery. Basel, Karger, 2008, pp 178–179

14.2 Practical Tips to Perform a Deltopectoral Flap

Roberto A. Lima[a, b], Fernando L. Dias[a, b], Jorge Pinho Filho[c]

[a] Head and Neck Service, Brazilian National Cancer Institute/INCA and,
[b] Catholic University of Rio de Janeiro, Rio de Janeiro,
[c] Memorial San Jose Hospital of Recife, Brazil

PEARLS

- Separate the fascia of the pectoral muscles in the subfascial plane, sparing the thin musculature investing the fascia to preserve the fine vascular network that supplies the random portion of the flap.
- Limited extension of the inferior incision does not compromise the length of the flap and assures the blood supply.

PITFALLS

- Good fixation prevents the flap from collapsing, compromising the suture on the recipient area.
- Tracheotomy fixation tape that is too tight compromises the blood supply.

Introduction

Bakamjian [1] introduced the deltopectoral skin flap in 1965, and thereafter it was used extensively for reconstructive surgery of the head and neck. Flap failure rates amount to 10–25% [2–5], and can exceed 50% in cases of pharyngoesophageal or oral cavity reconstruction [5]. Nevertheless, the deltopectoral flap remains a versatile and reliable tissue source that can be used simultaneously with the pectoralis major myocutaneous flap for a complex head and neck reconstruction.

The majority of complex head and neck reconstructions required more than one flap. The pectoralis major flap is most often combined with the deltopectoral flap in this setting. When used simultaneously, these two flaps are complementary.

Practical Tips

❶ Two nearly parallel lines running laterally from a parasternal base that spans the first four intercostals spaces mark the borders of the pectoral portion. The first is at the level of the inferior border of the clavicle and the second at the level of the apex of the anterior axillary fold. Continuing from these two lines the outline of the deltoid portion ends with a rounded linear margin that extends to the anterolateral, lateral or posterolateral line of the shoulder.

❷ The elevation of the flap should be done carefully, separating the fascia of the pectoral muscles sparing the thin musculature investing the fascia.

❸ Elevate the flap in the subfascial plane from lateral to medial. As the dissection proceeds into the parasternal region take care to not injure the perforating vessels of the internal mammary artery that supply the flap. The inferior incision is usually described as extending medially to the parasternal region to provide a maximal arc of rotation and length. Kingdom and Singer [6] reported that this is not necessary and can compromise the integrity of the third and fourth perforators. Hamaker [7] suggested that the extension of the inferior incision no further than the level of the nipple does not compromise the arc of rotation and length of the flap and blood supply is consistently preserved.

4 Provide postoperative care to avoid kinking or compression of the flap by dressings, drain tubes, or tape of the tracheotomy.

5 If the flap is to be passed beneath cervical flaps, the lower cervical incision must be horizontal and should be the same incision as the superior flap incision.

6 In cases of longer flaps, consider to autonomize the flap before the final reconstruction, also in the presence of arteriosclerosis, diabetes, or severe malnutrition. Some authors [5] suggested autonomizing the flap in cases of previous radiotherapy in the recipient area, reporting 49% of failures. We agree with the report of Bakamjian [2] that previous radiotherapy to the recipient site does not affect the flap viability. Kingdom and Singer [6] reported an 88% of successful reconstruction with deltopectoral flap in previously irradiated areas.

7 Use a larger flap base, usually with 4 perforating arteries, branches of the internal mammary artery, if the flap needs to reach the face and/or upper neck. This provides better blood supply.

8 Suture the inferior-medial incision pivot point and the superior cervical skin. This maneuver extends the arc of rotation, counteracts gravitational pull, and decreases the donor site defect [6].

9 In cases of peritracheostomal reconstruction, avoid fenestrating the flap [8]. It is preferable to rotate the distal end of the flap into the tracheal stump. In this setting, several centimeters of length can be provided and up to 360° of the tracheostoma reconstructed. Besides, this technique avoids the limited extensibility that occurs in the flap fenestration [6].

References

1 Bakamjian VY: A two-stage method for pharyngoesophageal reconstruction with a primary pectoral skin flap. Plast Reconstr Surg 1965;36:173–184.
2 Bakamjian VY, Long M, Rigg B: Experience with the medially based deltopectoral flap in reconstructive surgery of the head and neck. Br J Plast Surg 1971;24:174–183.
3 Mendelson BC, Woods JE, Masson JK: Experience with the deltopectoral flap. Plast Reconstr Surg 1977;59:360–365.
4 Tiwari RM, Gorter H, Snow GB: Experiences with the deltopectoral flap in reconstructive surgery of the head and neck. Head Neck Surg 1981;3:379–383.
5 Kirkby B, Krag C, Siemssen OJ: Experience with the deltopectoral flap. Scand J Plast Reconstr Surg 1980;14:151–157.
6 Kingdom TT, Singer MI: Enhanced reliability and renewed applications of the deltopectoral flap in head and neck reconstruction. Laryngoscope 1996;106:1230–1233.
7 Hamaker RC: Four chest flaps. Arch Otolaryngol 1978;104:437–438.
8 East CA, Flemming AF, Brough MD: Tracheostomal reconstruction using a fenestrated deltopectoral skin flap. J Laryngol Otol 1988;102:282–283.

Cernea CR, Dias FL, Fliss D, Lima RA, Myers EN, Wei WI (eds): Pearls and Pitfalls in Head and Neck Surgery. Basel, Karger, 2008, pp 180–181

14.3 Practical Tips for Performing a Pectoralis Major Flap

José Magrim, João Gonçalves Filho

Head and Neck Surgery and Otorhinolaryngology Department, Hospital AC Camargo, São Paulo, Brazil

PEARLS

- Design your flap in the donor area of the pectoralis at the beginning of the surgery; however, it should only be performed after resection.
- Use the maximum amount of muscle possible for providing a better supply to the skin.

PITFALLS

- Always start performing the flap by incising the skin of the inferior and lateral part.
- Avoid excessively manipulating the flap with your hands.
- Dissect the subclavicular tunnel between the clavicle and its posterior periosteum.

Introduction

Since it was described by Ariyan [1] in 1979, the pectoralis major myocutaneous flap (PMMF) has been one of the main methods of reconstruction in oncological surgery of the head and neck. The anatomical proximity of the donor area for performing the flap surgery to the resection location, the simplicity of the technique, its versatility and presence of a rich vascular pedicle have made the PMMF one of the most frequently used techniques in reconstruction of the head and neck.

The PMMF is widely used to repair surgical defects following treatment for tumors in the head and neck region, ranging from skin defects through to large reconstructions of the oral cavity and pharyngeal-esophageal tissues [1–3]. The main complications arising from its use, fistulas, dehiscence of the flap, partial or total ischemia of the skin and necrosis, have been described as occurring in 33–57% of cases [2, 4–6]. On the other hand, a major complication, such as the need for a new flap due to complete necrosis, occurs in 1–3% of cases [2, 4, 7].

Practical Tips

1. Design your flap in the donor area of the pectoralis at the beginning of the surgery; however, it should only be performed after resection and assessment of the extent of the receptor area, unless you are certain of the size of the resected area. When planning, it is important to observe the flap rotation arch, the dimensions and the location of the main vascular bundle.
2. Use the maximum amount of muscle possible, because the larger the muscular volume, the safer the flap, providing a better supply to the skin and avoiding ischemia.
3. Always start performing the flap by incising the skin of the inferior and lateral part (or distal extremity), avoiding the superior part of the pedicle. Its anterior face is then released at the suprafacial level of the skin and subcutaneous tissue; the posterior face is lifted from the thoracic wall, the entire course of main vascular pedicle being visualized, and the flap is raised in the inferior-superior direction. The vascular pedicle is dis-

sected between the clavipectoral fascia and the clavicular part of the pectoralis major muscle [4, 8].

4 We use a technical modification in which the clavicular bundle from the second to the third intercostal bundle and the lateral edge of the pectoralis major are preserved.

5 Avoid excessively manipulating the flap with your hands; place two stitches at the inferior extremity to lift it, preserving the integrity of the microcirculation.

6 After harvesting the flap and ligaturing collateral vessels of the pedicle, transfer it to the cervical region by the infraclavicular or supraclavicular route [8, 9].

7 The subclavicular tunnel (ST) is performed by dissecting the muscle down to the insertion and the inferior border of the subclavius muscle fascia. The neurovascular structure leading to the proximal portion of the pectoralis major muscle is identified and preserved. The ST is dissected between the clavicle and its posterior periosteum. During this maneuver, the subclavius muscle is deflected off the fascia and sectioned together with the posterior periosteum of the clavicle. By finger dissection, the tunnel is enlarged to accommodate passage of the flap. In difficult cases, such as in patients with bulky flaps, sterile liquid vaseline is used to lubricate the flap and the ipsilateral shoulder is raised to facilitate passage. During the procedure, a vasodilator substance (papaverine or lidocaine) is instilled over the flap pedicle.

Conclusion

The present technical modifications that preserve parts of the pectoralis major muscle are important, because they foresee functional deficits in the arm and are useful for manual laborers. The infraclavicular tunnel also provides an increase of around 2–3 cm to the flap rotation arch and it is important for alleviating the traction on the vascular pedicle.

References

1 Ariyan S: The pectoralis major myocutaneous flap. Plast Reconstr Surg 1979;63:73–81.
2 Milenovic A, Virag M, Uglesic V, Aljinovic-Ratkovic N: The pectoralis major flap in head and neck reconstruction: first 500 patients. J Craniomaxillofac Surg 2006;34:340–343.
3 Magrin J, Kowalski LP, Saboia M, Saboia RP: Major glossectomy: end results of 106 cases. Eur J Cancer B Oral Oncol 1996;32B:879–884.
4 Vartanian JG, Carvalho AL, Carvalho SM, Mizobe L, Magrin J, Kowalski LP: Pectoralis major and other myofacial/myocutaneous flaps in head and neck cancer reconstruction: experience with 437 cases at a single institution. Head Neck 2004;26:1018–1023.
5 Chepeha DB, Annich G, Pynnonen MA, Beck J, Wolf GT, Teknos TN, Bradford CR,Carroll WR, Esclamado RM: Pectoralis major myocutaneous flap vs revascularized free tissue transfer: complications, gastrostomy tube dependence, and hospitalization. Arch Otolaryngol Head Neck Surg 2004;130:181–186.
6 Mariani PB, Kowalski LP, Magrin J: Reconstruction of large defects postmandibulectomy for oral cancer using plates and myocutaneous flaps: a long-term follow-up. Int J Oral Maxillofac Surg 2006;35:427–432.
7 Shah JP, Haribhakti V, Loree TR, Sutaria P: Complications of the pectoralis major myocutaneous flap in head and neck reconstruction. Am J Surg 1990;160:352–356.
8 Azevedo JF: Modified pectoralis major myocutaneous flap with partial preservation of the muscle: a study of 55 cases. Head Neck Surg 1986;8:327–331.
9 Kerawala CJ, Sun J, Zhang ZY, Guoyu Z: The pectoralis major myocutaneous flap: is the subclavicular route safe? Head Neck 2001;23:879–884.

Cernea CR, Dias FL, Fliss D, Lima RA, Myers EN, Wei WI (eds): Pearls and Pitfalls in Head and Neck Surgery. Basel, Karger, 2008, pp 182–183

14.4 Practical Tips to Perform a Trapezius Flap

Richard E. Hayden

Mayo Clinic Arizona, Scottsdale, Ariz., USA

Pearls

- The superior trapezius flap is the most reliable but the least versatile. It is unaffected by previous neck surgery and damage to the transverse cervical vessels.
- The lower trapezius flap is the only pedicled musculocutaneous flap with an arc of rotation sufficient to reach the vertex or the frontal region.
- There is almost perfect reliability with the harvest of the lower trapezius flap if, instead of a distal skin island, the skin is maintained axially over the entire vertical extent of the flap. This allows flaps to be up to 8 × 38 cm. These skin paddles can extend up to 13 cm caudal to the trapezius muscle though sometimes requiring a second procedure to section the pedicle.

Pitfalls

- Intraoperative lateral decubitus positioning is required.
- Previous or contiguous neck surgery, especially radical neck dissection, may compromise the vascular pedicles of the lateral and lower flaps.
- Preoperative Doppler is recommended, but even if the arterial supply is noted, the venous drainage is difficult to assess.
- Seroma formation is common.
- Donor site skin grafts are unreliable.

Introduction

Trapezius musculocutaneous flaps are infrequently used in this era of advanced free flap reconstruction. However, they can provide simple and sometimes the best option for certain defects.

The flat trapezius muscle and overlying skin have three zones and three possible flaps with a very confusing vascular anatomy. The superior is supplied by the occipital and paraspinous perforating arteries. The middle is supplied by the superficial cervical artery (SCA; superficial branch of the transverse cervical artery). This artery leaves the lower posterior triangle of the neck to run under the trapezius usually near the accessory nerve. It runs over the levator scapulae and rhomboid vessels. The lower is supplied by the dorsal scapular artery (DSA; deep branch of the transverse cervical artery). The DSA leaves the lower posterior triangle by running deep to the levator and rhomboid muscles. It sends a nutrient branch through the space between rhomboid major and minor to supply the caudal or lower portion of the muscle.

The confusion stems mainly from the extreme variability of the origins of the vessels in the neck. The DSA can be a separate branch of the subclavian or costocervical trunk (45%) or form a common trunk with the SCA (33%), with the subscapular (3%) or with both (19%). The trunk formed by the DCA and the SCA is called the transverse cervical artery and in the 33% of cases where it is found, it originates from the subclavian in 19% and the thyrocervical trunk in 14%.

The lateral island flap from the middle zone which can carry the spine of the scapula is the least reliable flap. It is based on the SCA and SCV which drains into the external jugular vein in 80% of cases.

Practical Tips

❶ Consider superior flap for patients with large skin defect in the neck, when the muscle is already paralyzed after radical neck dissection.
❷ Extend caudad flap incision medially across the midline with a cephalad backcut to increase the arc of rotation.
❸ Consider extended lower flap for large scalp defects vertex to frontal.
❹ Line from acromion to T12 outlines the lower muscle border.
❺ 8-cm-wide skin paddle vertically oriented between spine and medial border scapula extends from level of scapular spine to 10–15 cm caudal to trapezius.
❻ Dissect distal to proximal superficial to rhomboids.
❼ Once visualized, temporarily occlude DSA with a vascular clip.
❽ If distal skin bleeding is unchanged, section DSA and pedicle flap on SCA for maximal arc of rotation.
❾ If distal skin is compromised, keep DSA as additional pedicle, section its caudal continuation deep to rhomboid major and section rhomboid minor to increase the arc of rotation.
❿ Divide upper trapezius only if necessary for adequate arc of rotation.
⓫ Close donor site primarily.

Conclusions

Trapezius flaps demand a thorough understanding of a variable anatomy. Avoid the lateral trapezius flap in patients with previously operated necks. Consider the superior flap for posterolateral neck defects after radical surgery. Consider the extended vertical (lower) flaps for large scalp defects and maximize the vertical length of the skin paddle to increase reliability.

References

1 Conley J: Use of composite flaps containing bone for major repairs in the head and neck. Plast Reconstr Surg 1972;49:522.
2 Demergasso F: The Lateral Trapezius Flap. Third International Symposium of Plastic and Reconstructive Surgery, New Orleans, 1979.
3 Panje WR: The Island (Lateral) Trapezius Flap. Third International Symposium of Plastic and Reconstructive Surgery, New Orleans, 1979.
4 Gregor RT, Davidge-Pitts KJ: Trapezius osteomyocutaneous flap for mandibular reconstruction. Arch Otolaryngol 1985;111:198–203.
5 Baek SM, Biller HF, Krespi YP, Lawson W: The lower trapezius island myocutaneous flap. Ann Plast Surg 1980;5:108–114.
6 Netterville JL, Wood D: The lower trapezius flap: vascular anatomy and surgical technique. Arch Otolaryngol Head Neck Surg 1991;117:73.
7 Urgurlu K, Ozcelik D, Huthut I, Yildiz K, Kiminc L, Bas L: Extended vertical trapezius myocutaneous flap in head and neck reconstruction as a salvage procedure. Plast Reconstr Surg 2004; 114:339–350.
8 Haas F, Weiglein A, Schwarzl F, Scharnagl E: The lower trapezius musculocutaneous flap from pedicled to free flap: anatomical basis and clinical applications based on the dorsal scapular artery. Plast Reconstr Surg 2004;113:1580–1590.

Cernea CR, Dias FL, Fliss D, Lima RA, Myers EN, Wei WI (eds): Pearls and Pitfalls in Head and Neck Surgery. Basel, Karger, 2008, pp 184–185

14.5 Latissimus Dorsi Myocutaneous Flap for Head and Neck Reconstruction

Gady Har-El[a, b], Michael Singer[b]

[a] Department of Otolaryngology – Head and Neck Surgery, Lenox Hill Hospital, New York, N.Y., and
[b] Department of Otolaryngology, State University of New York – Downstate Medical Center, Brooklyn, N.Y., USA

PEARLS

- The latissimus dorsi myocutaneous flap (LDMF) is a versatile flap that can be used to reconstruct large defects in the head, neck and scalp.
- Repositioning of the patient to inset the flap after harvest can be avoided in most cases.
- Maintaining the orientation of the flap is vital to prevent torsion of the vascular pedicle.

PITFALLS

- The exposed pedicle, which is not protected by a cuff of muscle, may be easily traumatized or compressed.
- Transferring the muscle through a narrow subcutaneous tunnel may expose the flap and pedicle to risk of obstruction and congestion.

Introduction

The LDMF is a reliable option for surgical reconstruction of virtually any region of the head, neck and scalp [2–4, 6, 9]. It is particularly useful for secondary reconstruction or cephalad defects. This is due to its large surface area, its long vascular pedicle which permits an extensive arc of rotation, its ease of dissection, and minimal donor site morbidity [8]. The vascular pedicle can extend 8–10 cm on average.

One factor that has limited the popularity of the LDMF is the repositioning of the patient. However, repositioning is usually not required. The patient can be placed in the supine position for the ablative segment of the surgery and then rotated into the lateral position for flap harvesting. Flap inset can often be accomplished with the patient remaining in the lateral position [10].

Practical Tips

1. Due to the branching nature of the thoracodorsal artery within the muscle, the cutaneous portion of the flap can be harvested as one or two skin paddles [1]. The more distal skin paddle has decreased viability due to fewer cutaneous perforators.
2. Division of the latissimus dorsi tendon increases the arc of rotation.
3. The skin paddle is stabilized by anchoring its dermal layer to surrounding muscle fascia with fine absorbable sutures.
4. Tagging the medial and lateral aspects of the LDMF with different sutures helps with orientation of the flap during transfer.
5. Flap elevation begins at the anterolateral muscle edge. Only after identifying the thoracodorsal vessels is medial and inferior elevation of the muscle performed.
6. Ligation and transection of the vascular branches to the serratus anterior muscle allow a greater arc of rotation.

7 Preservation of the circumflex scapular artery assists in maintaining flap orientation, but it can be divided to achieve greater pedicle length [7].
8 After transection of the tendon of the latissimus dorsi, the pedicle remains exposed without any muscular protection; then, it must be handled with extreme care. Excessively skeletonizing the vessels puts them at increased risk of vasospasm [5].
9 Care for the elevated muscle and skin flap should include wrapping them in warm, moist laparotomy pads.
10 Infiltration of the soft tissues around the pedicle with 2% lidocaine will prevent vasospasm.
11 Brachial plexus injury can be prevented by avoiding hyperabducting or overrotating the arm.
12 In order not to jeopardize flap viability the tunnel created for passing the LDMF is widened to at least 5–7 cm.
13 Most flaps are easily passed between the skin and clavicle. In some patients clavicular protrusion may result in an excessively tight tunnel. In these cases a subclavicular tunnel can be dissected and utilized.
14 The flap should not be rotated more than 180°.
15 After surgery, the arm is kept flexed across the chest for 5 days.
16 Postoperatively, avoid ipsilateral flexion of the neck, which can cause kinking of the pedicle.
17 Postoperatively, check the flap viability and capillary refill, and with Doppler ultrasound.
18 Rarely, the subcutaneous tunnel through which the flap passes can become swollen, risking flap viability. In this instance, the skin layer overlying the clavicle can be opened to allow for appropriate pedicle blood flow.
19 The vascular supply of the LDMF allows it to be harvested in a patient who has undergone a neck dissection. These patients are, however, at greater risk of shoulder dysfunction.

Conclusion

The LDMF is a dependable flap that should be considered when reconstructing defects in the head and neck. This flap can be easily elevated, has a large surface and long pedicle, and causes limited donor site morbidity.

References

1 Bartlett SP, May JW Jr, Yaremchuk MJ: The latissimus dorsi muscle: a fresh cadaver study of the primary neurovascular pedicle. Plast Reconstr Surg 1981;67:631–635.
2 Barton FE, Spicer TE, Byrd HS: Head and neck reconstruction with the latissimus dorsi myocutaneous flap. Anatomic observations and report of 60 cases. Plast Reconstr Surg 1983;71:199–204.
3 Maves MD, Panje WR, Sjagets FW: Extended latissimus dorsi myocutaneous flap reconstruction of major head and neck defects. Otolaryngol Head Neck Surg 1986;92:551–558.
4 Maxwell G, McGibbon B, Hoopes J: Experience with thirteen latissimus dorsi myocutaneous free flaps. Plast Reconstr Surg 1979;64:1–7.
5 Har-El G, Bhaya M, Sundaram K: Latissimus dorsi myocutaneous flap for secondary head and neck reconstruction. Am J Otolaryngol 1999;20:287–293.
6 Haughey BV, Fredrickson JM: The latissimus dorsi donor site – current use in head and neck reconstruction. Arch Otolaryngol Head Neck Surg 1991;117:1129–1134.
7 Hayden RE, Kirby SD, Deschler DG: Technical modifications of the latissimus dorsi pedicled flap to increase versatility and viability. Laryngoscope 2000;110:352–357.
8 Olivari N: Use of thirty latissimus dorsi flaps. Plast Reconstr Surg 1979;64:654–661.
9 Quillen CG, Shearin JC, Georgiade NG: Use of the latissimus dorsi myocutaneous island flap for reconstruction in the head and neck area. Plast Reconstr Surg 1978;62:113–117.
10 Urken ML, Sullivan MJ: Latissimus dorsi; in Urken ML, Cheney ML, Sullivan MJ, et al (eds): Atlas of Regional and Free Flaps for Head and Neck Reconstruction. New York, Raven Press, 1995, pp 237–259.

Cernea CR, Dias FL, Fliss D, Lima RA, Myers EN, Wei WI (eds): Pearls and Pitfalls in Head and Neck Surgery. Basel, Karger, 2008, pp 186–187

14.6 Transverse Rectus Abdominis Flap

Julio Morais Besteiro

São Paulo University Medical School, São Paulo, Brazil

Pearls

- One of the best and safest flaps for treatment of extensive soft tissue defects.
- Very versatile donor area.
- Constant and reliable pedicle.
- Hidden donor area scars specially in transverse rectus abdominis (TRAM) flap and muscle flap.

Pitfalls

- Risk of hernia or bulging in the lower abdomen.
- Risk of umbilicus deviation.
- Reduction of the muscular strength.
- Bulky flap in obese patients.
- Be aware of previous scars in the abdomen.

Introduction

The TRAM is among the most used free flaps for extensive soft tissue defects. The pedicle is constant, long and has a large diameter. The skin is supplied through a series of musculocutaneous perforators that are arranged in two parallel rows along the muscle. The distribution of the perforators permits different designs of the flap and a variety of patterns of the skin paddle.

Tips and Technical Details

Main perforators to the skin are around the umbilical area, so the design of the flap should include these vessels if a long flap is planned.

Large transverse or oblique previous abdominal scars are a relative contraindication for the TRAM. Previous abdominoplasty or extensive liposuction is an absolute contraindication for both TRAM and muscle-sparing flap [1].

The flap elevation should begin on the lateral border of the skin island, where the lateral row of perforators is encountered above the rectus fascia. As the medial perforators are identified, the rectus fascia is incised along its length and the dissection proceeds from medial to lateral until the medial row of perforators is reached again. Another vertical incision in the fascia, medial to the perforators, creates a thin strip of fascia that is included in the flap to preserve the perforator vessels. This strip should be thin enough to achieve direct closure of the anterior sheet of the aponeurosis without tension.

The lower part of the muscle is usually severed at the level of the arcuate line where the pedicle enters into the muscle. This preserves a distal stalk of muscle to be inserted in the arcuate line and to reconstruct the posterior sheet of the rectus fascia when closing the donor area.

Functionally, the closure of the aponeurotic layer is the main step in the donor area. A tight closure without excessive tension is mandatory.

The position of the umbilicus is important. As the harvesting of the muscle and aponeurosis is unilateral, the umbilicus will be displaced toward the donor site. It may be centered again through a row of stitches over the contralateral rectus fascia symmetric to the one on the donor site, or it may be rerouted through a stab wound adjacent to the vertical incision.

Potential Donor Site Complications

Previous abdominal transverse incisions or oblique incisions may cut the rectus muscle or the main perforator vessels. Even an extended appendectomy incision can sometimes cut the inferior epigastric pedicle. Extensive previous liposuction can also damage the perforator vessels.

The main drawback is the lower abdominal weakness and the development of hernias or abdominal bulging. For weak or lax fascia, Marlex™ mesh or other synthetic material should be used to reinforce the lower abdomen. Also, the smallest strip of fascia should be performed, to preserve the perforators when harvesting the flap.

Even partial resection of the muscle reduces the abdominus muscle strength, representing a problem in young and physically active patients [2, 3].

Reducing the Bulkiness

Patients have a different distribution of abdominal fat. Usually the oblique flap (the main axis of the skin paddle is from the umbilicus to the tip of the scapula) is thinner than other designs [4].

Defatting this flap is safe if done under the superficial fascia in the cutaneous portion. Some fat can also be removed with extreme care around the perforators. Secondary defatting with liposuction or sharp dissection is usually done and is safe [5, 6].

The muscular component of the flap can be reduced to a small cuff around the pedicle and the medial row of perforators.

Conclusion

This donor site provides a large amount of tissue in different types of design with an acceptable esthetic result in the donor area, allowing simultaneous dissection in donor and receptor areas. The long vascular pedicle with large-diameter vessels enables an easy and safe transfer. Variability of flap thickness must be considered.

References

1 Granzow JW, Levine JL, Chiu ES, Allen RJ: Breast reconstruction with the deep inferior epigastric perforator flap. J Plast Reconstr Aesthet Surg 2006;59:571–579.
2 Feller AM: Free TRAM. Results and abdominal wall function. Clin Plast Surg 1994;21:223–232.
3 Futter CM, Webster MH, Hagen S, Mitchell SL: A retrospective comparison of abdominus muscle strength following breast reconstruction with a free TRAM or DIEP flap. Br J Plast Surg 2000;53:578–582.
4 Taylor GI, Corlett R, Boyd JB: The extended inferior epigastric flap: a clinical technique. Plast Reconstr Surg 1983;72:751–764.
5 Hallock GG: Defatting of flaps by means of suction-assisted lipectomy. Plast Reconstr Surg 1985;76:948–952.
6 Taylor GI, Corlett RJ, Boyd JB: The versatile deep inferior epigastric (inferior rectus abdominis) flap. Br J Plast Surg 1984; 37:330–350.

Cernea CR, Dias FL, Fliss D, Lima RA, Myers EN, Wei WI (eds): Pearls and Pitfalls in Head and Neck Surgery. Basel, Karger, 2008, pp 188–189

14.7 Practical Tips to Perform a Microvascular Forearm Flap

Adam S. Jacobson, Mark L. Urken

Beth Israel Medical Center, New York, N.Y., USA

PEARLS

- Thin, soft, pliable, and easy to harvest.
- Two-team approach can be utilized.
- Harvest with or without an extended subcutaneous component for added bulk.
- Can be harvested with 7–9 cm of radius bone.
- Can be harvested with nerve for sensate flap reconstruction.

PITFALLS

- Usually requires a split-thickness skin graft for closure of donor site.
- If ulnar blood supply to hand is not adequate ischemia may result.
- Extremity requires splint for 7 days.
- Exposed tendon.
- Sensory loss over thumb and first finger due to injury to the superficial branch of radial nerve.
- Pressure ulceration from splint.

Introduction

The radial forearm fasciocutaneous free flap (RFF) was reported in the Chinese literature by Yang et al. [1] in 1981. It is a thin, pliable, highly reliable soft tissue flap.

This free flap is based on the radial artery and either the deep or superficial venous system. The superficial system has larger caliber vessels which have thicker walls, permitting an easier anastomosis. The blood supply to the thumb and index finger are most at risk following interruption of the radial artery if the superficial palmar arch is incomplete and there is a lack of communication between the superficial and deep arches. The coexistence of these two anomalies occurred in less than 12% of the specimens reported by Coleman and Anson [2].

The flap can be designed in a variety of geometric configurations and it can be harvested with vascularized bone (radius), vascularized tendon (palmaris longus), the brachioradialis muscle, and vascularized sensory nerves (medial and lateral antebrachial cutaneous nerves) [3].

Practical Tips

The Allen test is the most important preoperative test, to assess the adequacy of circulation to the hand through the ulnar artery. A more objective test is based on pulse oximeter readings.

The harvest is performed with a tourniquet for temporary occlusion of the radial artery.

We routinely perform an intraoperative assessment of the capillary refill of the thumb and index finger after interruption of the radial artery, following release of the tourniquet. Occasionally, when a patient has a questionable preoperative Allen test we have elected to proceed with the harvest and performed intraoperative assessment of the ulnar circulation. In this scenario, the distal incision is made in order to allow access to the radial artery. The radial artery is isolated and a temporary microvascular clamp is placed on the artery and the capillary refill of the hand is reassessed. If the refill time is acceptable, we safely proceed with the harvest.

We most frequently design the skin paddle to end distally at the flexor crease of the wrist, including the thinnest and the least hair-bearing forearm skin.

A skin monitor to provide postoperative access to buried flaps can be designed by creating a separate skin paddle over the proximal forearm [4].

A bilobed design can be utilized to reconstruct the tongue and floor of mouth separately [5].

If additional bulk is required, an extended component of subcutaneous tissue is harvested in continuity with the intermuscular septum and folded under the skin paddle.

Generally, we close the proximal limb of the donor site incision line primarily, but the location where the skin paddle was harvested often requires a split-thickness skin graft. Ulnar-based flaps can often be rotated into the defect to avoid a skin graft.

A volar splint is fashioned with meticulous attention paid to padding the hand and forearm to prevent pressure ulcerations.

Assess viability of a free flap with a 25-gauge needle prick. If bright red blood egresses in a timely fashion, one can feel comfortable that the circulation is adequate. If there is a delayed egress or the blood is too dark, one must quickly consider the possibility of a vascular compromise.

The donor site must be regularly assessed for adequate capillary refill. If the patient complains of pain at the donor site that is out of proportion to what is anticipated, one must remove the splint and assess the arm to rule out the possibility of pressure necrosis.

Conclusion

The RFF is an excellent soft tissue flap which can be used for a wide variety of defects, and is one of the most utilized free flaps in head and neck reconstruction today.

References

1 Yang G, Chen B, Gao Y: Forearm free skin flap transplantation. Natl Med J China 1981;61:139.
2 Coleman SS, Anson BJ: Arterial patterns in the hand based upon a study of 650 specimens. Surg Gynecol Obstet 1961;113:409–424.
3 Urken ML, Weinberg H, Vickery C, Biller HF: The neurofasciocutaneous radial forearm flap in head and neck reconstruction: a preliminary report. Laryngoscope 1990;100:161–173.
4 Urken ML, Futran N, Moscoso JF, Biller HF: A modified design of the buried radial forearm free flap for use in oral cavity and pharyngeal reconstruction. Arch Otolaryngol Head Neck Surg 1994;120:1233–1239.
5 Urken ML, Biller HF: A new bilobed design for the sensate radial forearm flap to preserve tongue mobility following significant glossectomy. Arch Otolaryngol Head Neck Surg 1994;120:26–31.

Cernea CR, Dias FL, Fliss D, Lima RA, Myers EN, Wei WI (eds): Pearls and Pitfalls in Head and Neck Surgery. Basel, Karger, 2008, pp 190–191

14.8 Mandible Reconstruction with Fibula Microvascular Transfer

Julio Morais Besteiro

São Paulo University Medical School, São Paulo, Brazil

PEARLS

- Carefully draw in the donor area the important anatomical elements and the skin island if necessary.
- On the upper part of the incision, identify and protect the common peroneal nerve as it courses around the neck of the fibula.
- During the dissection, flex the leg in order to relax the muscle of the posterior compartment of the leg.
- Excise a small piece of bone in the proximal osteotomy, in order to do a safer and easier dissection of the vascular pedicle.
- Spare 8 cm of the distal fibula to provide adequate ankle stability. In children, fix the distal fibula to the tibia with a lag screw, in order to prevent varus deformity.
- Carefully plan the osteotomies, the plate fixation and position of the recipient vessels.

PITFALLS

- The skin paddle of the osteocutaneous flap receives its vascular supply from the intermuscular septum, but sometimes the portion of the soleus or flexor hallucis longus must be included in the flap.
- Be aware of the absence of dorsalis pedis and posterior tibialis artery pulse. In about 1% of the patients, there is a single vessel in the leg and the transfer cannot be done.
- Avoid extensive periosteal dissection when multiple osteotomies are necessary.
- Be aware of deep varicose veins in the donor area. Although this does not prevent the transplant, it will make the flap dissection difficult.

Introduction

Since the first description of the fibular transplant for mandible, it became the gold standard in all mandibular reconstructions [1, 2]. Although it is a well-established technique it is still a complex surgery with many difficult steps.

Practical Tips

1. In the preoperative examination, check both dorsalis pedis and posterior tibialis pulse. When in doubt, it is safer to perform a radiographic evaluation of the vessels, because between 1 and 2% of the population has a single vessel in the leg (congenital peroneal magna artery) [3, 4]. Other aberrations can occur in up to 10% of the population.
2. Two teams work simultaneously, one in the donor area and the other in the recipient field.
3. The lateral approach is preferred, and a tourniquet is used in the thigh. If an osteocutaneous flap is indicated, the dissection should begin by the anterior border of the cutaneous island and the intermuscular septal vessels identified usually between the medial and distal third of the fibula [5]. The skin paddle has an unpredictable blood supply and may be lost in up to 5–10% of patients.
4. Identify septal vessels and the common peroneal nerve. The bone is isolated with a thin cuff of muscle all around. A small piece of bone should be excised in the proximal part and the peroneal vessels isolated. The distal osteotomy is then per-

formed and the distal fibular vessels are ligated. Cut the interosseous membrane and expose the vascular pedicle all along the fibula. Considerable additional length of the pedicle can be gained by harvesting a more distal segment of bone.

5 To fit the fibula to the mandible defect multiple osteotomies usually are performed. Osteotomies should be done opposite to the vessels, to avoid the risk of injury by the screws of the fixation plate. One single reconstruction titanium plate or several miniplates can be used.

6 Place the fibula in continuity with the inferior border of the remaining mandible to get a better contour result. If it is too thin and osseointegrated implants are anticipated, a bone graft or a double-barrel fibula can be done in part of the horizontal ramus of the neomandible. Osseointegrated implant placement as a secondary procedure is a worthwhile procedure [6, 7].

7 The mandible is maintained in occlusion and the defect is accurately measured. The fibula is then fixed in the defect, leaving enough space to insert a prosthesis between the fibula and the maxilla. Avoid inserting screws in the horizontal portion of the neomandible where the osseointegrated implants are supposed to be inserted.

8 Mandibular templates and measurements of the surgical specimen are useful.

9 When a reconstruction plate is used or the miniplates have a strong fixation, liquid or soft meal may be allowed from the very first days till the end of the third postoperative month. Usually, no intermaxillary fixation is used.

Conclusion

The fibular free flap can successfully restore mastication, dental occlusion and maintain adequate oral excursion. Good postoperative speech quality may be expected if no significant tongue resection is required. There is no significant morbidity related to the donor site.

References

1 Hidalgo DA: Fibula free flap: a new method of mandible reconstruction. Plast Reconstr Surg 1989;84:71.
2 Hidalgo DA, Pusic AL: Free-flap mandibular reconstruction: a 10-year follow-up study. Plast Reconstr Surg 2002;110:438.
3 Kim D, Orron DE, Skillman JJ: Surgical significance of popliteal arterial variants: a unified angiographic classification. Ann Surg 1989;210:776.
4 Astarci P, Siciliano S, Verhelst R, et al: Intra-operative acute leg ischaemia after fibula flap harvest for mandible reconstruction. Acta Chir Belg 2006;106:423–426.
5 Wei FC, Seah CS, Tsai YC, et al: Fibula osteoseptocutaneous flap for reconstruction of composite madibular defects. Plast Reconstr Surg 1994;93:294–306.
6 Gurlek A, Miller MJ, Jacob RF, Lively JA, Schusterman MA: Functional results of dental restoration with osseointegrated implants after mandible reconstruction. Plast Reconstr Surg 1998; 101:650.
7 Weischer T, Mohr C: Ten-year experience in oral implant rehabilitation of cancer patients: treatment concept and proposed criteria for success. Int J Oral Maxillofac Implants 1999;14:521.

Cernea CR, Dias FL, Fliss D, Lima RA, Myers EN, Wei WI (eds): Pearls and Pitfalls in Head and Neck Surgery. Basel, Karger, 2008, pp 192–193

14.9 Practical Tips to Perform a Microvascular Iliac Crest Flap

Mario S.L. Galvao

Reconstructive Microsurgery Unit, National Cancer Institute, Rio de Janeiro, Brazil

PEARLS

- Iliac crest offers excellent quality bone for mandibular reconstruction allowing osseointegrated implants.
- Reliable soft tissue paddle for oral reconstruction if needed.

PITFALLS

- Injury to ilioinguinal nerve may lead to important postoperative pain.
- This flap is contraindicated in obese or in very hairy patients.
- Hernia formation may be avoided by using mesh sheath.
- The compound flap (bone and skin) is contraindicated in obese patients, however, the flap is suitable for hairy patients as the skin overlying the iliac bone is always hairless.

Introduction

Several techniques have been described to reconstruct the mandible [1, 2], but the free iliac graft is undoubtedly the best one [3–5].

The main advantages to choose this bone are as follows:

• The thickness of the bone allows tridimensional reconstruction.

• Its normal curvature is ideal for hemimandible defects, allowing a reconstruction without fracturing the bone in order to obtain a normal contour.

• The bony structure is the best choice for osseointegrated implants.

• Compound graft has a reliable skin blood supply for intraoral reconstruction.

• Secondary defect and scarring are easily hidden by clothes, and the resulting linear scar is usually of good quality.

• The deep circumflex iliac vessels are of good caliber and reasonably long pedicle to reach the recipient vessels on the neck.

To achieve the best results, the mandible must be reconstructed immediately following resection, as the procedures in later reconstruction are more difficult due to retraction, fibrosis and displacement of the remaining mandible.

Furthermore, immediate reconstruction allows reattachment of the preserved masticatory muscles to the transplanted graft, improving the postoperative function.

The compound grafts (skin and bone) are indicated for mandible and intraoral lining defects. In some patients the defect involves the bone and also the soft tissue surrounding it. In these patients, the skin of the compound graft can be deepithelialized and used to fill defect contours, thus improving the esthetic appearance.

Practical Tips

Outlining the Flap

❶ The patient is operated on in the supine position with a cushion under his buttocks.
❷ The donor site must be ipsilateral.
❸ The skin is outlined about 1 cm above and parallel to the inguinal ligament, and over the iliac crest.

Dissecting and Carving the Flap

❶ The skin incision is made exposing the bone and the fascia above the inguinal ligament.
❷ About half way between the anterior superior iliac spine and the pubis, the external and internal oblique muscle fibers are dissected and the deep circumflex iliac vessels are found.
❸ A rubber band is passed around the vessels and dissection is carried out medially as far as the femoral vessels, and then, laterally close to the anterior superior iliac spine. The ascending branch of the deep circumflex iliac vessels and its small branches are ligated. These vessels must be preserved when dissecting compound flap.
❹ All muscles are detached from the outer border of the iliac crest, exposing the external part of the bone.
❺ The lateral cutaneous nerve of the thigh is found and preserved just bellow the anterior superior iliac spine. This is a very important guide as this nerve will cross the deep circumflex iliac vessels internally, behind the anterior superior iliac spine.
❻ The amount of bone necessary to be used is now carved using chisel and saw. It is mandatory to leave the anterior superior iliac spine intact in place with the inguinal ligament attached to it.
❼ The bone is fractured and dissection of the vessels is accomplished laterally passing the lateral nerve of the thigh.
❽ The muscles are cut internally close to the vessels and the bone is lifted on its pedicle.
❾ The same procedure is carried out for compound grafts. In these procedures about 12 × 4 cm of skin is left overlying the bone.
❿ Hemimandible defects do not require osteotomies. For central arch defects, miniplates are used following osteotomy.

Repairing the Secondary Defect

❶ The muscles are approximated with nonabsorbable stitches and a mesh graft is always used to avoid herniation.
❷ A corset is worn for 3 months.

Contraindications

❶ The compound graft (bone and skin) is not suitable for obese and hairy patients but it can be used in hairy patients as the skin overlying the iliac crest is always hairless.

References

1 Galvao MSL, Wance JR, Braga ACCR: A contribuição da microcirurgia no tratamento do paciente oncológico. Rev Brasil Cancerol 1984;30:29–34.
2 Galvao MSL, Sbalchiero J: Reconstrução mandibular. Cirurgia Plástica: Fundamentos e Arte. Rio de Janeiro, Editora Medsi, 2002, pp 949–962.
3 Sanders R, Mayou B: A new vascularized bone graft transferred by microvascular anastomosis as a free flap. Br J Surg 1979;66: 787–788.
4 Taylor GI, Townsend P, Corlett R: Superiority of the deep circumflex iliac vessels as the supply for free groin flaps. Experimental work. Plast Reconstr Surg 1979;64:595–604.
5 Taylor GI, Townsend P, Corlett R: Superiority of the deep circumflex iliac vessels and supply for free groin flaps. Clinical work. Plast Reconstr Surg 1979;64:745–759.

Cernea CR, Dias FL, Fliss D, Lima RA, Myers EN, Wei WI (eds): Pearls and Pitfalls in Head and Neck Surgery. Basel, Karger, 2008, pp 194–195

14.10 The Scapular Flap

Julio Morais Besteiro

São Paulo University Medical School, São Paulo, Brazil

PEARLS

- Indicated for complex three-dimensional defects of the mandible or the maxilla.

PITFALLS

- Two-team approach is difficult.
- Long lateral decubitus positioning is associated with morbidity of the brachial plexus.
- Possible decreased range of motion and weakness of the shoulder.

Introduction

The scapular donor area is unique in that it can provide a wide range of tissue types based in the same vascular pedicle [1]. Advantages of all these flaps include a long and constant pedicle (10–14 cm) with large-diameter vessels and abundant independent surface areas, which allows for freedom in a three-dimensional insetting. Up to 10 cm of bone can be removed from the lateral aspect of the scapula. This bone is not always thick enough to allow for osseointegrated implants [2, 3].

The main disadvantage of this donor site is its positioning that may prevent a two-team approach and increase operative time, that may provoke brachial plexus compression and the potential compromise in the range and power of the motion of the shoulder.

At present, these characteristics limit the indications to moderate mandible defects associated with extensive double-face tegumental defects or certain situations of maxilla reconstruction associated with extensive soft tissue defects

Practical Tips

As in all complex reconstructions, careful preoperative planning is mandatory. In this particular situation, the positioning of the patient must be considered. In some situations as in posterolateral defects, most of the operation can be done in lateral decubitus, although a simultaneous two-team approach may be necessary. The patient is positioned in a lateral or three-quarter lateral position, with the arm draped free with a stockinet, in such a way that it can be mobilized during flap dissection.

The transverse and descending branches of the circumflex scapular artery can preoperatively be identified with Doppler ultrasonography. If Doppler is not available, the flaps are centered over the triangular space of the lateral border of the scapula and the dissection begins distally in the cutaneous flap toward the triangular space, right over the deep fascia [4]. The vessels can be seen on the undersurface of the flap, especially with backward illumination.

The dissection proceeds toward the identification and isolation of the circumflex subscapular pedicle between the teres major and minor. The branch of the circumflex scapular artery to the lateral border of the scapula is identified and the dissection should preserve the connection between this artery and the periosteal vessels. If a long segment of bone, including the tip of scapula, or some osteotomy is necessary, the branch to the serratus muscle should also be included to assure the circulation of the tip of the scapula. The circumflex scapular artery can be traced to its origin in the triangular space at the subscapular artery by retracting the teres major and long head of the triceps [5]. The bone is cut with an oscillating saw parallel to the lateral border of the scapula and this is completed with a transverse osteotomy approximately 1 cm distal from the glenoid fossa. Some attachments of the serratus muscle and other muscles must be sharply divided to isolate the flap in the circumflex scapular pedicle [6].

To prevent complications each of the muscles that have been divided is reattached to the surrounding musculature using strong nonreabsorbable sutures. If no secure sutures can be obtained with muscle-to-muscle sutures, the muscles should be strongly reattached to the scapula through drill holes.

In the postoperative period, shoulder exercises are begun under the supervision of a physical therapist to restore shoulder elevation.

Potential Complications and Drawbacks

Functional recovery of the donor site is exceptionally good provided that the muscles are properly reinserted. Shoulder stiffness and decreased mobility have been seen in a minority of patients. The principal complication is the loss of the distal part of the bone, when distal osteotomies are done.

The extent of harvested bone is very limited and the positioning of the patient usually prevents the use of the two-team approach and increases operative time substantially.

References

1 Rowsell AR, Davis DM, Eisenberg N, et al: The anatomy of the subscapular-thoracodorsal arterial system: a study of 100 cadaver dissections. Br J Plast Surg 1984;37:574–576.
2 Frodel JL Jr, Funk GF, Capper DT, et al: Osseointegrated implants: a comparative study of bone thickness in four vascularized bone flaps. Plast Reconstr Surg 1993;92:449–455.
3 Roumanas ED, Markowitz BL, Lorant JA, et al: Reconstructed mandibular defects: fibula free flaps and osseointegrated implants. Plast Reconstr Surg 1997;99:356–365.
4 Teot L, Bosse JP, Moufarrege R, et al: The scapular crest pedicled bone grafts. Int J Microsurg 1981;3:257–262.
5 Swartz WM, Banis JC, Newton ED, et al: The osteocutaneous scapular flap for mandibular and maxillary reconstruction. Plast Reconstr Surg 1986;77:530–545.
6 Coleman JJ, Sultan MR: The bipedicle osteocutaneous scapula flap: a new subscapular system free flap. Plast Reconstr Surg 1991;87:682–692.

Cernea CR, Dias FL, Fliss D, Lima RA, Myers EN, Wei WI (eds): Pearls and Pitfalls in Head and Neck Surgery. Basel, Karger, 2008, pp 196–197

14.11 Reconstruction of Pharyngoesophageal Defects with the Jejunal Free Autograft

John J. Coleman, 3rd

Indiana University School of Medicine and Roudebush VAMC, Indianapolis, Ind., USA

Pearls

- Select a length of jejunum far enough away from the ligament of Treitz to allow for tube jejunostomy of the distal segment after anastomosis.
- Leave the graft in situ perfusing after jejunostomy until the neck is completely prepared for transfer of the segment.
- Perform the most difficult pharyngoenteric anastomosis first, then the microvascular anastomosis, then the second pharyngoenteric anastomosis to minimize ischemic time.

Pitfalls

- The mesenteric vessels particularly the vein are thin-walled and delicate. Careful dissection at the junction of the feeding branch to the superior mesenteric vessels and meticulous division of the venovenous branches of the venae comitantes is critical to avoiding damage to the vessels or mesenteric hematoma. This may be particularly difficult in obese patients.
- Positioning the segment and the donor and recipient vessels in the neck must account for the possibility of kinking the mesentery when the neck turns and causing vessel thrombosis. The carotid, jugular and pharyngoesophagus are all near midline structures and there is a finite length to the mesentery.

Introduction

The jejunal free autograft is a useful method of pharyngoesophageal reconstruction [1] that has shown in many large series to be reliable and versatile [2–4]. The bowel can be harvested by a second team of reconstructive surgeons working in the abdomen at the same time as the extirpative team works in the neck.

Practical Tips

(1) Through an upper midline incision the ligament of Treitz is identified. Moving distally along the jejunum, a segment of bowel is chosen that, when resected, will allow the remaining reanastomosed jejunum to reach without tension the abdominal wall, thus creating a feeding jejunostomy distal to the enteroenterostomy. When the appropriate segment has been identified, the branch of the superior mesenteric vessels that supplies that segment is isolated by carefully incising the serosa and separating the mesenteric fat from the vessels. By careful dissection from proximal (near the origin of the vessel from the superior mesenteric vessels) to distal (near the antimesenteric edge of the jejunum) the mesentery is divided proximal and distal and finally the bowel is divided with two lines of staples. It is important at this point to observe the ends of the reconstructive segment and the ends of the bowel remaining to assure that they are adequately perfused prior to harvest or enteroenterostomy. If the ends of the remaining bowel are viable enteroenterostomy is

performed and a tube jejunostomy placed distal to the anastomosis. The segment to be harvested is left in site perfused until the neck has been prepared for transfer since the jejunum tolerates a relatively short ischemia time.

❷ Preparation of the neck is critical. A branch of the external carotid and jugular vein or the transverse cervical artery and vein should be prepared under the microscope prior to dividing the mesenteric vessels. When the jejunum is brought to the neck the vessels must be arranged so that neither the vessels nor the mesentery will kink when the neck is turned. Usually it is best to perform the more difficult pharyngoenteric anastomosis (usually the jejunum to base of tongue) first, then the microvascular anastomosis, then the second pharyngoenteric anastomosis. An ischemia time of less than 2 h is desirable. Injection of saline through the nose under pressure will demonstrate possible sites of leak or potential fistula. The bowel segment should be sewn into the defect in an isoperistaltic orientation under slight tension because on reperfusion the jejunum will lengthen somewhat. Excessive graft length in the neck can result in swallowing difficulty.

❸ The flap can be monitored in a number of ways: by direct observation by leaving a small part of the neck flap incision open to observe the bowel serosa or by taking an extra small segment of jejunum separating it from the bowel conduit but leaving it perfused and exteriorizing it, by implantable Doppler or thermo probe, or by externally applied Doppler ultrasound. Continuity of the pharynx should be checked by contrast imaging 10 days after surgery [5].

Conclusion

The jejunal free autograft is a reliable method for pharyngoesophageal reconstruction, provided that some basic technical principles are strictly followed during its harvesting and positioning in the neck; carefully performed free-tension microvascular and visceral anastomoses are equally important.

References

1 Coleman JJ: Reconstruction of the pharynx after resection for cancer: a comparison of methods. Ann Surg 1989;209:554–561.
2 Carlson GW, Coleman JJ, Jurkiewicz MJ: Reconstruction of the hypopharynx and cervical esophagus. Curr Probl Surg 1993;30: 425–480.
3 Reece GP, Shusterman MA, Miller MJ: Morbidity and functional outcome of free jejunal transfer reconstruction for circumferential defects of the pharynx and cervical esophagus. Plast Reconstr Surg 1995;96:1307–1316.
4 Theile DR, Robinson DW, Theile DE, et al: Free jejunal interposition reconstruction after pharyngolaryngectomy: 201 consecutive cases. Head Neck 1995;17:83–88.
5 Torres WE, Fibus TF, Coleman JJ, et al: The radiographic evaluation of the free jejunal graft. Gastrointest Radiol 1987;12:226–230.

Cernea CR, Dias FL, Fliss D, Lima RA, Myers EN, Wei WI (eds): Pearls and Pitfalls in Head and Neck Surgery. Basel, Karger, 2008, pp 198–199

14.12 Practical Tips to Perform a Gastric Pull-Up

William I. Wei, Vivian Mok

Department of Surgery, University of Hong Kong Medical Centre, Queen Mary Hospital, Hong Kong, SAR, China

Pearls

- For adequate mobilization of the stomach to reach higher in the neck, the duodenum should be kocherized to the medial side of the inferior vena cava. The posterior wall of the oropharynx and nasopharynx should also be separated from the prevertebral muscle.
- The esophagus should be mobilized under direct vision through the assistance of the thoracoscope rather than transhiatally with blunt dissection.
- The fundus of the stomach is the highest point where it meets the oropharynx for pharyngogastric anastomosis. The incisions on the anterior stomach wall should be T-shaped, to allow the gastric wall to move up laterally to reduce the tension there. The base of the tongue moves inferiorly to meet the lowered anterior wall of the stomach.

Pitfalls

- During the transposition of the stomach transhiatally to the neck, the axis of the stomach tube should be maintained; twisting of the stomach will lead to necrosis.
- Pyloromyomectomy, removing a segment of the muscle at the pylorus, helps stomach emptying. A pyloroplasty, although equally effective, also shortens the stomach.
- For carcinoma of the cervical esophagus affecting the posterior tracheal wall the cuff of the tracheostomy tube should be lowered during the separation of these two walls to allow precise dissection.
- When the pharyngogastric anastomosis dehisced, there might not be significant signs to alert the clinician. Whenever leakage at the anastomosis is suspected, early drainage of the neck wound is essential to prevent extension of infection to the mediastinum.

Introduction

The gastric pull-up operation is one option of reconstruction for the hypopharynx after tumor extirpation. It was used before the era of myocutaneous flaps and microvascular free tissue transfer [1]. Recently, this operation has only been performed when the tumor is located in the lower portion of hypopharynx or in the cervical esophagus [2]. Removing the esophagus also eliminates the organ which might develop a second primary tumor [3].

This operation is indicated for patients who have dysphagia due to a tumor in the laryngopharyngeal region. The gastric pull-up operation, besides removing the tumor in a single operation, invariably relieves the disturbing dysphagia. The procedure however is still associated with hospital mortality and morbidity [4]. With technical improvements and better perioperative support, both morbidity and mortality rates have been reduced [5] and the associated long-term morbidities are acceptable [6].

Practical Tips

Preoperatively, patients should be given chest physiotherapy and enteric feeding with nasogastric tube or parenteral feeding to achieve a positive nitrogen balance.

The patient is positioned in the right lateral position for thoracoscopic mobilization of the esophagus. The sharp dissection under direct vision avoids damaging intrathoracic vessels and also reduces surgical trauma, and the patients in general have a smoother recovery [7]. After mobilizing the esophagus, the patient is then turned into the supine position; the neck and the abdomen are approached simultaneously by two surgical teams.

In the neck, soft tissue at the intrathoracic inlet is removed for the stomach to come up. When the posterior wall of the trachea is infiltrated by tumor in the cervical esophagus, it should be carefully dissected off the tumor. When the upper posterior tracheal wall is damaged, it can be repaired from the neck. If the injury is lower down, then thoracotomy is mandatory for direct closure of the defect [8].

In the abdomen, the stomach is mobilized into a tubular structure with the right and left gastric vessels running along lesser and greater curvatures. The adequately mobilized stomach should reach the posterior pharyngeal wall at the level of the tonsils. When the stomach is transposed orthotopically to the neck, the fundus is the highest point to reach the posterior pharyngeal wall. A 'T-shaped' incision is made on the anterior gastric wall, part of the anterior wall can be mobilized laterally to reduce the tension there and the base of the tongue can be pulled down towards the anterior wall of the stomach to complete the pharyngogastric anastomoses.

For a high anastomosis, a 'U-shaped' incision can be made on the anterior stomach wall. Turning this anterior gastric wall flap superiorly, it will reach the posterior pharyngeal wall and a myocutaneous flap can be used to close the defect in the anterior wall.

References

1. Lam KH, Wong J, Lim ST, Ong GB: Pharyngogastric anastomosis following pharyngolaryngoesophagectomy. Analysis of 157 cases. World J Surg 1981;5:509–516.
2. Lam KH, Choi TK, Wei WI, Lau WF, Wong J: Present status of pharyngogastric anastomosis following pharyngolaryngo-oesophagectomy. Br J Surg 1987;74:122–125.
3. Martins AS: Multicentricity in pharyngoesophageal tumors: argument for total pharyngolaryngoesophagectomy and gastric transposition. Head Neck 2000;22:156–163.
4. Sasaki CT, Salzer SJ, Cahow E, Son Y, Ward B: Laryngopharyngoesophagectomy for advanced hypopharyngeal and esophageal squamous cell carcinoma: the Yale experience. Laryngoscope 1995;105:160–163.
5. Wei WI, Lam LK, Yuen PW, Wong J: Current status of pharyngolaryngo-esophagectomy and pharyngogastric anastomosis. Head Neck 1998;20:240–244.
6. Wei WI, Lam KH, Choi S, Wong J: Late problems after pharyngolaryngoesophagectomy and pharyngogastric anastomosis for cancer of the larynx and hypopharynx. Am J Surg 1984;148:509–513.
7. Cense HA, Law S, Wei W, Lam LK, Ng WM, Wong KH, Kwok KF, Wong J: Pharyngolaryngoesophagectomy using the thoracoscopic approach. Surg Endosc 2007;21:879–884.
8. Wei WI, Lam KH, Lau WF, Choi TK, Wong J: Salvageable mediastinal problems in pharyngolaryngo-esophagectomy and pharyngogastric anastomosis. Head Neck Surg 1988;10:S60–S68.

Cernea CR, Dias FL, Fliss D, Lima RA, Myers EN, Wei WI (eds): Pearls and Pitfalls in Head and Neck Surgery. Basel, Karger, 2008, pp 200–201

15.1 Indications and Limitations of Fine Needle Aspiration Biopsy of Lateral Cervical Masses

Paulo Campos Carneiro, Luiz Fernando Ferraz da Silva

Department of Pathology, University of São Paulo School of Medicine, São Paulo, Brazil

PEARLS

- Fine needle aspiration biopsy (FNAB) is a powerful and accurate method to diagnose the majority of lateral cervical nodules.
- Imaging methods (IM) – ultrasound, CT scans and MRI – are helpful to define lesion topography. The ultrasound must always be the method of choice to guide FNAB.
- Immunocytochemistry of the FNAB sample increases the diagnostic precision.

PITFALLS

- Extensive representation is essential to avoid scant cytological material and to increase lesion sampling.
- Carefully sample cystic, calcified and fibrotic lesions.

Introduction

FNAB is the method in which puncturing with a fine needle (23–25 gauge) coupled to a syringe and a negative pressure device allows the assessment of cytological samples for diagnoses. It was first described in 1930 by Martin and Ellis [1], and has been increasingly used and improved with the help of IM. It is useful not only to differentiate malignant from benign processes, but also to determine the nature of the disease, including organ, microorganism and cell lineage identification [2]. When the lymph node is accessed by FNAB, it can commonly distinguish among reactional lymphadenitis (acute, chronic and granulomatous infectious process), Hodgkin and non-Hodgkin lymphoma, and metastases from different sites, including occult thyroid neoplasm. Yet, FNAB hardly differentiates, only on a morphological basis, among lymphoid proliferations, reactional lymphoid tissue or lymphoma. Immunocytochemical reactions are helpful tools in FNAB of lymph nodes [3].

FNAB of salivary glands is usually conclusive for acute and chronic inflammatory processes; benign neoplasm (pleomorphic adenoma, Warthin tumor); malignant neoplasm (mucoepidermoid, adenoid cystic, epidermoid, undifferentiated carcinomas and adenocarcinomas), and glandular ectopy in the low cervical region. Limitations: Sometimes, it is hard to differentiate between the benign and malignant characteristics of lesions with well-differentiated epithelial cell proliferation.

FNAB of cervical cysts, skin and its appendages usually confirms the clinical-radiological hypothesis of branchial cysts and thyroglossal duct cyst and defines skin and skin appendage neoplasms.

The identification of vascular structures with imaging exams, such as aneurisms, contraindicates FNAB.

Practical Tips

❶ Knowledge of previous IM is essential.

❷ When FNAB is not performed by the pathologist guided by the radiologist, an interaction among the patient's clinician, the physician who collects the sample and the pathologist may provide better results [4].

❸ Adequate sampling of each lesion is pivotal. Several strategies have been used to improve it, such as:

a) 2–4 biopsies from each region to be sampled.

b) Smears on 5–8 slides per biopsy for different stains (routinely, Papanicolaou and Giemsa stains).

c) Cell blocks with the remaining material in the syringe and needle (if there is too little, it is possible to pool it; if there is a large amount available, different cell blocks are preferred).

❹ Depending on the lesion characteristics, the FNAB method may be varied to ensure adequate sampling:

a) Partially cystic lesions: perform FNAB directed to solid areas, avoiding cystic ones. If not possible, drain the cystic content and then perform a new FNAB to sample the solid component.

b) Solid fibrotic/calcified lesions: increase the number of biopsies.

c) Hypervascularized lesions: increase the number of biopsies; use thinner needles (25 gauge); increase the needle movement speed, and decrease the total time of the procedure.

❺ Use of special techniques increases the diagnostic specificity. The commonly used ones are:

a) Cytochemical stainings: for microorganism identification such as acid-fast bacilli, fungi, and others.

b) Immunocytochemical reactions: identification of cell lineages, primary sites of neoplasms, clonality, prognostic markers, and other differential diagnoses [1].

c) Culture: for necrotic material and/or signs of infectious diseases.

Other useful techniques include in situ hybridization and polymerase chain reaction.

❻ The FNAB report should avoid simple classifications – such as positive, negative, suspect or inconclusive – as this restricts the range of diagnostic possibilities. When a single cytological diagnosis is not possible, it is essential to explore all diagnostic possibilities, preferentially ordering them from the most to the least probable differential diagnoses within the observed cytological aspect.

Conclusions

FNAB is a simple and easy method that can define the diagnosis in the majority of cervical lateral nodules. The knowledge of imaging methods is important to define the best approach and interpretation of FNAB. Special techniques, particularly immunocytochemistry, may improve the diagnostic potential of FNABs.

References

1 Martin HE, Ellis EB: Biopsy by needle puncture and aspiration. Ann Surg 1930;92:169–181.

2 Koss LG: Koss' Diagnostic Cytology and Its Histopathologic Bases, ed 5. New York, Lippincott Williams & Wilkins, 2005.

3 El Hag IA, Chiedozi LC, Al Reyess FA, Kollur SM: Fine needle aspiration cytology of head and neck masses. Seven years' experience in a secondary care hospital. Acta Cytol 2003;47:387–392.

4 Kocjan G, Feichter G, Hagmar B, Kapila K, Kardum-Skelin I, Kloboves V, Kobayashi TK, Koutselini H, Majar B, Schenck U, Schmitt F, Tani E, Totch M, Onal B, Vass L, Vielh P, Weynand B, Herbert A: Fine needle aspiration cytology: a survey of current European practice. Cytopathology 2006;17:219–226.

Cernea CR, Dias FL, Fliss D, Lima RA, Myers EN, Wei WI (eds): Pearls and Pitfalls in Head and Neck Surgery. Basel, Karger, 2008, pp 202–203

15.2 When and How to Perform an Open Neck Biopsy of a Lateral Cervical Mass

Pedro Michaluart, Jr., Sérgio Samir Arap

Head and Neck Service, Hospital das Clínicas da Faculdade de Medicina, Universidade de São Paulo, São Paulo, Brazil

PEARLS

- In patients older than 40 years and a with a neck mass, malignancy is the greatest concern.
- Fine-needle aspiration (FNA) biopsy usually precedes an open biopsy.
- When a metastatic carcinoma is suspected, evaluation of the upper aerodigestive tract mucosa is indicated.
- In case of suspicion of well-differentiated metastatic thyroid cancer, thyroglobulin should be put on the FNA material.
- Frozen-section examination during open biopsy aims to confirm that the tissue sample is adequate.
- Metastatic cancer in a supraclavicular mass should raise the suspicion of a thoracic or abdominal primary.

PITFALLS

- Do not substitute physical examination by image diagnosis.
- Do not perform open biopsy before complete head and neck evaluation.
- Open biopsy of neck mass as the first investigative procedure is rarely recommended as it may interfere with future treatment strategies.
- Do not realize open biopsy within the parotid topography without being sure that the node is extraglandular.
- The spinal accessory nerve (SAN) is superficial in the posterior triangle of the neck and its injury is the most frequent complication of surgeries at this site.

Introduction

Evaluation of neck masses is one of the most common situations in the head and neck surgeon's daily clinical practice. Inflammatory, congenital or neoplastic diseases may present with a neck mass and may affect neck organs other than lymph nodes (LN) [1–3]. It is crucial to have in mind all the differential diagnoses while evaluating the patient. It is very important to obtain a careful clinical history and a complete physical examination. Imaging studies should be used when necessary. Ultrasound and CT scan are the most helpful exams and can differentiate LN enlargements from other masses and show important characteristics, for example, whether the mass is within the parotid gland or not. To define the etiology, a tumor sample is needed. In case of metastatic squamous cell carcinoma, the primary tumor is often found within the upper aerodigestive tract mucosa and a biopsy can easily be done. Biopsies of neck masses should start routinely with cytology obtained by FNA. In most instances the cytology is able to confirm a diagnosis and definitive treatment can be planned. Sometimes though, the diagnosis cannot be made on the basis of cytology and an open biopsy is needed [1–5]. This is the case for lymphomas when routinely an LN should be evaluated for accurate diagnosis and treatment planning [1]. When cytology suggests metastatic carcinoma and an LN biopsy is indicated, general anesthesia should be considered, so that a pan endoscopy can also be done at the same time.

Practical Tips

Performing an LN Biopsy

1 The first step is to determine a target node. It is important to determine if the LN is superficial or deep to the sternocleidomastoid muscle.

2 The target LN should be the most easily accessible with characteristics of disease involvement like enlargement, stiffness or necrotic center.

3 Nodes may become less palpable after infiltration of anesthesia so it is helpful to mark the skin incision before.

4 Several factors should be considered for definition of the anesthesia. The size, location and mobility of the node are important. Patients' characteristics are also relevant, for instance, age and capacity to collaborate.

5 Posterior superficial LNs may be of the SAN chain. Caution needs to be exercised with the incision and elevation of skin flaps in the posterior triangle because of the superficial course of the nerve and absence of the platysma. The incision should allow for adequate exposure of the nerve [6, 7].

6 Every effort should be made to excise the LN without rupture of the capsule so that its architecture is preserved. Grabbing the node with clamps should be avoided. For traction a nylon 3-0 stitch that transfixes the node may be helpful.

7 Frozen section of the LN should be performed to make sure that there is enough material for the diagnosis.

8 When there is a possibility of infectious diseases, material should be collected for cultures.

Conclusion

Although LN biopsy is usually considered a simple procedure, complications may be disabling and should be prevented with careful preoperative evaluation and selection of the best anesthesia for each case. The surgeon has to have profound knowledge of the anatomy of the neck and should be prepared to perform a bigger operation if needed.

References

1 Karen M, Close LG: Mass in the neck; in Close LG (ed): Essentials of Head and Neck Oncology. Stuttgart, Thieme, 1998, pp 243–251.

2 Frank DK, Sessions RB: Physical examination of the head and neck; in Harrison LB, Sessions RB, Hong WK, Kies MS, Medina JE, Mendehall WM, Mukherji SK, O'Malley BB, Wenig BM: Head and Neck Cancer: A Multidisciplinary Approach, ed 2. Baltimore, Lippincott Williams & Wilkins, 2004, pp 4–10.

3 Schwetschenau E, Keley DJ: The adult neck mass. Am Fam Physician 2002;66:831–838.

4 Gleeson M, Herbert A, Richards A: Regular review: management of lateral neck masses in adults. BMJ 2000;320:1521–1524.

5 Batthacharyya N: Predictive factors for neoplasia and malignancy in neck mass. Arch Otolaryngol Head Neck Surg 1999;125:303–307.

6 Nason RW, Abdulrauf BM, Stranc MF: The anatomy of the accessory nerve and cervical lymph node biopsy. Am J Surg 2000;180:241–243.

7 Weisberger EC, Lingeman RE: Cable grafting of the spinal accessory nerve for rehabilitation of shoulder function after radical neck dissection. Laryngoscope 1987;97:915–918.

Cernea CR, Dias FL, Fliss D, Lima RA, Myers EN, Wei WI (eds): Pearls and Pitfalls in Head and Neck Surgery. Basel, Karger, 2008, pp 204–205

15.3 Practical Tips in Managing Radiation-Associated Sarcoma of the Head and Neck

Thomas D. Shellenberger[a, b], Erich M. Sturgis[c, d]

[a] Head and Neck Surgical Oncology, M.D. Anderson Cancer Center Orlando, Orlando, Fla.,
[b] The University of Texas M.D. Anderson Cancer Center and Departments of [c] Head and Neck Surgery and
[d] Epidemiology, The University of Texas M.D. Anderson Cancer Center, Houston, Tex., USA

PEARLS

- Management of radiation-associated sarcoma (RAS) depends on prompt diagnosis/evaluation, defined treatment goals, and multimodal therapy.
- Despite the poor prognosis of RAS, the combination of surgery, chemotherapy, and rarely additional radiotherapy can offer a chance for disease cure.

PITFALLS

- Failing to consider the possibility of RAS delays diagnosis.
- RAS must be differentiated from more common sarcoma to optimize treatment.

Introduction

Sarcoma can arise as a rare secondary malignancy within radiation treatment fields, and the double-strand DNA damage induced by ionizing radiation appears to underlie RAS pathogenesis. The etiology of RAS may include the effects of other carcinogens such as chemotherapy alkylating agents, genetic susceptibility, or other unknown factors. Therefore, the terms RAS and postirradiation sarcoma may be more descriptive than radiation-induced sarcomas.

RAS occurs in head and neck cancer patients less frequently than in other cancer patients with more prolonged survival probabilities. The estimated incidence of RAS ranges from 0.03 to 2.2% in those surviving more than 5 years after head and neck radiotherapy [1, 2]. The criteria for RAS include: development of a sarcoma within the radiation field and at least 5-year latency between radiation and RAS diagnosis [3]. RAS appears to occur in a dose-dependent manner with the majority of cases occurring after therapeutic doses (median 50 Gy) [4, 5]. The histology is frequently of high grade, including pleomorphic sarcoma (malignant fibrous histiocytoma or undifferentiated sarcoma) and osteosarcoma [2, 4].

Practical Tips

(1) The risk of RAS is low; therefore, RAS risk should not have a major influence on treatment decisions for patients with head and neck cancer [6]. However, the incidence of RAS may increase as improvements in head and neck cancer treatment and changing demographics result in prolonged survival.

(2) New symptoms/signs or changes in the character of chronic symptoms, such as pain, should prompt investigation. Fine needle aspiration is often adequate for initial diagnosis, but histologic typing will usually require core needle or open biopsy, which should be approached with further surgery in mind. All specimens from current and previous biopsies, along with clinical and radiographic features, must be reviewed by a patholo-

gist with experience in sarcoma. Immunohistochemical stains and cytogenetic studies can assist pathologic subtyping.

3 Old records and dosimetry data may not be available; nonetheless, evidence of the extent of the radiated field may come from tattoo marks, cutaneous radiation changes, and histologic findings of radiation injury in tissues adjacent to the RAS.

4 For RAS, 5-year overall survival ranges from 10 to 30% [7–9]. Grade and tumor size are the most important prognostic factors. Prognosis for RAS appears worse than that for sarcomas of a similar stage arising de novo. Patel et al. [10] offer the following explanations: (1) delay in diagnosis caused by the unreliability of clinical examination due to postradiation induration and fibrosis, (2) proximity of tumor to major neurovascular structures constraining surgical resection, (3) limited treatment options, (4) relatively poor chemosensitivity, (5) more aggressive biology, and (6) immunodepression caused by the first tumor and/or its treatment.

5 Surgical resection with adequate margins, in combination with neoadjuvant or adjuvant chemotherapy, provides the best chance for RAS cure in the absence of metastatic disease (and for palliation in selected cases). By the time of detection, many tumors have extended beyond their local confines limiting the probability of complete en bloc resection. Moreover, tissue changes in the radiated field impose technical difficulties at surgery, challenge the pathologic analysis of margins, and affect wound healing.

6 High-grade tumors of borderline resectability should be considered for neoadjuvant chemotherapy followed by complete resection whenever possible. Resectable high-grade tumors and all low-grade tumors should be treated surgically whenever possible followed by adjuvant chemotherapy when a negative margin is difficult or impossible. Because of the high risk for distant failure, adjuvant chemotherapy should be considered even in those completely resected high-grade tumors [1].

7 While further external beam radiotherapy is rarely possible, brachytherapy or intraoperative radiotherapy may be applied in selected cases.

Conclusion

Detection of RAS at an early stage is paramount, and favorable outcomes depend on a high index of suspicion in patients with a history of radiation exposure. RAS presents unique challenges; nonetheless, complete surgical resection offers the only realistic chance for long-term survival.

References

1 Patel SR: Radiation-induced sarcoma. Curr Treat Options Oncol 2000;1:258–261.
2 Ko JY, Chen CL, Lui LT, Hsu MM: Radiation-induced malignant fibrous histiocytoma in patients with nasopharyngeal carcinoma. Arch Otolaryngol Head Neck Surg 1996;122:535–538.
3 Cahan WG, Woodward HQ, Higinbotham NL, Stewart SW, Coley BL: Sarcoma arising in irradiated bone: report of eleven cases. Cancer 1948;1:3–29.
4 Brady MS, Gaynor JJ, Brennan MF: Radiation-associated sarcoma of bone and soft tissue. Arch Surg 1992;127:1379–1385.
5 Kuttesch JF, Wexler LH, Marcus RB: Second malignancies after Ewing's sarcoma: radiation dose-dependency of secondary sarcomas. J Clin Oncol 1996;14:2789–2795.
6 Mark RJ, Bailet JW, Poen J, Tran LM, Calcaterra TC, Abemayor E: Postirradiation sarcoma of the head and neck. Cancer 1993;72:887–893.
7 Robinson E, Neugut AI, Wylie P: Clinical aspects of postradiation sarcomas. J Natl Cancer Inst 1988;80:233–240.
8 Davidson T, Westbury G, Harmer CL: Radiation induced soft-tissue sarcoma. Br J Surg 1986;73:308–309.
9 Wiklund TA, Blomqvist CP, Raty J, Elomaa I, Rissanen P, Miettinen M: Postirradiation sarcoma: analysis of a nationwide cancer registry material. Cancer 1991;68:524–531.
10 Patel SG, See AC, Williamson PA, Archer DJ, Rhys Evans PH: Radiation induced sarcoma of the head and neck. Head Neck 1999;21:346–354.

Cernea CR, Dias FL, Fliss D, Lima RA, Myers EN, Wei WI (eds): Pearls and Pitfalls in Head and Neck Surgery. Basel, Karger, 2008, pp 206–207

15.4 Practical Tips for Performing Transoral Robotic Surgery

Gregory S. Weinstein, Bert W. O'Malley, Jr.

Department of Otorhinolaryngology – Head and Neck Surgery, University of Pennsylvania, Philadelphia, Pa., USA

PEARLS

- Transoral robotic surgery (TORS) is performed via mouth gags and never tubular laryngoscopes.

PITFALLS

- Attempting TORS without both general da Vinci robot certification as well as a standardized animal and operating observational course specifically focused on TORS is inadvisable.

Introduction

The feasibility of TORS using the da Vinci® Robotic Surgical System (Intuitive Surgical, Sunnyvale, Calif., USA) was first demonstrated, by our surgical team at the University of Pennsylvania, in mannequin, cadaver and canine models [1–3]. TORS utilizes a readily available robotic system in which there is a bedside robotic cart which has a minimum of three arms that can be inserted via a variety of mouth gags to perform the transoral surgery. The robotic arms are under the control of the surgeon who sits at a console and sees a three-dimensional video view of the operative field. In TORS two instrument arms are utilized as well as the central double video endoscope. The surgeon has full control of the miniaturized robotic instruments via manipulators in the console. Our team has published numerous preclinical reports as well as reports from our TORS patient study including the TORS approach to supraglottic partial laryngectomy, tongue base resections and radical tonsillectomy [4–8].

Practical Tips

1 As in all oncologic surgery, patient selection is paramount. With some exceptions we recommend preoperative assessment both in the outpatient setting as well as at the time of preoperative endoscopy under general anesthesia at which time the patient may be triaged between nonsurgical treatment, open surgical resection, transoral laser surgery, and TORS.

2 Intraoperative efficiency is significantly improved if there is a dedicated team of operating room personnel trained in robotic and operating room setup for TORS.

3 Since with rare exceptions the same set of robotic instruments and nonrobotic instruments are needed for TORS cases, the room setup and instrument setup should be standardized and the same for every case which yields improved efficiency and decreased operative times.

4 Never attempt to do TORS via a tubular laryngoscope. Mouth gags must be used to provide access for instruments and the most commonly used is the Davis-Crow mouth gag (tongue base and tonsil) and FK-Laryngo-Pharyngoscope sys-

tem (Feyh-Kastenbauer retractor) from Gyrus ACMI (www.gyrus-ent.com)/Explorent GmbH, Tuttlingen, Germany (www.explorent.de; larynx and hypopharynx).

5 The bedside assistant plays key roles in TORS including retraction, suctioning and applying clips to blood vessels for hemostasis.

6 The 5-mm spatula tip electrocautery instrument is the most common 'cutting' tool and works very well in all anatomic locations.

7 All blood vessels with a lumen large enough to visualize should have two to three clips applied to each end prior to transection. We have found it more efficient to apply clips with the handheld Storz Laryngeal clip applier (Karl Storz, Tuttlingen, Germany).

8 If at the end of the case the surgeon is concerned about the potential for significant airway edema then the patient should remain intubated for a period of 24–48 h with both intravenous steroids and antibiotics.

9 Neck dissection, when it is indicated, is staged and performed 1–3 weeks following TORS. The rationale for staging the neck dissection has been discussed elsewhere [7].

10 In patients in whom aspiration is a possible risk, a percutaneous gastrostomy is performed preoperatively.

Conclusion

In this chapter the reader was exposed to the key points for successfully performing TORS. Our experience with over 150 TORS procedures has allowed us to not only describe reproducible surgical approaches but also summarize the common features of all TORS cases that if followed will improve the chance for excellent outcomes [5–8].

References

1 Weinstein GS, O'Malley BW Jr, Hockstein NG: Transoral robotic surgery (TORS): supraglottic laryngectomy in the canine model. Laryngoscope 2005;115:1315–1319.
2 Hockstein NG, O'Malley BW Jr, Weinstein GS: Assessment of intraoperative safety in transoral robotic surgery. Laryngoscope 2006;116:165–168.
3 O'Malley BW Jr, Weinstein GS, Hockstein NG: Transoral robotic surgery (TORS): glottic microsurgery in a canine model. J Voice 2006;20:263–268.
4 O'Malley BW Jr, Weinstein GS, Snyder W, Hockstein NG: Transoral robotic surgery (TORS) for base of tongue neoplasms. Laryngoscope 2006;116:1465–1472.
5 Weinstein GS, O'Malley BW Jr, Snyder W, Hockstein NG: Transoral robotic surgery: supraglottic partial laryngectomy. Ann Otol Rhinol Laryngol 2007;116:19–23.
6 O'Malley BW Jr, Weinstein GS: Robotic anterior and midline skull base surgery: preclinical investigations. Int J Radiat Oncol Biol Phys 2007;69(2 Suppl):S125–S128.
7 Weinstein GS, O'Malley BW, Snyder W: Transoral robotic surgery (TORS) radical tonsillectomy. Arch Otolaryngol Head Neck Surg, in press.
8 O'Malley BW, Weinstein GS: Robotic skull base surgery: preclinical investigations to human clinical application. Arch Otolaryngol Head Neck Surg, in press.

Corresponding Authors by chapters

1.1
Dr. Orlo H. Clark, MD
UCSF/Mt. Zion Medical Center
Department of Surgery
1600 Divisadero St., Box 1674
Hellman Building, Room C-347
San Francisco 94143-1674 CA, USA
E-Mail clarko@surgery.ucsf.edu

1.2/7.2/7.10/8.9/8.10
Prof. Claudio R. Cernea
Department of Head and Neck Surgery
Univ. of São Paulo Medical School
Alameda Franca, 267-cj 21
Jd. Paulista
01422-000 São Paulo, SP, Brazil
E-Mail cerneamd@uol.com.br

1.3
Dr. Gregory W. Randolph, MD
243 Charles Street
Boston 02114 MA, USA
E-Mail
Gregory_Randolph@meei.harvard.edu

1.4/1.6
Prof. Ashok R. Shaha
Head and Neck Service
Memorial Sloan-Kettering Cancer Ctr.
Cornell Univ. Med. Center
1275 York Ave.
New York 10021 N.Y., USA
E-Mail shahaa@mskcc.org

1.5
Prof. Jean-François Henry, MD
University Hospital Marseille
Department of Endocrine Surgery
264, rue Saint-Pierre
Marseille 13385 Cedex 05, France
E-Mail
jean-francois.henry@mail.ap-hm.fr

1.7
Dr. Jeremy L. Freeman, MD, FRCSC, FACS
Mount Sinai Hospital
600 University Avenue 401
Toronto M5G 1X5, Canada
E-Mail jfreeman@mtsinai.on.ca

1.8
Dr. Erivelto M. Volpi, MD
R. das Figueiras, 551
09080-370 Santo Andre, SP, Brazil
E-Mail eriveltovolpi@hotmail.com

1.9
Dr. William B. Inabnet, MD, FACS
Chief, Section of Endocrine Surgery
Co-Director of New York Thyroid Center
Associate Professor of Clin. Surgery
College of Physicians and
Surgeons of Columbia University
161 Fort Washington Ave.
New York 10032 NY, USA
E-Mail wbi2102@columbia.edu

1.10
Prof. Keith S. Heller, MD, FACS
Professor and Chief of Endocrine Surgery
New York University, School of Medicine
530 First Avuene, Suite 6H
New York 10016 NY, USA
E-Mail keith.heller@med.nyu.edu

1.11
Dr. Fábio Luiz de Menezes Montenegro, MD
Rua Apeninos, 1118 APT 62
Paraiso
04104-021 São Paulo, SP, Brazil
E-Mail fabiomonte@uol.com.br

1.12
Dr. Alfred Simental, MD
Chief Otolaryngology,
Head and Neck Surgery
11234 Anderson St. Suite 2584
Loma Linda 92354 CA, USA
E-Mail asimenta@ahs.llumc.edu

1.13/8.1/8.4
Dr. Dan M. Fliss, MD
Department of Otolaryngology
Head and Neck Surgery
Tel-Aviv Sourasky Medical Center
6 Weizmann St.
Tel Aviv 64239, Israel
E-Mail fliss@tasmc.health.gov.il

1.14
Dr. Marcos R. Tavares, MD
Department of Head and Neck Surgery
University of São Paulo
Medical School
Rua Joaquim Floriano, 101
Conj. 601
04534-010 São Paulo, SP, Brazil
E-Mail Tavares.mr@uol.com.br

1.15
Dr. Patrick Sheahan
125 Pier View Street, No. 109
Daniel Island
Charleston 29492 SC, USA
E-Mail sheahan.patrick@gmail.com

1.16
Prof. Thomas V. McCaffrey, MD, PhD
Professor and Chair
Department of Otolaryngology
Head and Neck Surgery
University of South Florida
12902 Magnolia Drive
Suite 3057
Tampa 33612-9497 FL, USA
E-Mail Thomas.McCaffrey@Moffitt.org

2.1
Dr. Michiel van den Brekel, MD, PhD
Netherlands Cancer Institute
Plesmanlaan 121
1066 CX Amsterdam, The Netherlands
E-Mail m.vd.brekel@nki.nl

2.2
Dr. Yoav P. Talmi, MD, FACS
Chief of Head and Neck Service
The Chaim Sheba Med. Center
Tel Hashomer, Israel 52621
E-Mail yoav.talmi@sheba.health.gov.il

2.3/7.1/7.9/8.5
Prof. Fernando L. Dias, MD, FACS
Chief, Head & Neck Surgery Dept.
Brazilian National Cancer Institute
Professor of Surgery
Post Graduation School of Medicine
Av. Alexandre Ferreira, 190
Lagoa
2270220 Rio de Janeiro, SP, Brazil
E-Mail fdias@inca.gov.br

2.4
Prof. Francisco Civantos, MD, FACS
Co-Director, Head and Neck Surgery
Associate Professor
Department of Otolaryngology
University of Miami
Sylvester Comprehensive Cancer Ctr.
1475 NW 12 Ave. No. 4027
Miami 33136 FL, USA
E-Mail FCivanto@med.miami.edu

2.5
Prof. Jesus E. Medina, MD
Department of Otorhinolaryngology
University of Oklahoma
Health Sciences Center
P.O. Box 26901
Oklahoma City 73190 OK, USA
E-Mail jesus-medina@ouhsc.edu

2.6
Dr. John C. O'Brien, Jr., MD
Sammons Cancer Center
Baylor University Medical Center
1004 North Washington Avenue
Dallas 75204-6416 TX, USA
E-Mail job8223@aol.com

2.7
Prof. K. Thomas Robbins, MD
Simmons Cooper Cancer Institute
at Southern Illinois University
P.O. Box 19677
Springfield 62794-9677 IL, USA
E-Mail trobbins@siumed.edu

2.8
Dr. Jonas T. Johnson
Dept. of Otolaryngology
University of Pittsburgh
Suite 500, 203 Lothrop Street
Pittsburgh 15213 PA, USA
E-Mail johnsonjt@upmc.edu

2.9a
Prof. James Cohen, MD, PhD
Department of Otolaryngology
Head and Neck Surgery
Oregon Health Sci. University
3710 SW US Veterans Hospital Road
Portland 97239 OR, USA
E-Mail James.Cohen2@VA.gov

2.9b/7.3
Dr. Randal S. Weber, MD, FACS
Department of Head and Neck Surgery
University of Texas
M.D. Anderson Cancer Center
1515 Holcombe Boulevard
Box 441
Houston 77030-4009 TX, USA
E-Mail rsweber@mdanderson.org

2.10
Dr. Rod P. Rezaee, MD, FACS
University Hospital
Case Medical Center
1110 Euclid Avenue
4th Floor Lakeside Bldg.
Cleveland 44106 OH, USA
E-Mail rod.rezaee@uhhospitals.org

2.11
Prof. Gary L. Clayman, DMD, MD
Department of Head and Neck Surgery
The University of Texas
M.D. Anderson Cancer Center
1515 Holcombe Boulevard, Unit 441
Houston 77030 TX, USA
E-Mail gclayman@mdanderson.org

2.12/4.10
Dr. Bhuvanesh Singh MD, PhD, FACS
Laboratory of Epithelial Cancer Biology
Head and Neck Service
Memorial Sloan-Kettering Cancer Ctr.
1275 York Avenue
New York 10065 NY, USA
E-Mail singhb@mskcc.org

3.1
Prof. Charles René Leemans, MD, PhD
Professor and Chairman
Department of Otolaryngology
Head and Neck Surgery
VU University Medical Center (VUmc)
P.O. Box 7075
1007 MB Amsterdam, The Netherlands
E-Mail chr.leemans@vumc.nl

3.2
Dr. Neal D. Futran, MD, DMD
Department of Otolaryngology
Head and Neck Surgery
Uni. of Washington School of Medicine
1959 NE Pacific Street, Room BB 1165
Seattle 98195-6515 WA, USA
E-Mail nfutran@u.washington.edu

3.3
Dr. Richard J. Wong, MD
Memorial Sloan-Kettering Cancer Center
Head and Neck Service, C-1069
Department of Surgery
1275 York Avenue
New York 10021 NY, USA
E-Mail wongr@mskcc.org

3.4
Dr. Matthew M. Hanasono, MD
Department of Plastic Surgery
The University of Texas
M.D. Anderson Cancer Center
1515 Holcombe Boulevard, Unit 443
Houston 77030 TX, USA
E-Mail mhanasono@mdanderson.org

3.5
Dr. Jacob Kligerman, MD
Av. Rui Barbosa 870 apto. 901
22250-020 Rio de Janeiro-Flamengo,
SP, Brazil
E-Mail jkligerman@uol.com.br

3.6
Dr. Sheng-Po Hao
14 F, No. 16, Alley 4, Lane 137
Min-Sheng E. Road
Taipei, Taiwan (ROC)
E-Mail shengpo@adm.cgmh.org.tw

4.1
Dr. F. Christopher Holsinger, MD, FACS
Department of Head and Neck Surgery
The University of Texas
M.D. Anderson Cancer Center
1515 Holcombe Boulevard
Box 441
Houston 77030-4009 TX, USA
E-Mail holsinger@mdanderson.org

4.2
Dr. Steven M. Zeitels, MD, FACS
Director
Center for Laryngeal Surgery and
Voice Rehabilitation
Massachusetts General Hospital
One Bowdoin Square
11th floor
Boston 02114 MA, USA
E-Mail steven@mgh.harvard.edu

4.3
Dr. Onivaldo Cervantes
Rua Estela, 515.
Bloco G – cj. 81
04011-002 Viala Mariana
São Paulo, SP, Brazil
E-Mail ocervantes@uol.com.br

4.4/4.9/13.1
Dr. Eugene N. Myers
Distinguished Prof. and Emeritus Chair
Department of Otolaryngology
University of Pittsburgh
School of Medicine
The Eye & Ear Insitute, Suite 519
200 Lothrop Street
Pittsburgh 15213 PA, USA
E-Mail myersen@msx.upmc.edu

4.5/14.2
Dr. med. Roberto A. Lima, MD
Av. Armando Lombardi, 1000 Bloc2 107
22640-000 Rio de Janeiro, SP, Brazil
E-Mail rlimamd@uol.com.br

4.6/15.4
Prof. Gregory S. Weinstein, MD, FACS
Professor and Vice Chair
The Department of Otorhinolaryngology
Head and Neck Surgery
The University of Pennsylvania
3400 Spruce Street
Philadelphia 19035 PA, USA
E-Mail
gregory.weinstein@uphs.upenn.edu

4.7
Prof. Javier Gavilán, MD
Servicio de ORL
Hospital Unviersitario La Paz
Paseo de la Castellana, 261
28046 Madrid, Spain
E-Mail jgavilan.hulp@salud.madrid.org

4.8/5.2
Prof. Dennis H. Kraus, MD
Memorial Sloan-Kettering Cancer Center
Head and Neck Service
1275 York Avenue
New York 10065 NY, USA
E-Mail krausd@mskcc.org

5.1
Dr. Abrao Rapoport
Head and Neck Surgeon
Hospital Heliopolis
Rua Congeo Xavier, 276 – 10 andar
04231-030 São Paulo, SP, Brazil
E-Mail arapoport@terra.com.br

5.3
Dr. Frans JM Hilgers, MD, PhD
Netherlands Cancer Institute
Plesmanlaan 121
1066 CX Amsterdam, The Netherlands
E-Mail f.hilgers@nki.nl

5.4/6.1/6.2/6.3/14.12
Prof. William I. Wei
Li Shu Pui Professor of Surgery
Chair in Otorhinolaryngology
Department of Surgery
University of Hong Kong Med. Ctr.
Queen Mary Hospital
Hong Kong, People's Republic of China
E-Mail hrmswwi@hkucc.hku.hk

7.4
Prof. Peter C. Neligan, MB, FRCS
University of Washington Med. Ctr.
Division of Plastic Surgery
1959 NE Pacific St.
Box 356410
Seattle 98195-6410 WA, USA
E-Mail pneligan@uwashington.edu

7.5
Dr. Richard V. Smith, MD, FACS
Department of Otorhinolaryngology
Head and Neck Surgery
3400 Bainbridge Avenue
Bronx 10467 NY, USA
E-Mail rsmith@montefiore.org

7.6
Prof. Bruce J. Davidson, MD, FACS
Professor and Chairman
Department of Otolarynology
Head and Neck Surgery
Georgetown University Medical Center
Washington 20007 DC, USA
E-Mail davidsob@georgetown.edu

7.7
Prof. Alfio José Tincani, MD
Professor of Head & Neck Surgery
State University of Campinas – UNICAMP
Rua Geraldo Trefiglio 140
13083-793 Campinas, SP, Brazil
E-Mail alfio.jt@gmail.com

7.8
Dr. Randall P. Morton, MB, BS, MSc, FRACS
Counties-Manukau DHB, and
Auckland University
PO Box 98 743
South Auckland Mail Centre
Manukau 2240
Auckland, New Zealand
E-Mail rpmorton@middlemore.co.nz

7.11
Dr. Jeffrey D. Spiro, MD
Division of Otolaryngology/
Head and Neck Surgery
University of Connecticut Health Ctr
263 Farmington Avenue MC-6228
Farmington 06030-6228 CT, USA
E-Mail spiro@nso.uchc.edu

7.12
Dr. Kwang Hyun Kim, MD
Department of Otolaryngology
Head and Neck Surgery
Seoul National University
College of Medicine
28, Yeongeon-dong, Jongno-gu
110-744 Korea, South Korea
E-Mail kimkwang@plaza.snu.ac.kr

8.2
Dr. Fernando Walder, MD
Federal University of São Paulo
UNIFESP
Rua Joaquim Floriano, 397/3rd floor
04534-011 São Paulo, SP, Brazil
E-Mail fernandowalder@terra.com.br

8.3
Dr. Eduardo Vellutini
Paça Amadeu Amaral 27/71
01327-010 São Paulo, SP, Brazil
E-Mail evellu@terra.com.br

8.6
Prof. Ehab Hanna MD, FACS
Professor and Vice Chairman
Director of Skull Base Surgery
Medical Director Head and Neck Ctr.
Department of Head and Neck Surgery
University of Texas
M.D. Anderson Cancer Center
1515 Holcombe Boulevard, Unit 441
Houston 77030-4009 TX, USA
E-Mail eyhanna@mdanderson.org

8.7
Dr. Marcos Q.T. Gomes
Praca Amadeu Amaral 27/71
01327-010 São Paulo, SP, Brazil
E-Mail marcos@dfvneuro.com.br

8.8
Dr. Patrick J. Gullane, MB
Department of Otolaryngology
Head and Neck Surgery
200 Elizabeth Street, 8N-800
Toronto M5G 2C4, Canada
E-Mail Patrick.gullane@uhn.on.ca

9.1/9.2
Prof. James Y. Suen, MD
Professor and Chairman
Department of Otolaryngology
Head and Neck Surgery
4301 W. Markham St.
Little Rock 72205 AR, USA
E-Mail suenjamesy@uams.edu and
suenjamesy@exchange.uams.edu

9.3
Dr. Eduardo Noda Kihara
Hospital Albert Einstein
Neuro Interventional Department
Avenida Albert Einstein, 701
Hemodinamica 4° andar
05651-091 São Paulo, SP, Brazil
E-Mail kihara@einstein.br

10.1
Dr. Marcelo D. Durazzo, MD
Praça Amadeu Amaral 47, suite 41
01413-000 São Paulo, SP, Brazil
E-Mail durazzo@attglobal.net

10.2
Dr. Nilton T. Herter, MD
Av. Independência 1211 Sala 201
90035-075 Porto Alegre, SP, Brazil
E-Mail nherter@uol.com.br

11.1
Dr. Nadir Ahmad
Department of Otolaryngology
Head and Neck
Vanderbilt University Medical Center
7209 Medical Center East, South Tower
1215 21st Avenue South
Nashville 37232-8605 TN, USA
E-Mail nadirahmad@hotmail.com

11.2
Dr. Ziv Gil, MD
Department of Otolaryngology
Head and Neck Surgery
Tel-Aviv Sourasky Medical Center
6 Weizmann Street
64239 Tel-Aviv, Israel
E-Mail ziv@baseofskull.org

11.3
Dr. Kerry D. Olsen, MD
Mayo Clinic Rochester
200 First Street Southwest
Rochester 55905 MN, USA
E-Mail olsen.kerry@mayo.edu

12.1
Prof. Flávio C. Hojaij, MD
Rua Padre João Manuel 450, cj 18
01411-001 São Paulo, SP, Brazil
E-Mail fchojaij@uol.com.br

12.2
Dr. Dorival De Carlucci, Jr., MD
Rua Padre João Manuel 45, room 18
Cerqueira César
01411-001 São Paulo, SP, Brazil
E-Mail decarlucci@uol.com.br

13.2
Dr. Carlos N. Lehn, MD
Chief of the Head and Neck Surgery
Service
Hospital Heliópolis, São Paulo
Rua Joaquim Floriano 636 ap 22
04534-002 São Paulo, SP, Brazil
E-Mail cnlehn@terra.com.br

13.3
Prof. David W. Eisele, MD, FACS
Professor and Chairman
400 Parnassus Avenue
Suite A-730
San Francisco 94143-0342 CA, USA
E-Mail deisele@ohns.ucsf.edu

14.1
Dr. Luiz Carlos Ishida, MD
Plastic Surgery Division of the
Faculty of Medicine of the
University of São Paulo
Rua Itamiami, 35
Vila Mariana
04120-100 São Paulo, SP, Brazil
E-Mail lci@uol.com.br

14.3
Dr. José Magrim, MD, PhD
Head and Neck Surgery and
Otorhinolaryngology Department
Hospital AC Camargo
Rua Professor Antonio Prudente, 211
01509-900 São Paulo, SP, Brazil
E-Mail jgon13@terra.com.br

14.4
Prof. Richard E. Hayden, MD
Professor and Chair
Department of Otolaryngology
Head and Neck Surgery
5777 East Mayo Boulevard
Phoenix 85054 AZ, USA
E-Mail hayden.richard@mayo.edu

14.5
Prof. Gady Har-El, MD, FACS
Chairman, Dept. of Otolaryngology
Head and Neck Surgery
Lenox Hill Hospital, New York
Prof. of Otolaryngology & Neurosur.
State University of New York
Downstate Medical Center
Brooklyn 11201 NY, USA
E-Mail gadyh@aol.com

14.6/14.8/14.10
Dr. Julio Morais, MD, PhD
Assistant Professor of Plastic Surgery
São Paulo University Medical School
Rua Baronesa de Bela Vista, 196
04612-000 São Paulo, SP, Brazil
E-Mail jmorais@br2001.com.br

14.7
Dr. Mark L. Urken, MD
Beth Israel Medical Center
10 Union Square East, Suite 5B
New York 10003 NY, USA
E-Mail murken@chpnet.org

14.9
Dr. Mario S.L. Galvao, MD
Reconstructive Microsurgery Unit
National Cancer Institute
Rua Visconde Silva 52/suite 1006
Botafogo, Rio de Janeiro, SP, Brazil
E-Mail galvaorj@iis.com.br

14.11
Prof. John J. Coleman, 3rd, MD
Professor of Surgery
Chief of Plastic Surgery
Indiana University School of Med.
Roudebush VAMC- Indianapolis
Indianapolis 46204 IN, USA
E-Mail jjcolema@iupui.edu

15.1
Dr. Paulo Campos Carneiro, MD, PhD
University of São Paulo
School of Medicine
Department of Pathology
Av. Rebouças 353 cj. 114
05401-000 Cerqueira Cesar,
São Paulo, SP, Brazil
E-Mail p.carneiro@saudetotal.com.br

15.2
Dr. Pedro Michaluart, Jr., MD
Head and Neck Service
Hospital das Clinicas da Faculdade
de Medicina da Universidade
de São Paulo
R. Dr. Enéas de Carvalho Aguiar, 255
No. 8 andar, Sala 8074
0540 3900 São Paulo, SP, Brazil
E-Mail pemic@uol.com.br

15.3
Dr. Erich M. Sturgis, MD, MPH
Department of Head and Neck Surgery
and Epidemiology
The University of Texas
M.D. Anderson Cancer Center
1515 Holcombe Boulevard, Unit 441
Houston 77030-4009 TX, USA
E-Mail esturgis@mdanderson.org

Subject Index

Abscess, deep neck abscess surgical planning 166, 167
Arteriovenous malformation (AVM)
  bleeding emergency management 154, 155
  management of extensive malformations 150, 151
AVM, *see* Arteriovenous malformation

Bilateral neck dissection (BND) 48, 49
BND, *see* Bilateral neck dissection
Branchial cleft, cyst and fistula management 156, 157

Carotid body tumor (CBT), management 160, 161
Cavernous sinus, extradural approach in skull base tumor surgery 142, 143
CBT, *see* Carotid body tumor
Completion thyroidectomy (CT)
  facilitation 10
  indications 10
  technique 11
Computed tomography (CT)
  carotid body tumor 160
  chemoradiotherapy node-positive neck patients 55
  deep neck abscess surgical planning 166, 167
  laryngeal cancer 73
  skull base tumors 130
Cricothyroidectomy, indications versus tracheotomy 172, 173
CT, *see* Completion thyroidectomy; Computed tomography

da Vinci Robotic Surgical System, transoral robotic surgery 206, 207
Deep neck abscess, surgical planning 166, 167
Deltopectoral flap, technique 178, 179

EBSLN, *see* External branch of superior laryngeal nerve
External branch of superior laryngeal nerve (EBSLN), injury avoidance 4, 5

Facial nerve
  main trunk identification 106, 107
  parotid surgery intraoperative decisions 110, 111
  reconstruction in parotid surgery 112, 113
  retrograde approach indications and technique 108, 109

Fibula microvascular transfer, mandible reconstruction 190, 191
Fine needle aspiration biopsy (FNAB)
  lateral cervical masses 200, 201
  salivary gland tumors 118, 119, 126
FNAB, *see* Fine needle aspiration biopsy

GAN, *see* Great auricular nerve
Gastric pull-up, technique 198, 199
Glottis, reconstruction after partial vertical laryngectomy 76, 77
Goiter, intrathoracic goiter surgery 12, 13
Great auricular nerve (GAN), sparing in parotid surgery 120, 121

Head and neck squamous cell carcinoma, preoperative workup 34, 35
Hyperparathyroidism, secondary hyperparathyroidism surgical management 22, 23
Hypoparathyroidism, management 9
Hypopharyngeal cancer
  N3 neck patient management 92, 93
  reconstruction
    total laryngectomy/partial pharyngectomy defect 94, 95
    total pharyngolaryngectomy 98, 99
  voice rehabilitation after pharyngolaryngectomy 96, 97

ILN, *see* Inferior laryngeal nerve
Inferior laryngeal nerve (ILN)
  anatomy 2, 3
  injury avoidance 2, 3
  intrathoracic goiter surgery 12, 13
  monitoring with NIM 2 system 6, 7
  well-differentiated thyroid cancer management with recurrent nerve invasion 50, 51
Intrathoracic goiter, surgery 12, 13
Invasive thyroid cancer, *see* Well-differentiated thyroid cancer

Jejunal free autograft, pharyngoesophageal defect reconstruction 196, 197

Laryngeal cancer, laser resection 72, 73
Laryngectomy
glottis reconstruction after partial vertical laryngectomy 76, 77
hypopharyngeal cancer
reconstruction
total laryngectomy/partial pharyngectomy defect 94, 95
total pharyngolaryngectomy 98, 99
voice rehabilitation after pharyngolaryngectomy 96, 97
pharyngocutaneous fistula prevention 84, 85, 90, 91
supracricoid partial laryngectomy 82, 83
supraglottic laryngectomy and functional outcome improvement 80, 81
total laryngectomy and functional outcome improvement 84, 85
tracheostomal recurrence management 86, 87
tracheostomal stenosis prevention 88, 89
Lateral cervical mass
fine needle aspiration biopsy 200, 201
open biopsy 202, 203
Latissimus dorsi myocutaneous flap, technique 184, 185
LM, *see* Lymphatic malformation
Lymphatic malformation (LM), management of extensive malformations 152, 153

Magnetic resonance imaging (MRI)
carotid body tumor 160
laryngeal cancer 73
suprahyoid pharyngotomy planing 78
Mandibular osteoradionecrosis, management 70, 71
Mandibular resection
anterior mandibular reconstruction 66, 67
reconstruction with fibula microvascular transfer 190, 191
surgical margins in oral cavity squamous cell carcinoma 64, 65
Marginal mandibular nerve (MMN), management in neck dissection 46, 47
Maxillary swing approach, nasopharyngeal cancer 102, 103
Medullary thyroid cancer (MTC), lymph node management 28, 29
Microvascular anterolateral thigh flap, technique 176, 177
Microvascular forearm flap, technique 188, 189
Microvascular iliac crest flap, technique 192, 193
MMN, *see* Marginal mandibular nerve
MRI, *see* Magnetic resonance imaging
MTC, *see* Medullary thyroid cancer

Nasopharyngeal cancer
maxillary swing approach 102, 103
neck metastasis management 104, 105
surgical indications 100, 101
Neck dissection
bilateral neck dissection 48, 49
chemoradiotherapy node-positive neck patients 54, 55
functional modified neck dissection 58, 59
marginal mandibular nerve management 46, 47
medullary thyroid cancer and lymph node management 28, 29
oral cancer
N0 neck
elective neck dissection 38, 39
sentinel lymph node biopsy 40, 41
wait and watch policy 36, 37
N+ neck dissection 42, 43
paratracheal neck dissection 26, 27
parotid cancers and elective neck dissections 122, 123
spinal accessory nerve management 44, 45
Necrotizing fasciitis (NF), management 168, 169
Neurogenic tumor (NT), management of extensive tumors 162, 163
NF, *see* Necrotizing fasciitis
NIM 2, recurrent laryngeal nerve monitoring 6, 7
NT, *see* Neurogenic tumor

OE, *see* Orbital exenteration
Oral cancer
mandibular resection surgical margins 64, 65
N0 neck
elective neck dissection 38, 39
sentinel lymph node biopsy 40, 41
wait and watch policy 36, 37
N+ neck dissection 42, 43
reconstructive surgery
large defects 62, 63
small defects 60, 61
Orbital exenteration (OE), skull base tumor surgery 140, 141
Osteoradionecrosis, *see* Mandibular osteoradionecrosis

Parapharyngeal space tumor, surgical approach selection 164, 165
Parathyroid glands
autotransplantation 9
hypoparathyroidism management 9
limited parathyroidectomy 20, 21
preservation in thyroid surgery 8, 9

reoperative parathyroidectomy 24, 25
secondary hyperparathyroidism surgical management 22, 23
video-assisted parathyroidectomy 18, 19
Parathyroid hormone (PTH), intraoperative measurement 20, 21, 25
Paratracheal neck dissection (PTND)
indications 26
tips 26, 27
Parotid surgery, *see* Salivary gland tumors
Partial horizontal laryngectomy, functional outcome improvement 80, 81
Partial vertical laryngectomy (PVL), glottis reconstruction 76, 77
PCF, *see* Pharyngocutaneous fistula
PDT, *see* Percutaneous dilatational tracheotomy
Pectoralis major flap, technique 180, 181
Percutaneous dilatational tracheotomy (PDT), complication avoidance 174, 175
PET, *see* Positron emission tomography
Pharyngectomy, hypopharyngeal cancer
reconstruction
total laryngectomy/partial pharyngectomy defect 94, 95
total pharyngolaryngectomy 98, 99
voice rehabilitation after pharyngolaryngectomy 96, 97
Pharyngocutaneous fistula (PCF), prevention in total laryngectomy 84, 85, 90, 91
Positron emission tomography (PET)
chemoradiotherapy node-positive neck patients 55
skull base tumors 130
PTH, *see* Parathyroid hormone
PTND, *see* Paratracheal neck dissection
PVL, *see* Partial vertical laryngectomy

Radiation-associated sarcoma (RAS), management 204, 205
RAS, *see* Radiation-associated sarcoma
Reconstruction
anterior mandibular 66, 67
cranial base defect 144, 145
facial nerve in parotid surgery 112, 113
flaps
deltopectoral flap 178, 179
latissimus dorsi myocutaneous flap 184, 185
microvascular anterolateral thigh flap 176, 177
microvascular forearm flap 188, 189
microvascular iliac crest flap 192, 193
pectoralis major flap 180, 181
scapular flap 194, 195
transverse rectus abdominis flap 186, 187
trapezius flap 182, 183
gastric pull-up 198, 199
glottis after partial vertical laryngectomy 76, 77
hypopharyngeal cancer
total laryngectomy/partial pharyngectomy defect 94, 95
total pharyngolaryngectomy 98, 99
jejunal free autograft for pharyngoesophageal defect reconstruction 196, 197
mandible reconstruction with fibula microvascular transfer 190, 191
oral cancer surgery
large defects 62, 63
small defects 60, 61
Recurrent laryngeal nerve, *see* Inferior laryngeal nerve
Retropharyngeal lymph node metastasis, management in thyroid cancer
transcervical approach 52, 53
transoral approach 50, 51

Salivary gland tumors
deep lobe parotid tumor approaches 114, 115
diagnosis 118, 119
elective neck dissections in parotid cancers 122, 123
facial nerve
main trunk identification 106, 107
parotid surgery intraoperative decisions 110, 111
reconstruction in parotid surgery 112, 113
retrograde approach indications and technique 108, 109
great auricular nerve sparing in parotid surgery 120, 121
parotid tumor surgery indications 126, 127
recurrent parotid pleomorphic adenoma management 116, 117
submandibular gland excision 126, 127
tactical parotidectomy in nonsalivary lesions 124, 125
SAN, *see* Spinal accessory nerve
Sarcoma, *see* Radiation-associated sarcoma
Scapular flap 194, 195
SCPL, *see* Supracricoid partial laryngectomy
Sentinel lymph node biopsy (SLNB), N0 oral cancer 40, 41

Skull base tumors
cavernous sinus and extradural approach 142, 143
contraindications for resection 138, 139
cranial base defect reconstruction 144, 145
craniofacial diaphragm sealing 136, 137
facial translocation approach 132, 133
fibro-osseous lesion management 148, 149
large dural defect management 134, 135
orbital preservation and exenteration 140, 141
recurrent tumor management 146, 147
subcranial approach 130, 131
SLNB, *see* Sentinel lymph node biopsy
SMG, *see* Submandibular gland
SP, *see* Suprahyoid pharyngotomy
Spinal accessory nerve (SAN), management in neck dissection 44, 45
Squamous cell carcinoma, *see* Head and neck squamous cell carcinoma; Oral cancer
Stoma, creation 85
Submandibular gland (SMG), excision 126, 127
Substernal goiter, *see* Goiter
Superior laryngeal nerve, *see* External branch of superior laryngeal nerve
Supracricoid partial laryngectomy (SCPL) 82, 83
Suprahyoid pharyngotomy (SP) 78, 79

TD, *see* Thoracic duct
TEP, *see* Tracheoesophageal puncture
TGDC, *see* Thyroglossal duct cyst
Thoracic duct (TD), injury avoidance in left level IV lymph node resection 56
Thyroglossal duct cyst (TGDC), management 158, 159
Thyroid cancer, *see* Medullary thyroid cancer; Retropharyngeal lymph node metastasis; Well-differentiated thyroid cancer
Thyroidectomy
completion thyroidectomy
facilitation 10
indications 10
technique 11
extent for benign disease 14, 15
minimally invasive video-assisted surgery 16, 17
Tongue carcinoma
resection margins 68, 69
suprahyoid pharyngotomy 78, 79
TORS, *see* Transoral robotic surgery
Tracheoesophageal puncture (TEP), speech rehabilitation after total laryngectomy 85
Tracheostomal recurrence, management after laryngectomy 86, 87
Tracheostomal stenosis, prevention after laryngectomy 88, 89
Tracheotomy
complication minimization 170, 171, 174, 175
indications versus cricothyroidectomy 172, 173
percutaneous dilatational tracheotomy 174, 175
Transoral robotic surgery (TORS) 206, 207
Transverse rectus abdominis flap, technique 186, 187
Trapezius flap, technique 182, 183

Upper airway obstruction, *see* Cricothyroidectomy; Tracheotomy

Vocal fold, phonomicrosurgical treatment of benign lesions 74, 75
Voice rehabilitation, pharyngolaryngectomy 96, 97

WDTC, *see* Well-differentiated thyroid cancer
Well-differentiated thyroid cancer (WDTC)
invasive thyroid cancer management 32, 33
management with recurrent nerve invasion 50, 51